New Frontiers in Veterinary Medicine

New Frontiers in Veterinary Medicine

Edited by **Mel Roth**

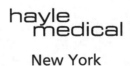

New York

Published by Hayle Medical,
30 West, 37th Street, Suite 612,
New York, NY 10018, USA
www.haylemedical.com

New Frontiers in Veterinary Medicine
Edited by Mel Roth

International Standard Book Number: 978-1-63241-295-9 (Hardback)

Printed in the United States of America.

Contents

Preface

Veterinary medicine is a branch of science that deals in the treatment of animals. It is developing at a fast pace, specifically given the width of the discipline. This book analyzes recent advances covering a broad area of concern from health and welfare in livestock, pets, and wild animals to public health supervision and biomedical research. Research chapters in the book have been compiled by specialists with a glimpse into analyzing developments in the veterinary profession and veterinary science, while looking at particular forms of applied veterinary medicine: general aspects and clinical attention in pets. It offers a precise, summarized and interesting analysis of the entire science of veterinary medicine.

Significant researches are present in this book. Intensive efforts have been employed by authors to make this book an outstanding discourse. This book contains the enlightening chapters which have been written on the basis of significant researches done by the experts.

Finally, I would also like to thank all the members involved in this book for being a team and meeting all the deadlines for the submission of their respective works. I would also like to thank my friends and family for being supportive in my efforts.

Editor

Part 1

Veterinary Medicine: General Aspects

How Experience Can Be Useful in Veterinary Pathological Anatomy

Paulo Tomé[1] and Helena Vala[2]
[1]*Algoritmi Research Center/Polytechnic Institute of Viseu*
[2]*Center for Studies in Education, and Health Technologies,*
CI&DETS, Polytechnic Institute of Viseu
Portugal

1. Introduction

Veterinary anatomical pathology is a medical specialty which is very similar to human anatomical pathology. This specialty consists in diagnosing diseases based mainly on gross and microscopic examination of organs and tissues obtained by surgical procedure or necropsy. It consists in applying criteria based on knowledge of gross and histological lesions in order to obtain a final pathological diagnosis. The aim of this specific diagnosis is, generally speaking, to find which disease is affecting the animal, if it is alive, or what caused its death.

The main difficulties in veterinary pathological diagnosis are related to the various animal species a pathologist has to deal with, the use of exhaustive classifications of different types, costs, subjectivity, including disagreement between the clinical and pathological diagnoses, and the urgency in issuing the report. So, the urgent need to compile all available information to obtain a diagnosis in a short time is the constant challenge professional experts face.

Pathology consists in using scientific methods to study structural and functional changes in cells, tissues and organs that underlie disease (Cotran et al., 1999). It is divided into two branches: anatomical pathology, dedicated to examining organs, tissues and cadavers and clinical pathology, dedicated to laboratory analysis of body fluids and/or tissues. The pathologist has the professional expertise devoted to the practice of both, anatomical and clinical pathology (Langone Medical Center, Department of Pathology, 2011).

Past knowledge is an important resource in veterinary pathological anatomy. Professionals often use their previous experience (Dungworth et al., 1999; Goldschmidt et al., 1998; Head et al., 2003; Hendrick et al., 1998; Kennedy et al., 1998; Kiupel et al., 2008; Koestner et al., 1999; Maxie, 2007; Meuten et al., 2004; Misdorp et al., 1999; Scott et al., 2001; Slayter et al., 1994a; Valli et al., 2002; Wilcock et al., 2002)[1].

This chapter will be devoted to veterinary anatomical pathology, not in terms of further development of its study methods, extensively detailed in the specialty bibliography, but from a different approach, with the aim of better understanding routine work in the pathology lab.

---

[1] The twelve books: (Dungworth et al., 1999; Goldschmidt et al., 1998; Head et al., 2003; Hendrick et al., 1998; Kennedy et al., 1998; Kiupel et al., 2008; Koestner et al., 1999; Meuten et al., 2004; Misdorp et al., 1999; Slayter et al., 1994a; Valli et al., 2002; Wilcock et al., 2002) were published by World Health Organization (WHO).

Emphasis will be given to the difficulties faced by the veterinary pathologist every day, in order to justify the development of new solutions to support the issuance of more accurate diagnoses.

The authors describe a framework and a software system that can be useful for diagnosing diseases. The developed framework is based on analysis of the bibliography in this field. Both proposals can be useful to yield better diagnoses. Pathological diagnosis is a supplementary diagnostic test usually ordered by the veterinarian clinician, in order to direct treatment to administer to the sick animal, or living members of a group of animals (e.g. cattle), in which a death occurred. Thus, although the methods used are similar to those used in human medicine, the ends are quite different.

As far as is known, no artificial intelligence system has ever been applied or implemented to areas of diagnosis in veterinary medicine. The system proposed in this chapter is applied to generating solutions for real clinical cases, submitted to complementary pathological diagnosis exams.

In the following sections it will be described pathological diagnosis, as well as the main re-using knowledge mechanisms created in the field of Artificial Intelligence, framework system and the software application. Finally, in section 5 are reported final conclusions and beliefs about the framework and software application.

2. Pathological diagnosis

Veterinary anatomical pathology is quite similar to human anatomical pathology, usually referred as anatomical pathology. It is a medical specialty which diagnoses diseases, based on gross, microscopic, chemical, immunologic and molecular examination of organs and tissues, obtained by surgical procedure and by necropsy (in animal species; autopsy refers to Human species) (Miller et al., 2009).

Anatomical pathology is itself divided in subspecialties, the main ones being:

- surgical pathology, which is the subspecialty pathologists devote more time to. It consists in gross and microscopic examination of surgical specimens, as well as biopsies, submitted mostly by clinicians, dermatologists and surgeons (Grzybicki et al., 2004);
- cytopathology, the branch of anatomical pathology, dedicated to the microscopic examination of cytological specimens, obtained from smears or fine needle aspirates from organs, masses or cysts, used mostly as a complementary diagnosis of the histological exam, since it has more interpretative limitations (Meyer, 2001);
- forensic pathology, whose main aim is to determine cause of death of the animal and is applied mostly in cases of death without previous disease, including criminal causes. This subspecialty is applied to legal purposes. In veterinary medicine, the forensic pathologists are required mainly due to suspicious death by criminal causes (almost always attributed to acts of revenge by neighbors) but in reality, the outcome of most cases culminates in the diagnosis of natural causes, mainly diseases of dietary, infectious or parasitic aetiology, which is very common in domestic animals (Williams et al., 1998);
- necropsy pathology (equivalent to autopsy pathology in human medicine) consists in performing necropsies, i.e. complete and careful examination of the animal cadaver or post-mortem examination, assessing body cavities, liquid presence,

position of organs, gross appearance of organs, sampling injured organs, focus on the transition between normal and injured aspect, in each organ, in order to determine disease factors which caused animal's death and to contribute to pre-diagnosis of disease.

This subspecialty has a greater importance in veterinary medicine, since it allows other cohabitants of a group (herd or flock) to be saved or an infected animal to be eliminated, acting preventatively to avoid transmission to other animals or humans, contributing favourably to public health. Also, euthanasia is acceptable and legally provided in veterinary medicine, which reinforces the appeal and importance of this branch of anatomical pathology.

In all subspecialties, additional tests from other medical specialities could be required to determine the cause of death or to obtain a definite diagnosis. The most commonly required tests are linked to toxicology, virology, bacteriology and genetics.

Pathological diagnosis is the medical specialty that deals with the examination of gross and microscopic lesions (Miller et al., 2009). It also consists in the further microscopic study of tissues and cells, in order to provide a complementary means for diagnosis. The solid background of expertise is constructed based on medical literature, educational programs, training activities, meetings, technical rules and the cognitive skills of the pathologist which allows him to describe lesions, interpret histological slides and make decisions. In this long and complex process, the pathologist takes into account the animal data, clinical history (including physical exam), results of other complementary exams (including biochemical analysis and x-rays), using a strategy to arrive at a diagnosis which is not qualitatively different from those used by clinicians (Pena & Andrade-Filho, 2009).

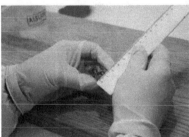 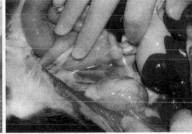

(a) Description and measurement of a surgical specimen (b) Post-mortem exam of dead animal cadaver

Fig. 1. Gross examination

The most commonly used procedures in the pathological diagnosis processes include gross examination, histopathology or microscopic examination, evaluating histological aspects, including cellular characteristics and organizational patterns, immunohistochemistry and cytopathology, among other more specific tests. Gross examination consists in describing the specimen with the naked eye. It is based on observation, description and measurement of gross lesions, found in a surgical specimen, submitted to the pathology lab (figure 1 a)), or found in animal cadavers, if such is the case, during the meticulous post-mortem exam (figure 1 b)), especially if the animal is injured. It is also during this step, that the pathologist decides which areas and specimens need to be processed for histopathology and microscopic evaluation (University of Utah of Spencer S. Eccles, 2011; Zarbo & Nakhleh, 2009).

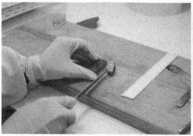
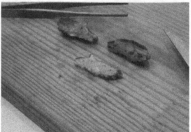

(a) Cut of formalin fixed specimens   (b) Selection of areas to be processed

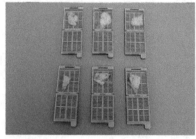
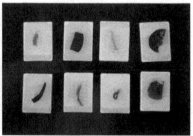

(c) Placing the specimen in standard   (d) Paraffin blocks
plastic histological cassettes

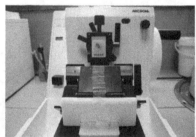
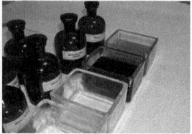

(e) Execution of histological sections (f) Staining by standard haematoxylin
with a rotary microtome   and eosin

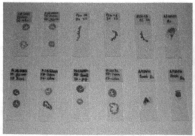
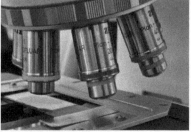

(g) Final preparations   (h) Microscopic observation

Fig. 2. Routine histological technique

To perform tissue observations under the microscope, a complex and relatively time consuming procedure is performed, in order to obtain very thin sections that can be traversed by the microscope condenser's light. The microscope is an extension of the pathologist's vision. It is a fundamental instrument throughout the process of diagnosis and with which the pathologist must feel very comfortable, spending many hours of his life at the microscope. Without a microscope the pathologist is blind and incomplete.

The basis of routine histological technique (figure 2) culminates obtaining histological sections (with 3 μm) that will subsequently be stained by standard haematoxylin and eosin or other more specific methods, to obtain a more accurate histopathological diagnosis, namely histochemistry. Histochemistry consists in using chemical reactions to localize chemical compounds of cells and tissues (figure 3 a) and b)) (Pellicciari, 2009) and immunohistochemistry, a technique for identifying cellular or tissue constituents (antigens) by means of antigen-antibody interactions (figure 3 c) and d)). These methods are performed in the pathological diagnostic field, mainly in oncology diagnosis (Miller, 2002).

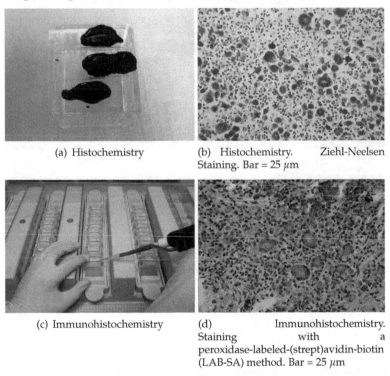

(a) Histochemistry

(b) Histochemistry. Ziehl-Neelsen Staining. Bar = 25 μm

(c) Immunohistochemistry

(d) Immunohistochemistry. Staining with a peroxidase-labeled-(strept)avidin-biotin (LAB-SA) method. Bar = 25 μm

Fig. 3. Specific histological techniques

Finally, the professional veterinary pathologist produces an understandable and grammatically correct report (Pena & Andrade-Filho, 2009) which includes a complete description of macroscopic and histological observations and a definite diagnosis issued based on the specific knowledge of these observations and statements.

The pathological report must be understood directly by the clinician which operates under the same system of rules (Pena & Andrade-Filho, 2009), without triggering an array of interpretive questions which will increase the time spent on a particular case. Also, misinterpretation of a pathological diagnosis may lead to an incorrect or surgical therapeutic approach to the lesion concerned (Pena & Andrade-Filho, 2009). So, the development of a system of rules will also help to solve this problem.

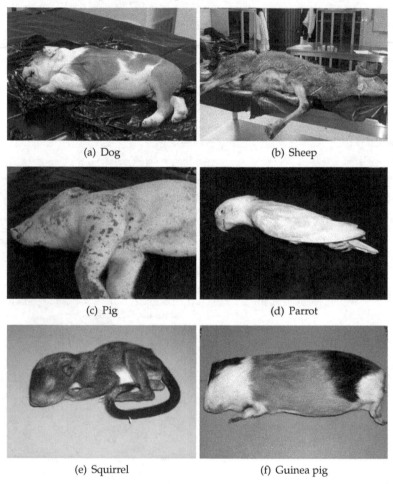

(a) Dog   (b) Sheep

(c) Pig   (d) Parrot

(e) Squirrel   (f) Guinea pig

Fig. 4. Different species of animals to necropsy

One of the major difficulties associated with veterinary medicine is, that unlike human medicine, which is dedicated to a single species, its target is a number of different species of animals to study/diagnose. To overcome this difficulty, the animal species are usually grouped into specialties, based in their affinity (e.g. pets - dogs and cats, ruminants - cows, sheep and goats, swine, equine species, exotic species, etc.) (figure 4). In parallel, veterinary anatomical pathology deals with different animal species, which requires knowledge of the anatomy of each species, species-specific diseases, their lesions and lesion patterns. To achieve a correct and definitive diagnosis per species, the ideal situation would be the constitution of multidisciplinary teams, in which each expert would focus on a single species or group of species. This may, however, be impossible for smaller institutions wishing to offer a diagnosis service in the field of veterinary pathology.

Also, pathological anatomy uses different types of exhaustive classifications (e.g. infectious diseases, metabolic diseases, endocrine diseases, neoplasm, etc.). It can be highlighted, as reference books to the veterinary pathologist's diagnostic decisions: Dungworth et al. (1999); Goldschmidt et al. (1998); Head et al. (2003); Hendrick et al. (1998); Kennedy et al. (1998); Kiupel et al. (2008); Koestner et al. (1999); Maxie (2007); Meuten (2002); Meuten et al. (2004); Misdorp et al. (1999); Scott et al. (2001); Slayter et al. (1994a); Valli et al. (2002); Wilcock et al. (2002), among several others dedicated to the pathology of different animal species.

If, on the one hand, not following a clinical case directly or contacting the owner or veterinary clinician personally may be beneficial, in terms of exemption in reaching conclusions, on the other hand, the summary of the clinical information in the requested analysis, may omit crucial information to the final conclusion/diagnosis.

Furthermore, reading that the animal is two years old and has intense itching, is not the same as visiting a young animal that that is constantly scratching itself. So, during the long process of making a diagnosis, this type of information may easily lose its proper influence, which would not happen if it had been obtained by direct observation, especially if the pathologist is seeing abnormal cells in the microscope, i.e. with features of high malignancy, which would tend to overlap, in terms of influencing the summary of the clinical history reported indirectly.

Often, the pathologist has no notice knowledge of the outcome, performed treatments or results of outside consultations, which prevents him from verifying the authenticity of his diagnosis and evaluate eventual failures, when he fails, making it difficult to improve and learn from their mistakes (Pena & Andrade-Filho, 2009).

For these reasons, pathologists may enhance their diagnostic abilities, acquiring specific abilities related to other fields by means of expressing relevant warrants and backings to their conclusions, deducing and expressing intrinsic rules that guide the different actions related to the diagnostic task (Pena & Andrade-Filho, 2009).

In complex cases, if the pathologist needs to use additional analytical methods to reach a definitive diagnosis, such as histochemistry, immunohistochemistry or other medical speciality tests, the authors propose a prior consultation with the client, as these additional studies increase diagnostic costs, and thus, should be subjected to client discretion. This information should be included in the first report, with the explanation for the necessity of more diagnostic procedures, along with the budget of all the expected costs. Procedures and respective costs must, preferably, be presented in a phased and sequential manner. As an example, a report for an undifferentiated round cell tumour should describe macroscopic and microscopic features, the preliminary diagnosis as "consistent with round cell tumour", and a detailed account for the need of additional diagnostic workup: "to determine definitive histogenesis, further protocols are recommend to rule out possible differential diagnosis: toluidine blue for mast cell (cost value), CD1a for histiocytoma (cost value) and CD3 and CD79α for lymphoma (cost value). These protocols will be realized in this order and executed only to the point needed to reach a definitive diagnosis.

Although the pathologist is protected in his lab from contact with the owner and patient (animal), he should be sensitive to their economic difficulties, especially in the absence of health insurance for animals. In addition, he must be aware that the diagnosis is only a precursor to the stage of healing, i.e. the treatment stage remains indispensable and is also expensive. For these reasons, and according to proper medical conduct, the proposed plan

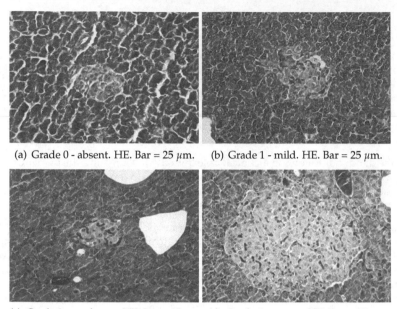

(a) Grade 0 - absent. HE. Bar = 25 μm.   (b) Grade 1 - mild. HE. Bar = 25 μm.

(c) Grade 2 - moderate. HE. Bar = 25 μm   (d) Grade 3 - severe. HE. Bar = 25 μm

Fig. 5. Semi-quantitative access to congestion

must hereinafter follow one of the following two rules: from the lowest to highest cost or from the most likely diagnosis to the less likely. The goal is that customers do not have to go through the whole plan outlined by the pathologist, and achieve a definitive diagnosis as early as possible, thereby providing savings to owners, who still have to invest heavily in the therapeutic approach/process that follows.

In recent literature (Pena & Andrade-Filho, 2009), the pathologic diagnosis was envisioned as a human task, involving people - the pathologist which can make a diagnosis, based on the strategy called pattern recognition. In other words, pattern recognition is the realization that the histological picture conforms to a previously learned picture of a certain disease, which produces a diagnosis interpretation. Also, other kinds of diagnosis strategies, usually adopted by pathologists, were described in this paper, some leading to pathological difficulties or errors, which need to be compensated with new action plans.

Faced with clinical information that a mass located in the mammary gland was punched, the pathologist will inevitably direct his diagnosis to one of the multiple hypotheses included in the classification of mammary tumours available. He is being driven by location and can hardly be impartial and independent from the information provided. If instead, the clinician punched a herniated organ placed at this location, it is not impossible to get a diagnosis of a mammary adenoma, as the pathologist's brain was already formatted to diagnose of one of the several types of mammary tumours.

Recent reports showed disagreement between clinical and pathologic diagnoses, except in necropsy, which is the best method to assess overall diagnostic accuracy (Kent et al., 2004; Vos et al., 2005). Also, autopsy is still the most accurate method of determining the cause of death and auditing accuracy of clinical diagnosis, diagnostic tests and death certification

(Roulson et al., 2005). Increased availability of teaching funds may promote efforts to have necropsies performed in veterinary teaching hospitals (Kent et al., 2004). However, in this aspect the problem is getting worse in human medicine, in which the number of autopsies has shown a tendency to decline (Roulson et al., 2005).

The pressure of having to issue a diagnosis that will help save the animal's life combined with deterioration of the clinical situation increases the responsibility of having to make decisions quickly and can shorten the long and complex process that the pathologist needs to go through to be in possession of the necessary information to make decisions. So, the pathologist is already under sufficient pressure.

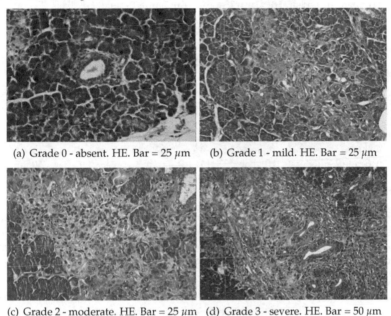

(a) Grade 0 - absent. HE. Bar = 25 μm   (b) Grade 1 - mild. HE. Bar = 25 μm

(c) Grade 2 - moderate. HE. Bar = 25 μm   (d) Grade 3 - severe. HE. Bar = 50 μm

Fig. 6. Semi-quantitative access to fibrosis

More pressure can be caused by the phone ringing continuously in the lab, which will not help to reach an accurate pathological diagnosis. The pathology lab must be a sacred place, where silence and peace must prevail. It is the only way to bring information together, to interpret the observed images correctly. Only then will the images seen on macroscopic exam interact with those observed under the microscope and in the pathologist brain come together to form a conclusion. We must be aware that the pressure clinicians or owners place on the pathologist may precipitate a insufficiently accurate diagnosis.

Nowadays several semi-quantitative and quantitative methods to access macroscopic and microscopic lesions, namely congestion (figure 5), fibrosis (figure 6), inflammatory infiltrate (figure 7), cellular degeneration, mitosis rate, malignancy degrees, among several others, have been developed and published to promote international uniformity, reducing the subjectivity of descriptions depending on the observer, and also to allow statistical studies. Just as a reference, it can be mentioned two: classification and grading of canine mammary tumours (Goldschmidt et al., 2011) and classification of diabetic nephropathy (Tervaert et al., 2010).

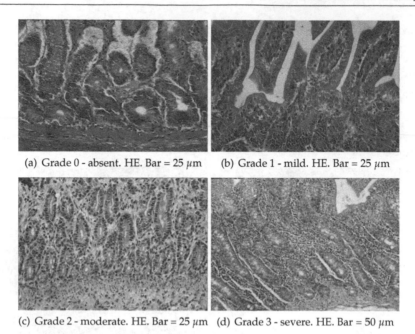

(a) Grade 0 - absent. HE. Bar = 25 μm   (b) Grade 1 - mild. HE. Bar = 25 μm

(c) Grade 2 - moderate. HE. Bar = 25 μm   (d) Grade 3 - severe. HE. Bar = 50 μm

Fig. 7. Semi-quantitative access to inflammatory infiltrate

In research projects two or more observers are required to score lesions independently, in order to enhance the credibility of the results, which is time consuming, expensive and fastidious. Also, some authors defend a standardization of the pathological diagnosis, as a measure to minimize diagnostic variability and error (Foucar, 2000).

The pathologist cannot be reduced to a cognitive instrument for assessing a diagnosis (Pena & Andrade-Filho, 2009) but needs useful instruments to improve his performance.

So the urgent need to compile all available information to obtain a diagnosis in a short period of timeframe, which will help to save the animal's life, is the constant challenge set before the professionals.

A system of rules that allows pathologists to standardize descriptions, easily interpreted by clinicians, will permit an association of descriptions to a conclusive final diagnosis, which would simplify stages in the complex system of diagnosis, thus increasing accuracy. So, the authors propose a model that provides less variability, discrepancies and uncertainties.

3. The re-using knowledge mechanisms

The Artificial Intelligence research community has already proposed some techniques that can be used in several domains to re-use experience. These techniques are described in several bibliographic sources, such as Bratko (2000); Cawsey (1998); Nilsson (1998); Russel & Norvig (2003); Shapiro (1987). In this section, only will be described techniques that have been used in related areas, namely Rule-Based, Pattern and Case-Based Reasoning (CBR).

Rule-Based is the oldest technique. This mechanism emerged from early work on practical and intuitive systems for logical inference (Russel & Norvig, 2003). The rule-based systems have three properties: locality, detachment and truth-functionality. Proposals by Bachmann et al. (2004); Lloyd-Williams (1994); Tauzovich (1990) are examples of Rule-based systems.

Pattern techniques (Shapiro, 1987), not pattern recognition which is described for example in Duda et al. (2001), are used in many areas. They generally involve the definition of patterns and the use of pattern-matching algorithms. A pattern is a structural sketch of an item with some pieces left undefined. Pattern matching is the process of comparing patterns to see if they are similar. In the Information Systems domain there are several works, such as Batra (2005); Conte et al. (2004); Rieu et al. (2002); Seruca & Loucopoulos (2003), which use pattern techniques.

Finally, the CBR method uses past resolved situations to solve new problems (Aamodt & Plaza, 1994; Kolodner, 1993; Mantaras et al., 2006; Riesbeck & Schank, 1989; Watson, 1999). According to Althoff et al. (1995), CBR is a good method to apply in ill situations, such as modelling tasks. CBR comprises two main elements: Case and Process model.

The *case* is formed by the problem and its solution (Kolodner, 1993). The objective and the characteristics of the situation are described by the problem. The solution consists of the solution itself, the solution evaluation and reasoning. Identification of case types constitutes the major step forward in the development of the CBR system. The set of cases of the CBR system is called case memory. An important issue related to cases is indexing. The index is a label associated with the case that will allow us to remember it.

The solving process (or process model), usually called CBR Cycle, begins with the problem description and ends with the solution. The CBR cycle has two main models: 4Rs proposed by Aamodt & Plaza (1994) and the one proposed by Kolodner (1993). The CBR cycle, as illustrated in figure 8, generally involves the following activities:

- case search to find similar cases;
- similarity evaluation to measure the level of similarity between the problem that needs solving and the stored ones;
- adaptation to adjust one or several solutions to the current problem;
- case retain to store the newly resolved problem.

Case search is based on problem description. Similarity evaluation is based on similarity functions (Althoff et al., 1995). Consequently, the new solution is built by adapting old solutions to the needs of the current problem. The last task of the CBR cycle is the inclusion of the case in the case memory. Given the fact that a new case is added to the system, the CBR systems could be said to have the ability to learn. It is worth mentioning, that there are a lot of domains where the CBR methodology has been used (Kolodner, 1993; Mántaras & Plaza, 1997; Watson, 1996). CBR application areas consist of software development, health, architectural design (Pearce et al., 1992), meal planning and legal reasoning systems, for example.

4. The framework and the system

It is important to say that this work was developed after a first approach (published in Tomé & Vala (2010)) of applying CBR to a set of 641 with good results. As shown in table 1, 47.1% of the solutions have a similarity greater than 40% of the solution proposed by the veterinary pathologists. Only 16.8% of cases have solutions in the range 0 to 20%. Although

---

[2] Adapted from (Leake, 1996).

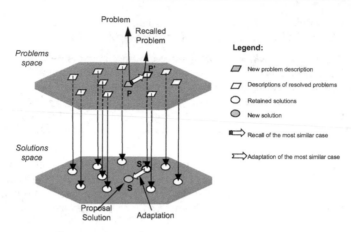

Fig. 8. The CBR method[2]

these results are positive, it is important to mention that the cases are described by regular text which constrains the searching process.

Level of solutions' similarities	[0 , 0.2[	[0.2 , 0,4[	[0.4 , 0.6[	[0.6 , 0.8 [	[0.8 , 1]
	108	231	166	80	56

Table 1. Analysis of level of similarity between solutions

As previously mentioned, several authors proposed a diagnosis system (also called a classification schema) based on some animals aspects. These diagnosis systems are used in disease diagnosis by veterinarian pathologists. The WHO proposed a classification schema for animal tumours in twelve, published three books with a classification schema for animal disease based on most affected organs.

The veterinary pathologists, faced with a disease in a particular species, with a certain clinical information, assess which of the body system, and/or specific organ, is most affected. The specialists process a set of likely differential diagnoses, directing the gross and microscopic diagnosis in order to exclude the less likely, until the possession of a set of information consistent with a pathologic diagnosis of a specific aetiology, mostly grouped in bibliography in: congenital and hereditary; abnormalities of development and growth; degenerative; circulatory; traumatic; foreign bodies; metabolic; nutritional; endocrine; toxic; immune-mediated; inflammatory (viral; bacterial; fungal; protozoal; parasitic; miscellaneous); unknown cause (Maxie, 2007).

The veterinary pathologists, faced with a neoplastic disease in a particular species (mostly pets whose lifetime is longer, having a higher predisposition to this pathologic entity) with a certain clinical information, assess in which body system, and/or specific organ, the tumour is primary located, directing the gross and microscopic diagnosis to exclude the less likely diagnosis, using international histopathological classifications. These provided a widely accepted standard nomenclature of domestic animals tumours, promoting advancements in veterinary pathology and facilitating communication between veterinary and medical pathologists, clinicians and researchers. These classifications also pretended to cross geographic and academic boundaries and establish an international consensus pertaining to the nomenclature of domestic animal tumours (Kiupel et al., 2008).

These classifications include a preliminary assessment of the mass, equivalent to gross examination (measurements; superficial and cut section aspects - colour, consistency of the tissues; evaluation of local invasion; attachment to surrounding tissues; evaluation of possible regional lymph node involvement) and then the evaluation of histological criteria which includes cellular phenotype which includes, in turn, nuclear characteristics - shape, colour and staining characteristics, type of chromatin, nucleoli and cytoplasmic characteristics - shape, colour and staining characteristics, intercellular unions); presence or absence of extracellular matrix and its type, when present; cellular pattern organization and cellular differentiation - anaplasia, anysocariosis, anysocytosis, pleomorphism; mitotic rate.

Based on these cellular features and differentiation degree, the tumours are subdivided primarily into benign and malignant groups and then subdivided, based on phenotype and amount of cellular matrix, in mesenchymal or epithelial neoplasias. The third major sub-division consists in the determination of the specific subtype from the classification for the specific target organ. In general, to determine the specific subtype of a given classification of mesenchymal neoplasias, the specialists must take into account the predominant cellular type recognized and the type of cellular matrix produced by the cells (Slayter et al., 1994b). In a given classification of epithelial neoplasias, the veterinary pathologists must take into account the predominant cell type recognized and the cellular organizational pattern.

Based on the previous descriptions, it can be concluded that each diagnosis:

- is applied for a specific type of disease;
- is based on a set of characteristics;
- is related to a specific type of animal/part..

Based in the previous aspects, it can be concluded that the framework for classification of animal diseases can have the structure illustrated in figure 9.

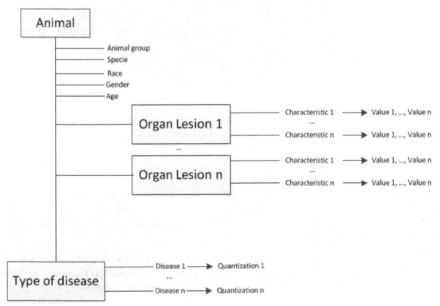

Fig. 9. Classification Schema

For instance, the Adenoma disease (defined in (Meuten et al., 2004)) is characterized by:

"... rare tumor in domestic animals. ... . Adenonomas are discrete, solitary, tan-white masses confined to the renal cortex. They are small (usually < 2cm) in dogs and cats."

Based on the previous description it can be concluded that Adenoma is characterized by the following attributes: *Size, Color, Number, Place, Aspect, Shape, Differentiation, Pattern, Cellular Phenotype, Cytoplasm, Nuclei, Nucleoli, Mitotic Rate* and *Stroma*. The value of each of each attribute is *< 2 cm, Tan-White, Solitary, Renal cortex, Discrete and Masses, Well-differentiated, Tubular, Cuboidal epithelial, Ample, Single, Single, Rare* and *Poor*. How these attributes and values are stored in a software application is shown in figure 11.

The way the attributes and values of each type of disease are structured improves the search of previous cases of the animal's disease. As mentioned at the beginning of this section, searching previous situations with diagnostics described in regular text it is not an easy task because similar situations can be described with the slightest differences.

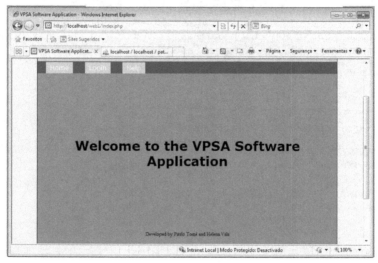

Fig. 10. Software Application

As previously mentioned, it was developed a software application, of which the main window is shown in figure 10 that can be used for storing knowledge about diseases and cases of animal diseases. The first part of the application - knowledge about diseases - is a library of descriptions of animal diseases described in the bibliography of the domain (such as (Dungworth et al., 1999; Goldschmidt et al., 1998; Head et al., 2003; Hendrick et al., 1998; Kennedy et al., 1998; Kiupel et al., 2008; Koestner et al., 1999; Meuten et al., 2004; Misdorp et al., 1999; Slayter et al., 1994a; Valli et al., 2002; Wilcock et al., 2002)). The second part of the application stores data about cases of animal diseases. In this part it is applied the CBR method described in section 3.

In the CBR part (the structure is shown in figure 12) the four phase cycle of Aamodt and Plaza was implemented (Aamodt & Plaza, 1994). The system implements the retrieve, reuse, revise and retain phases and has a repository with cases and knowledge domain.

As shown in figure 12, the system has components that store data and components that do some of the systems tasks. The components: case memory, vocabulary of domain, adaptation

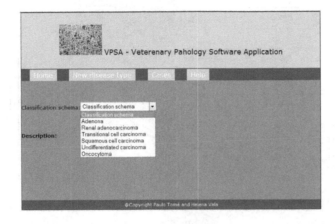

(a) Definition of Disease types

(b) Adenoma Disease

Fig. 11. Definition of Diseases types

rules, case description, inference rules and metric system, store data; while the components: retrieve, reusing, revision and retaining, implement the system tasks.

Each case is stored as a frame (Minsky, 1974). Each case is divided according the Kolodner (1993) proposal into: objective, characteristics and solution. The characteristics and the solutions are pairs of name x value.

In the domain vocabulary module the most frequent expressions used to describe cases of the domain are stored.

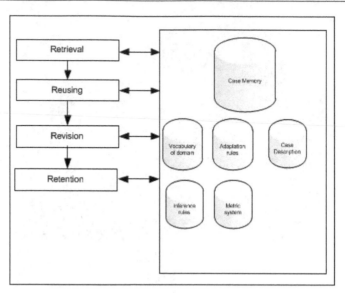

Fig. 12. Structure of the CBR part

The adaptation rules module stores information about how diagnosis can be adapted. In this module if-then rules [3] can be stored which define how diagnosis can be adapted based on the case's characteristics.

The Inference rules module is also built out of if-then rules. These rules are based on the knowledge defined in the books of the domain (such as (Dungworth et al., 1999; Goldschmidt et al., 1998; Head et al., 2003; Hendrick et al., 1998; Kennedy et al., 1998; Kiupel et al., 2008; Koestner et al., 1999; Meuten et al., 2004; Misdorp et al., 1999; Slayter et al., 1994a; Valli et al., 2002; Wilcock et al., 2002)).

In figure 13 the process of definition of a new case disease is shown. As can be seen in the figure, the first three elements (dropdowns of the figure) are elements of the Classification Schema illustrated in figure 9. The elements *Values usually used* and *Attributes also used* were designed to help the user in the process of defining a new case.

The element *Values usually used* can be used for retrieving values that are frequently used for a specific attribute. For instance, in the Adenoma situation the attribute size is usually characterized by the value < 2cm. The use of this facility reduces the chance of defining equal values by different ways.

The element *Attributes also used* aims to help the veterinary pathologist in the definition of the characteristics of the case. Every time the veterinary pathologist defines an attribute, the set of *Attributes also used* shows the attributes which were not defined but may defined regarding the diseases where they appear. For instance, consider the disease and attributes shown in table 2. If the veterinary pathologist already defined the attributes x and y the attributes shown in *Attributes also used* are z,w,a and b. The attributes c,d,e,f,g and h do not appear because they are not in diseases where the attributes x and y appear.

---

[3] Stored according Cawsey (1998).

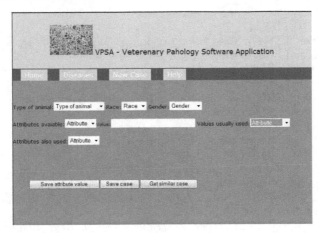

Fig. 13. Definition of Disease types

Diseases	Attributes
A	x,y,z,w
B	x,y,a,b
C	a,b,c,d
D	e,f,g,h

Table 2. Example of Diseases and attributes

Finally, it will be explained the functionality of solution finding based on previously resolved/solved cases. This functionality applies CBR to get a case which is the most similar to the current one. The system searches in the Case memory for a case with similarities to the current one. For all the cases in the Case memory the similarity to the current one based on the values of the attributes and on the knowledge of the domain is determined. The case with highest similarity value is selected.

5. Conclusion and future remarks

In this chapter, it is proposed a framework (Conceptual schema) that can be used to structure knowledge about causes of animal death. The framework was developed based on the analysis of the bibliography of the field.

The framework can be used to develop new databases to store data about animal's death diagnosis and also to improve applications that use previous knowledge of causes of animal death in order to make new diagnoses.

The use of previous knowledge about animal death can improve the task of making diagnoses. First the veterinarian is able to diagnose quickly because he can easily retrieve information about how a similar past situation was diagnosed. Besides that, past knowledge can be considered a library of information where the veterinarian can get useful help or information.

Finally, it is important to highlight that the framework is supported (and was tested) by a software application. Through the developing and testing of the software application, it can be guaranteed that the framework fits into aim for which it was developed.

6. References

Aamodt, A. & Plaza, E. (1994). Case-based reasoning: Foundational issues, methodological variations and systems approaches, *AI-Communications* 7(1): 39–52.

Althoff, K. D., Auriol, E., Barletta, R. & Manago, M. (1995). A review of industrial case-based reasoning tools, *Technical report*, AI Intelligence.

Bachmann, F., Bass, L., Klein, M. & Shelton, C. (2004). Experience using an expert system to assist an architect in designing for modifiability, *Fouth Working IEEE/IFIP Conference on Software Architecture*.

Batra, D. (2005). Conceptual data modeling patterns: Representation and validation, *Journal of Database Management* 16(2): 84–106.

Bratko, I. (2000). *Prolog Programming for Artificial Intelligence*, 3th edn, Addison-Wesley.

Cawsey, A. (1998). *The Essence of Artificial Intelligence*, Prentice-Hall.

Conte, A., Hassine, I., Rieu, D. & Tasted, L. (2004). An information system development tool based on pattern reuse, *ICEIS*, Porto.

Cotran, R., Kumar, V. & Collins, T. (1999). *Robbins Pathologic Basis of Disease (6th ed.)*, W.B. Saunders, Philadelphia.

Duda, R. O., Hart, P. E. & Stork, D. G. (2001). *Pattern Classification*, second edn, John Wiley & Sons, Inc.

Dungworth, D. L., Hauser, B., Hahn, F. F., D.W., W. & Haenichen, T. andHarkema, J. (1999). *International classification of tumours of domestic animals histological classification of tumors of the respiratory system of domestic animals*, Vol. VI, Armed Forces Institute of Pathology.

Foucar, E. (2000). Individuality in the specialty of surgical pathology: self-expression or just another source of diagnostic error?, *Am J Surg Pathol* 24: 1573–1576.

Goldschmidt, M., Dunstan, R., Stannard, A., von Tscharner, C., Walder, E. & Yager, J. (1998). *International classification of tumours of domestic animals histological classification of epithelial and melanocytic tumors of skin of domestic animals*, Vol. III, Armed Forces Institute of Pathology.

Goldschmidt, M., Peña, L., Rasotto, R. & Zappulli, V. (2011). Classification and grading of canine mammary tumors, *Vet Pathol* 48: 117–131.

Grzybicki, D., Vrbin, C., Reilly, T., Zarbo, R. & Raab, S. (2004). Use of physician extenders in surgical pathology practice, *Archives of Pathology & Laboratory Medicine* 128(2).

Head, K., Cullen, J. M., Dubielzig, R., Else, R.W. andMisdorp, W., Patnaik, A., Tateyama, S. & Van der Gaag, I. (2003). *International classification of tumours of domestic animals histological classification of tumors of the alimentary system of domestic animals*, Vol. X, Armed Forces Institute of Pathology.

Hendrick, M., Mahaffey, E., Moore, F. & Vos, J.H. andWalder, E. (1998). *International classification of tumours of domestic animals. Histological classification of mesenchymal tumors of skin ande soft tissues of domestic animals*, Vol. II, Armed Forces Institute of Pathology.

Kennedy, P., Cullen, J., Edwards, J., Goldschmidt, M. H. andLarsen, S., Munson, L. & Nielsen, S. (1998). *International classification of tumours of domestic animals histological classification of tumors of the genital system of domestic animals*, Vol. IV, Armed Forces Institute of Pathology.

Kent, M., Lucroy, M., Dank, G., Lehenbauer, T. & Madewell, B. (2004). Concurrence between clinical and pathologic diagnoses in a veterinary medical teaching hospital: 623 cases (1989 and 1999), *Journal of the American Veterinary Medical Association* 224(3): 403–406.

Kiupel, M., Capen, C., Miller, M. & Smedley, R. (2008). *International classification of tumours of domestic animals histological classification of tumors of the Endocrine System of domestic animals*, Vol. Second Series; XII, Armed Forces Institute of Pathology.

Koestner, A., Bilzer, T., Fatzer, R., Schulman, F., Summers, B. A. & Van Winkle, T. (1999). *International classification of tumours of domestic animals histological classification of tumors of the nervous system of domestic animals*, Vol. V, Armed Forces Institute of Pathology.

Kolodner, J. (1993). *Case-Based Reasoning*, Morgan Kaufmann Publishers.

Langone Medical Center, Department of Pathology (2011). For patients: Practice of pathology. Consulted in July of 2011.
    URL: *http://pathology.med.nyu.edu/patient-care/for-patients/practice-of-pathology*

Leake, D. B. (1996). Cbr in context: The present and future, *in* D. B. Leake (ed.), *Case-Based Reasoning - Experiences, Lessons, & Future Directions*, AAAI Press/The MIT Press, pp. 3 – 30. ISBN - 0-262-62110-X.

Lloyd-Williams, M. (1994). Expert system support for object-oriented database design, *International Journal of Applied Expert Systems* 1(3).

Mantaras, R. L., Mcsherry, D., Bridge, D., Leake, D., Smyth, B., Craw, S., Faltings, B., Maher, M. L., Cox, M. T., Forbus, K., Keane, M., Aamodt, A. & Watson, I. (2006). Retrieval, reuse, revison and retention in case-based reasoning, *The Knowledge Engineering Review* 20(3): 215–240.

Maxie, M. G. (2007). *Jubb, Kennedy & Palmer's Pathology of Domestic Animals*, Vol. I, II, III, fifth edn, Elsevier Saunders, Edinburgh.

Meuten, D. (2002). *Tumors in domestic animals*, 4th edn, Blackwell Publishing Company.

Meuten, D. J., Everitt, J., Inskeep, W., Jacobs, R. M., Peleteiro, M. & Thompson, K. (2004). *International classification of tumours of domestic animals histological classification of tumors of the urinary system of domestic animals*, Vol. XI, Armed Forces Institute of Pathology.

Meyer, D. (2001). The acquisition and management of cytology specimens, *in* R. Raskin, D. Meyer, R. Raskin & D. Meyer (eds), *Atlas of canine and feline cytology*, W.B. Saunders Company, pp. 1 – 5.

Miller, F. P., Vandome, A. F. & McBrewster, J. (2009). *Anatomical Pathology*, VDM Publishing House Ltd.

Miller, K. (2002). Immunocytochemical techniques, *in* J. Bancroft, M. Gamble, J. Bancroth & M. Gamble (eds), *Theory and pratice of histological techniques*, 5th edn, Churchill Livingstone, pp. 421–424.

Minsky, M. (1974). A framework for representing knowledge, *Technical report*, Massachusetts Institute of Technology.

Misdorp, W., Else, R., Hellmén, E. & Lipscomb, T. (1999). *International classification of tumours of domestic animals histological classification of mammary tumors of the dog and cat*, Vol. VII, Armed Forces Institute of Pathology.

Mántaras, R. L. & Plaza, E. (1997). Case-based reasoning: An overview, *AI Comunication* 10(1): 21–29.

Nilsson, N. J. (1998). *Artificial Intelligence: a New Synthesis*, Morgan Kaufmann Publishers.

Pearce, M., Goel, A. G., Kolodner, J. L., Zimring, C., Sentosa, L. & Billington, R. (1992). Case-based design support: A case study in architectural design, *IEEE Expert* October: 14–20.

Pellicciari, C. (2009). Histochemistry through the years, browsing a long-established journal: novelties in traditional subjects, *Eur J Histochem* 54(4).

Pena, G. & Andrade-Filho, S. (2009). How does a pathologist make a diagnosis?, *Arch Pathol Lab Med* 133: 124–132.

Riesbeck, C. K. & Schank, R. C. (1989). *Inside Case-Based Reasoning*, Lawrence Erlbaum Associates, Publishers.

Rieu, D., Conte, A. & Giraudin, J. P. (2002). Pattern-based environments for information systems development, *The Sciences of Design*, Lyon, France.

Roulson, J., Benbow, E. & Hasleton, P. (2005). Discrepancies between clinical and autopsy diagnosis and the value of post mortem histology; a meta-analysis and review, *Histopathology* 47: 551–559.

Russel, S. & Norvig, R. (2003). *Artificial Intelligence, a Modern Approach*, Prentice Hall.

Scott, D., Miller, W. & Griffin, C. (2001). *Muller and Kirk's Small Animal Dermatology*, 6th edn, Saunders, Philadelphia.

Seruca, I. & Loucopoulos, P. (2003). Towards a systematic approach to the capture of patterns within a business domain, *The Journal of Systems and Software* 67: 1–18.

Shapiro, S. C. (1987). *Encyclopedia of Artificial Intelligence*, Vol. 1 e 2, John Wiley & Sons.

Slayter, M. V., Boosinger, T. R., Pool, R. R., Dämmrich, K., Misdorp, W. & Larsen, S. (1994a). *International classification of tumours of domestic animals histological classification of bone and joint tumors of domestic animals*, Vol. I, Armed Forces Institute of Pathology.

Slayter, M. V., Boosinger, T. R., Pool, R. R., Dämmrich, K., Misdorp, W. & Larsen, S. (1994b). *International classification of tumours of domestic animals histological classification of bone and joint tumors of domestic animals animals*, Vol. Second Series , Vol. I, Armed Forces Institute of Pathology.

Tauzovich, B. (1990). An expert system for conceptual data modelling, *8th International Conference on the Entity-Relationship Approach*, Toronto, Canada.

Tervaert, T., Mooyaart, A., Amann, K., Cohen, A., Cook, H. & Drachenberg, C. (2010). Pathologic classification of diabetic nephropathy, *J Am Soc Nephrol* 21: 556–63.

Tomé, P. & Vala, H. (2010). Cbr technique in veterinary pathological anatomy, *in* J. E. Q. Varajão, M. M. Cruz-Cunha & G. D. Putnik (eds), *Enterprise Information Systems*, Vol. 2, Springer, Viana do Castelo - Portugal, pp. 401–405.

University of Utah of Spencer S. Eccles (2011). For patients: Practice of pathology. Consulted in March of 2011.
    URL: *http://library.med.utah.edu/WebPath/HISTHTML/HISTOTCH/HISTOTCH.html*

Valli, V., Jacobs, R.M. andParodi, A. a. W. & Moore, P. (2002). *International classification of tumours of domestic animals histological classification of hematopoietic tumors of domestic animals*, Vol. VIII, Armed Forces Institute of Pathology.

Vos, J., Borst, G., Visser, I., Soethout, K., de Haan, L. & Haffmans, F. (2005). Comparison of clinical and pathological diagnoses in dogs, *Vet Q* 27(1): 2–10.

Watson, I. (1996). Case-based reasoning tools: an review, *2nd UK Workshop on Case-Based Reasoning*, AI-CBR/SGES Publications, University of Salford, pp. 71–78.

Watson, I. (1999). Cbr is a methodology not a technology, *Knowledge Based Systems Journal* 12(5-6).

Wilcock, B., Dubielzig, R. R. & Render, J. A. (2002). *Histological classification of ocular and otic tumors ofdomestic animals*, Vol. IX, Armed Forces Institute of Pathology.

Williams, D. J., Ansford, A. J. S. D. & Forrest, A. S. (1998). *Colour Guide Forensic Pathology*, Churchill Livingstone.

Zarbo, R. & Nakhleh, R. (2009). Surgical pathology specimens for gross examination only and exempt from submission, *Archives of Pathology & Laboratory Medicine* 123(2): 133–139.

2

The Veterinary Business Landscape: Contemporary Issues and Emerging Trends

Colette Henry and Lorna Treanor
Royal Veterinary College,
University of London,
Hatfield (Herts),
UK

1. Introduction

The veterinary sector has witnessed considerable change in recent years, and this has had a significant impact on the wider veterinary business landscape. Most noteworthy, perhaps, has been the change at the global level in the focus of animal welfare, with a growth in small/companion animal care and a reduction in large animal work (Lowe, 2009). This has resulted in increased competition amongst veterinary practices and the recognition that veterinary services need to be appropriately marketed. Furthermore, it has been noted that the increase in and improved access to on-line veterinary pharmacies is beginning to 'squeeze' practices' profit margins on the sale of veterinary medicines, prompting the realisation that pricing structures for core veterinary services may need to be significantly revised in order to compensate.

With specific regard to large animal work, equine services now tend to be handled by specialists, and farm animal work is considered to be in decline, with the latter prompting particular concern. Indeed, significant changes to the farming sector (i.e. declining livestock populations, a reduction in the number/size of farm holdings, new legislation and a radical change in the relationship between government and veterinarians) mean that farm animal veterinary practices now face significant competitive and sustainability issues.

There have also been significant changes to existing veterinary business models, with a marked decrease in the number of small private, independent practices and a drive toward partnerships, groups and large corporate structures with shared resources and strengthened buying powers. As a result of the latter, new management career opportunities have opened up within the corporate sector for appropriately trained and entrepreneurially motivated veterinarians to run individual clinics or sites as semi-independent business units.

Collectively, the above changes have created an extremely dynamic and highly competitive veterinary business landscape. Indeed, it is now widely recognised that managers within the broader veterinary industry need to be much more commercially aware than in the past, prompting the recognition of a significant skills gap in business and management (Lowe, 2009). This skills gap is recognised beyond the traditional practice management role, with some acknowledgement that managers in the veterinary science, diagnostics and genetics areas of the pharmaceutical, bio-science and pet food industries are experiencing similar difficulties. Recent literatures further platform the need for other veterinary professionals, such as advisors in government departments and those responsible for intensive livestock production units, to acquire business and management skills. Such trends, are not confined to the UK, rather, they would appear to be global phenomena.

Against this backdrop, and by way of providing valuable context for some of the more clinically oriented chapters in this book, our chapter considers some of the recent changes and emerging trends within the broader veterinary sector and the actual and potential impact of these on the veterinary business landscape. In particular, we focus our discussion on changes and trends within three key areas related to veterinary medicine: firstly, the recent changes within the agricultural sector; secondly, the global gender shift toward a predominately female profession and, finally, the evolving veterinary educational curriculum with an emerging trend toward the incorporation of business and management topics. We argue that, collectively, changes in these areas will have a considerable impact on the veterinary sector from a business perspective, and that such impact will be both positive and negative in nature. Given that the extent of the changes and emerging trends in these particular areas is only beginning to gain recognition, little by way of robust academic attention has been paid to their potential impact from a business perspective. As a consequence, there is a dearth of research at both the conceptual and empirical level in these areas, with a clear need for extant literature to be developed and expanded.

In this conceptual chapter, we explore the above issues by reviewing relevant literatures, identifying current trends and discussing the potential impact of these on the veterinary profession. With few studies in this particular area, the authors adopt an inductive approach, designed to generate new understanding and propositions for further research (Rosa & Dawson, 2006). Following this introductory section, we examine some of the recent changes within the agricultural sector and the impact of these on the veterinary profession. This is followed by a discussion of the gender shift currently being experienced within the profession and, subsequently, the emerging trend within veterinary curricula to include business and entrepreneurship modules. With regard to the latter, the potential impact of such curricula developments on employable skills is explored. The chapter concludes with a discussion on the implications of all these changes for the veterinary sector and offers some suggestions for future research. Thus, the authors lay the theoretical foundation for future empirical work in this field by debating some key concepts and generating hypotheses for future study. Specifically, the authors posit that veterinary curricula will need to continue to adapt to ensure graduates are equipped with the relevant skills and abilities to enable them to keep pace with the dynamic and highly competitive industry in which they will eventually work. In this regard, the incorporation of business and entrepreneurship education will be critical.

2. The agricultural sector

According to Lincoln (2004), the veterinary profession of old was primarily concerned with horses and other large working animals; this was not surprising, given the strong agricultural basis of earlier local economies. However, as national economies moved away from dominant agricultural bases, the mass manufacture of farm machinery made life somewhat less laboursome for farming communities, reducing the dependence on large working animals and manual labour. Eventually, modernization processes led to the industrialization of both arable and livestock farming (Ilbery & Maye, 2010), with assembly-line production systems incorporated into farming practice to help boost production and lower costs. Through a combination of mechanisation, genetics and artificial inputs, farmers were able to improve yields (Boulton, Rushton, Wathes & Wathes, 2011). As a result, in the dairy sector, milk quotas had to be introduced in the '80s to address overproduction, and this was followed by the deregulation of milk markets in the '90s. Dairy producer numbers declined, lactation yields per cow increased and there was a significant reduction in the number of dairy cattle (Boulton et al; 2011). The impact of such a radical change on the veterinary profession was becoming clear - fewer dairy cattle would eventually mean fewer 'patients' for farm animal vets. Indeed, the gradual reduction in veterinary 'patient' numbers has not been confined to the diary sector. The pig population has also halved over the past fifteen years resulting from a combination of factors including the Euro-pound exchange rate, changes to animal welfare regulations and disease problems (Henry, Baillie & Rushton, 2011). The 'Foot and Mouth' (FMD) epidemic of 2001, in conjunction with changes to EU subsidy payments, has also resulted in a reduced sheep population. According to the Department for Environment, Food and Rural Affairs (Defra), the gradual decline in livestock numbers witnessed by the agricultural sector has been developing over recent decades (Defra, 2010). The net effect of this raft of changes and events has been a reduction in the number of family-run, working farms in the UK, whilst a growth in larger corporate holdings and 'hobby-style' or supplementary-income farms has been noted (Defra, 2009; Rushton & McLeod, 2006; Henry et al., 2011).

EU enlargement, the CAP reform, changing consumer demands and globalization have also impacted negatively on the agricultural sector (Rudmann, 2008), with the scale of support provided to farmers drastically reduced (Alsos, Carter, Ljunggren & Welter, 2011). A gradual decline in income from traditional farming activities has forced many farming businesses to diversify in order to remain viable. Diversification requires farmers to combine other, typically non-agricultural activities with their core farm business. In this regard, conversion of farm buildings for alternative, tourism-related product offerings became a popular choice. Indeed, about 50% of farms in the UK have supplemented traditional incomes through some type of farm diversification (Defra, 2008, as cited by McElwee & Bosworth, 2010: 820). Again, all of this has had a negative impact on the veterinary community, as the trend toward smaller farms with fewer livestock and diversified activities has resulted in less demand for veterinary services overall.

3. The gender shift

The veterinary profession has traditionally been a male domain, however, in recent years, there has been an unprecedented increase in the number of women entering veterinary medicine (BVA/AVS, 2008; Lowe, 2009). By way of example, in 1998, one in three vets in the UK were female, with 57% of those under thirty being women; by 2002, 37% of vets registered with RCVS were female (RCVS, 2002), whereas in 2010, seventy one percent of UK vets under 40 were female (RCVS, 2010: viii). The recent '2010 Survey of the UK Veterinary and Veterinary Nursing Professions' (RCVS, 2010) highlighted that fifty-four percent of respondent veterinarians working in practice were women; furthermore, eighty-four percent of respondents in veterinary practice were employed within clinical veterinary practice and fifty-seven percent of those were women. Indeed, in 2011, women outnumber men as working veterinarians in the UK; moreover, eighty percent of veterinary undergraduates are female (RCVS, 2010). This significant shift in the gender make-up of both the student and practicing professional veterinary populations raises a number of important issues relating to educational strategies, career orientation, pay, working practices, and the general future direction of the profession. All of these, as will be discussed in section five of this chapter, will have a direct impact on the future veterinary business landscape.

Not surprisingly, perhaps, the trend toward a predominantly female profession is not restricted to the UK. According to statistics from the American Veterinary Medical Association (AVMA), the number of female veterinarians in the US more than doubled between 1991 and 2002 (Zhao, 2002). Whereas only 5% of applications to US vet schools were from females in the late 1960s, by the end of the 1990s, over seventy percent of applications were from young women.

The increasing numbers and dominance of women within the veterinary profession have also been discussed in several other countries (see, for example, Heath (2007) in relation to Australia; Lofstedt (2003) in relation to Canada, and Basagac Gul et al. (2008) with regard to Turkey). Collectively, such data suggest that the 'feminization' of the veterinary profession is not only a global phenomenon but also looks set to continue for some time.

With regard to the 'cause' of this phenomenon, several explanations have been offered, including improvement in chemical restraints available for large animals, the elimination of gender-based admission discrimination and the generally caring portrayal of veterinarians in both the literature and on television (Lofstedt, 2003:534). Controversially, perhaps, the marked increase in women entering the veterinary profession and, in parallel, the decline in men's participation, may also be attributed to the relatively lower salary levels of veterinary professionals (Lofstedt, 2003). This hypothesis builds on Tuchman's (1989) argument that professions deemed to be lacking in appropriate economic incentives and, by association, cultural legitimacy, may quickly lose their attraction for men. It must be noted, however, that despite the increasing number of women entering veterinary medicine and the fact that women now make up more than half the veterinary workforce, most veterinary businesses, whether based on traditional practice or the commercialisation of scientific research, are still led by men. Thus, to date, women have not featured prominently as business leaders within the veterinary profession, nor have they been perceived as potential entrepreneurs or innovators. This point is particularly important, because based on what we know about women and business ownership/entrepreneurship generally (see, for example, Brush, 1997; Brush, Carter, Gatewood, Green & Hart, 2001; Henry & Treanor, 2010), it is unlikely that current levels of veterinary entrepreneurship will be maintained or, indeed, increased in a female dominated veterinary sector.

As with the majority of professional disciplines, veterinary colleges are the 'gatekeepers to the profession' (Andrews, 2009). However, the merit-based admission system now in place, whilst undoubtedly facilitating women's entry into the profession, means that it is veterinary 'applicants', rather than veterinary 'students' who should be profiled to gauge the attractiveness of (or barriers to) veterinary medicine (Andrews 2009; Lincoln, 2004). For example, in the US, Zhao (2002) reports that both vet students and veterinarians consider the salary to be off-putting to male students. The salary of veterinary practitioners is significantly less than that of their human medicine counterparts and, therefore, men may be more inclined to train in human medicine. Zhao (2002) indicates that males and females choose their careers for different reasons – women will select something they are passionate about and think they will enjoy, whereas financial reward tends to shape the options considered by men. Zhao (2002) points to anecdotal evidence that men consider their longer-term futures and ability to provide for their families; similarly, he posits that an attraction for women to veterinary medicine is the ability to work part-time when raising young children, an option that has not traditionally been open to medical professionals to the same extent.

Interestingly, Lincoln (2010) found that young males were more likely to be deterred from applying to veterinary schools where faculty is predominately female. Research also suggests that men are dissuaded from entering female dominated professions as 'women's work' tends to attract lower salaries (Reskin & Roos, 1990; Lincoln 2004). It certainly seems that the veterinary profession is likely to become increasingly feminised in the medium to long term, and that the implications of such feminisation for future veterinary businesses now need to be given serious consideration.

4. Veterinary education

Admission to veterinary programmes around the globe is a highly competitive process, with candidates typically required to attain top grades in science-based subjects to qualify for entry. Owing to the large number of applicants to veterinary schools, interviews often form part of the selection process. Although curricula will vary from provider to provider, veterinary programmes are extremely intensive courses of study and typically include pre-clinical, para-clinical and clinical components. In addition, as part of their extramural study (EMS), veterinary students are required to spend a considerable amount of time over the course of their degree in a range of veterinary practices and hospitals to gain practical clinical experience. In the UK, course duration is typically five years, although it can be longer elsewhere.

In addition to an in-depth knowledge and understanding of the scientific and clinical aspects, veterinary students also need to have a grasp of the legal, ethical and social elements of veterinary practice. Thus, communication and interpersonal skills; responsible and professional behaviour, and an understanding of the business context of veterinary practice are now recognized as important areas that should be incorporated into veterinary curricula. With particular regard to the latter, it was a group of women veterinary surgeons in the UK who, in 1941, first called for business training to be included within veterinary programmes (Aitken, 1994). While such calls are gaining momentum, the Lowe Report (2009) highlights that UK veterinary graduates remain insufficiently prepared for effective business management or leadership, this despite the fact that most will probably work within or lead a small veterinary business at some stage in their careers. More specifically, Lowe (2009) called for the inclusion of business planning, marketing, human resource management and an awareness of the veterinary business environment to be provided to veterinary students as part of their undergraduate training so that, upon entering the workplace, they would be equipped to offer clients treatments and prevention strategies that are both cost-effective and aligned with the needs of the individual veterinary business within which they work (Lowe, 2009: 55). Similar calls have been made for the inclusion of such business and management training in North America (Ilgen, 2002; Kogen et al., 2005).

Currently, where business and management topics are included in the veterinary curriculum, they tend to be incorporated under the banner of 'Professional Studies', a strand of education running though most veterinary degrees, which, as its label suggests, covers the professional behaviour aspects of veterinary medicine. This strand typically includes the non-clinical skills and abilities associated with working as a veterinary professional, thus, communications, legal and ethical considerations, insurance, veterinary certification and compliance issues, all form part of this element of the programme. With particular regard to business and management, a range of topics are taught, including enterprising skills and abilities (i.e. creativity and idea generation), practice management (i.e. marketing, finance and human resource management for existing veterinary practices) and entrepreneurship (i.e. new venture creation or the development of a new service/clinic within the veterinary practice sector). Indeed, there appears to be growing recognition that any type of entrepreneurship education can be extremely beneficial for students regardless of their discipline area. Such education not only prepares individuals for starting new businesses but, in increasingly competitive environments, equips students with the knowledge, skills and competences to engage in a more enterprising, innovative and flexible manner (Hynes & Richardson, 2007: 733), preparing them for a world where they will increasingly need to manage their own careers in an entrepreneurial way (Hytti & O'Gorman, 2004: 11-12) and add value to their employers' businesses (Henry & Treanor, 2010).

Notwithstanding the above, the incorporation of business education, including entrepreneurship education, within veterinary curricula is still relatively new, despite the long-standing recognition that the provision of business skills will benefit both veterinary graduates and employers. However, the typical positioning of business topics within the professional studies strand of the veterinary curriculum has been somewhat problematic, with anecdotal evidence suggesting that such non-clinical topics tend to be viewed by students as peripheral rather than core. While this is, to some degree, understandable, given the already overcrowded veterinary curriculum, it does pose a number of problems for veterinary business educators tasked with preparing students for the competitive business environments in which they will eventually work.

While pedagogical approaches to veterinary education will vary from provider to provider, most veterinary schools tend to employ a combination of formal lectures, directed learning sessions, tutorials, practicals and case-based learning (QAA, 2002), with assessment methodologies ranging from multiple-choice questions (MCQs) through to portfolios and objective structured clinical examinations (OSCEs) (Baillie and Rhind, 2008). Veterinary business topics also tend to be examined in the traditional MCQ or EMQ (extended matching questions) format, however, the more practical and reflective assessment methods normally associated with mainstream business education are beginning to be introduced. While the current trend within veterinary curricula is clearly toward the inclusion rather than the exclusion of business education, it is widely acknowledged that the business curriculum is still evolving and is undergoing continuous refinement as a result of student feedback and industry consultation.

5. Discussion and implications

The changes discussed above under the three headings of the agricultural sector, the gender shift and veterinary education have significant implications for the veterinary business landscape across the broader veterinary sector, impacting beyond the practice wing of the profession. As mentioned at the outset of this chapter, to date, robust academic attention has not been paid to the implications of changes in these areas. Such implications will now be discussed under the relevant headings below.

5.1 Implications of changes within the agricultural sector

A review of the literature highlights a number of changes within the agricultural sector, all of which have a direct impact on the provision of farm animal veterinary services. In the first instance, and at the fundamental level, reduction in livestock numbers, farm holdings and farm sizes mean that there are going to be significantly fewer farm 'patients' requiring veterinary services. Although it is now recognised that farm animal veterinary practice is in decline (Lowe, 2009), there is still a substantial farming community around the globe, and thus this valuable specialist service still needs to be provided to those who require it. As a result, farm animal veterinary practices are coming under increasing pressure to review their operational business model to ensure their practice is both viable and sustainable.

In parallel, with reduced government support, a decline in income from traditional farming activities, and forced to diversify to sustain their own businesses, farmers now have less disposable income to spend on veterinary services. As a result, with regard to veterinary work, there is a growing trend toward farmers doing more for themselves rather than immediately referring work to the vet. Therefore, the average spend on veterinary services per farm holding is going to reduce. The business implications of this for rural farm animal veterinary practice are quite serious: turnover and profit margins will be affected. As a result, farm animal veterinary practices will need to revisit their operational costs to ensure the service they are offering is both viable and aligned with their clients' needs. In this regard, future veterinary graduates interested in farm animal work will need to have a thorough understanding of their clients' needs; appreciate the changes taking place within the farming sector and be able to advise farmers on the more strategic issues related to farm animal health and welfare.

It would appear too that marketing will be crucial to the survival of farm animal veterinary practice. With reduced demand for services but increased competition from existing providers, farm animal vets will need to engage more closely with their client base to determine farmers' needs, adapt their service and market it appropriately. It seems inevitable that, in the future, farmers will look for a more holistic veterinary service offering. It would appear, therefore, that in parallel with farming enterprises themselves, farm animal veterinary practices will need to explore diversification strategies if they are to remain viable from a business perspective.

5.2 Implications of the gender shift

Interestingly, the global trend towards a predominately female veterinary profession, as discussed above, has raised a number of serious concerns that will directly impact on the future veterinary business landscape. Such concerns range from a potential reduction in mean salaries for veterinarians overall (as evidence from other sectors suggests that women tend to accept lower salaries), through to potential ramifications for large animal practice (as women tend to favour small, companion animal work (Lowe, 2009)). There are also fears that women will remain less likely to own practices than their male counterparts (RCVS, 2006, 2010), which may result in larger corporate chains becoming increasingly commonplace.

Rubin (2001: 1753) cites a succinct list of 'critical issues or concerns' set out by the Gender Issues Task Force (GITF), established by the National Commission on Veterinary Economic Issues (NCVEI) in 2000, as:

- Women's income lags that of men
- Women work fewer hours
- Women may be less likely to own practices; may achieve practice ownership later
- Women may define job satisfaction more subjectively, with less objective rewards
- Women may price services lower than men
- Women's business acumen may lag that of men
- Women may be more highly satisfied with lower income levels
- Women's income may be negatively influencing income levels for all veterinarians
- Women tend to bear more of the burden of balancing home, childcare, and eldercare responsibilities with professional responsibilities
- Women may be more reluctant to take on job or management responsibilities in the face of home management responsibilities.

By way of example of the potential negative impact of the 'feminization' of the veterinary profession, Smith (2002) highlights the gender shift that has occurred in the United States since the 1980s and outlines the parallel decline in veterinarians' economic standing over that period. In a similar vein, other commentators have reported that male veterinary graduates in the USA have received more offers of employment, larger salaries and, typically, greater benefit packages than their female counterparts (Gehrke, 1997; Slater & Slater, 2000; Lincoln, 2004). Similarly, the Brakke Management and Behaviour Study conducted in the USA in 1998 showed that women earned significantly less than their male peers even when factors such as ownership status, years experience and hours worked were the same.

Similar concerns relating to reduced salaries and pay gaps between genders have been voiced in the UK. For example, the Inter-Professional Group study of 'Women Professionals in the EC' (1993) highlighted unfavourable salary trends for UK women vets (Aitken, 1994). This issue was further highlighted in the RCVS Survey of the Profession (2010), which highlighted that: "females account for 59% of those who are leaving [the profession] on grounds of pay" (RCVS, 2010: 40). Thus, the veterinary sector could face significant staff shortages in the future, with veterinary businesses unable to deliver the range of services required by their clients.

As women come to dominate the profession numerically, the lower pay they receive ultimately means that the average salary for veterinarians may fall in real terms. For women in particular, the impact is greater, with existing pay gaps and potentially lower salary levels restricting women from amassing the requisite capital to buy into a partnership or establish their own practice. This will have a direct impact on the veterinary business landscape, with potentially fewer independent practices and a continued growth in large corporate structures.

5.3 Implications of changes within veterinary education

In contrast with the two areas discussed above, the trend in veterinary education toward the incorporation of business and management topics within the curriculum should have a significant positive impact on the veterinary business landscape. Regardless of their discipline area, graduates in the 21st century face an increasingly competitive and volatile employment market and it is critical that they are equipped with skills that enable them to maximise their full potential (HEA, 2005). Future graduates will need to have greater ownership of their employable skills and be able to cope with economic upheavals to capitalise on career opportunities (McNair, 2003, as cited in HEA, 2005:12). Universities are under pressure to demonstrate how they are enhancing graduate employability (Dearing, 1997; BIS, 2009) and, in this regard, veterinary schools are no exception. According to BIS (2009), employable skills are modern workplace skills such as team working, business awareness and communication skills; essentially, they are skills that prepare students for the world of work. Thus, interpersonal, leadership and team skills; confidence, motivation and networking skills; problem-solving and business acumen are all deemed critical to enhancing graduate employability (Hawkins, 1999). In this regard, business and management education, more specifically, entrepreneurship education will have a particularly valuable role to play in veterinary curricula in the future. Indeed, there is already evidence in the literature to show that employers recruiting postgraduates place considerable value on such skills in the context of leadership, analytical thinking, problem-solving and idea generation in addition, of course, to actual work experience (CIHE, 2010).

Due to the highly competitive nature of the current veterinary business landscape, veterinary practices need to operate as viable business entities more so than ever before. Thus, veterinary graduates will need to have at least some foundation in marketing and finance. Furthermore, the new career opportunities created by the corporate sector will require entrepreneurially minded individuals who have an understanding of the broader veterinary business sector in addition to their veterinary degree. Through joint venture partnership arrangements, appropriately oriented veterinary graduates will have the opportunity to run their own business without all of the costs and risks associated with setting up a new independent practice or raising the finances required to buy into an existing partnership. If current trends in veterinary (business) education continue, then future veterinary graduates should be well equipped to not only exploit such opportunities as they emerge, but also to add value to the business dimension of all types of existing veterinary practice by helping to develop effective marketing strategies, contributing toward financial sustainability and enhancing the overall veterinary service offering. Furthermore, given that the majority of veterinary graduates take up roles within traditional practice settings, there would appear to be considerable scope for the commercialisation of research and new venture creation outside of this realm. In this regard, increasing the entrepreneurship dimension of the veterinary business curriculum will have obvious benefits.

6. Conclusions

This chapter has considered some of the recent changes and emerging trends within the broader veterinary sector and the actual and potential impact of these on the veterinary business landscape. Focusing our discussion on three key areas: the agricultural sector, the gender shift toward a predominately female profession and the evolving veterinary educational curriculum we reviewed the relevant literatures and explored the implications involved for the veterinary business landscape. Essentially, given the dearth of research in these particular areas, our primary contribution in this chapter has been to raise awareness of the potential impact of recent changes on the broader veterinary business landscape. In so doing, we enhance understanding of the business dimension, platform concerns, and encourage debate around future potential strategies that could help alleviate the negative impact of some of the changes we have discussed. This is important, given that little by way of concerted academic attention has been paid to the business dimension of the broader veterinary sector.

We demonstrated that the above changes have created an extremely dynamic and highly competitive veterinary business landscape. In the first instance, changes to the agricultural sector have had a significant negative impact on farm animal veterinary businesses, with fewer 'patients' for farm animal vets. Rural veterinary service providers will have to rethink their service offering and, possibly, diversify to ensure business viability in what is essentially a declining but still competitive marketplace. To some degree, this parallels the measures that farming clients have had to implement in order to sustain their own farm business. Undoubtedly, in the future, we will see significantly fewer farming enterprises and fewer farm animal veterinary practices in the veterinary business landscape. However, those farm animal veterinary service providers remaining in the sector will be offering a much more holistic service much more aligned to the changing needs of their farming clients.

The gender shift toward a predominately female veterinary profession will, as highlighted above, have a considerable impact on the veterinary business landscape. This area, however, has been particularly slow to gain attention in the literature and now requires urgent action if some of the potential negative impacts outlined in the earlier part of our chapter are to be avoided. The impact of career breaks, maternity leave, lower pay and, potentially, a continued trend toward companion animal care only, all suggest a future veterinary business landscape that fails to appropriately cater for farm animal, exotic species or specialist services and procedures. Furthermore, if women make up the majority of the veterinary workforce in the future, then their needs, working behaviours and career aspirations will need to be appropriately catered for and managed. This will have to lead to the introduction of new, more family-friendly working practices. In addition, if, as our discussion suggests, women remain less likely to pursue business leadership roles, then the veterinary business landscape will be 'stocked' with corporate enterprises managed, very possibly, by non-veterinary business managers. While further exploration is clearly needed, this could potentially be detrimental for the veterinary profession as a whole.

With regard to the veterinary curriculum, while the case for business and entrepreneurship education within veterinary medicine has never been stronger, the challenge now for educationalists is to figure out *what* exactly should be taught and *how* best to teach it. In what is already a crowded curriculum with large student groups to cater for, prioritizing the business and enterprise agenda over the more clinical topics or 'ologies' (i.e. immunology, pathology, epidemiology, etc) is not an easy task. Given all the changes that are taking place in the broader veterinary sector, we argue the case for including the full spectrum of business and entrepreneurship education - 'enterprise skills for life', core elements of 'practice management' and opportunities for 'new venture creation' within the five-year veterinary medicine degree programme. Given that relatively few graduates work outside the pure practice wing of the profession, the opportunities to encourage entrepreneurship are significant. Indeed, while a full discussion on this particular topic is outside the scope of this chapter, the potential for innovation and new venture creation in the context of commercialisation of veterinary clinical research, development of new drugs and treatments, and the creation of new products and services for supply to veterinary practices to date has not been fully explored. Developments in these areas could only serve to enhance the veterinary business landscape in the future.

6.1 Future research

Looking to the future, collaboration and partnership arrangements amongst veterinary service and education providers, both nationally and internationally, is likely to offer considerable mutual benefit for all those involved in the veterinary sector. In this regard, future research should consider how such partnerships might be encouraged and where they might be most beneficial. In addition, and with specific regard to the gender shift, future research should focus on increasing the business leadership and entrepreneurial intentions of female veterinary students. This is particularly important if the veterinary business landscape is to continue to include practices led by veterinary professionals. Finally, from our discussion in this chapter, we posit that there is considerable potential within veterinary educational curricula to enhance students' understanding of the business dimension of the veterinary sector, to ensure they are fully aware of the changes taking place within the sector and how these will impact on the veterinary businesses in which they will work in the future. In this regard, the evolving veterinary educational curriculum needs to continue its trend toward a business orientation.

7. References

Aitken, M.M. (1994) "Women in the Veterinary profession" The Veterinary Record, 134, 546-551.

Alsos, G. A., Carter, S., Ljunggren, E. and Welter, F. (2011), "Introduction: researching entrepreneurship in agriculture and rural development", in G.A Alsos., S. Carter., E. Ljunggren and F. Welter (eds), *The handbook of research in entrepreneurship in agriculture and rural development*, Cheltenham: Edward Elgar, pp.1-18.

Andrews, F.M. (2009) 'Veterinary School admissions in the United Kingdom: attracting students to veterinary careers to meet the expanding needs of the profession and of global society', Rev. Sci. Tech., 28 (2): 699-707.

Baillie, S. and Rhind, S. (2008), "A guide to assessment methods in veterinary medicine," A 'Blue Sky' project funded by the RCVS Trust, available from http://www.live.ac.uk/documents/assessment_guide.pdf, last accessed 20th May 2010.

Basagac Gul, R.T., Ozkul, T., Ackay, A. & Ozen, A. (2008) 'Historical Profile of Gender in Turkish Veterinary Education' JVME, 35 (2), pp. 305-309.

BIS – Department for Business Innovation and Skills. (2009). "Higher ambitions: The future of universities in a knowledge economy," available from www.bis.gov.uk

Boulton, A., Rushton, J., Wathes, C. M. & Wathes, D. C. (2011). "Three decades of change: a review of the UK dairy industry", Royal Agricultural Society Journal (forthcoming).

Brush, C. (1997). Women owned businesses: Obstacles and opportunities. *Journal of Developmental Entrepreneurship*, 2(1), 1–25.

Brush, C., Carter, N., Gatewood, E., Green, P., & Hart, M. (2001). "The Diana Project, women business owners and equity capital: the Myths dispelled." Insight Report, Kansas City, MO: Kauffman Center for Entrepreneurial Leadership.

BVA - British Veterinary Association / AVS - Association of Veterinary Students. (2008). "Survey 2008," available from:
http:www.bva.co.uk/student_centre/Student_survey.aspx, last accessed 9th April 2010.

CIHE – Council for Industry and Higher Education. (2010), "Talent fishing: What businesses want from postgraduates," A CIHE report for the Department of Business Innovation and Skills, CIHE: London (www.cihe.co.uk)

Dearing, R. (1997), "The Dearing Report," available from:
https://bei.leeds.ac.uk/Partners/NCIHE

Defra. (2009), "Agriculture in the United Kingdom", available from:
http://www.defra.gov.uk/evidence/statistics/foodfarm/general/auk/latest/index.htm
(last accessed 17 May 2011).

Defra. (2010), "June Census of Agriculture and Horticulture - UK", 25 May, available from:
http://archive.defra.gov.uk/evidence/statistics/foodfarm/landuselivestock/june
survey/documents/June-labour-2010.pdf (last accessed 30 May 2011).

Gehrke, BC. (1997) 'Employment of Male and Female Graduates of US veterinary medical colleges" Jamva, 212: 208-209

Hawkins, P. (1999), "The art of building windmills: Career tactics for the 21st century

HEA – Higher Education Academy (2005), "Embedding employability in the curriculum: enhancing students' career planning skills," report available from
http://www.heacademy.ac.uk, last accessed 10th May 2010.

Heath TJ., (2007) "Longitudinal study of Veterinary Students and veterinarians: The First 20 Years", Australian Veterinary Journal, Vol 85 No. 7, pp. 281-289

Henry, C. & Treanor, L. (2010). Entrepreneurship education and Veterinary Medicine: Enhancing Employable Skills. Education & Training, Vol. No. (December, 2010), pp. 607-623.

Henry, C., Baillie, S. & Rushton, J. (2011). Exploring the future sustainability of farm animal veterinary practice, paper presented at the Rural Enterprise Conference, Nottingham Trent University, June.

Hynes, B. & Richardson, T. (2007), "Creating an entrepreneurial mindset: getting the process right for information and communication technology students", in Lowry, G. (Ed.), Information Systems and Technology Education: From the University to the Workplace, IGI Global, Hershey, PA.

Hytti, U. & O'Gorman, C. (2004), "What is 'enterprise education'? An analysis of the objectives and methods of enterprise education programmes in four European countries", Education & Training, Vol. 46 No. 1, pp. 11-23.

Ilbery, B. & Maye, D. (2010), "Agricultural Restructuring and Changing Food Networks in the UK," in N. Coe and A. Jones, (eds), The Economic Geography of the UK, London: Sage, pp. 166-180.

Ilgen, D.R. (2002), "Skills, knowledge, aptitudes and interests for veterinary practice management: fitting personal characteristics to situational demands", JVME, Vol. 29 No. 3, pp. 153-6.

Kogan, L.R., McConnell, S.L. & Schoenfeld-Tacher, R. (2005), "Perspectives in professional education: response of a veterinary college to career development needs identified in the KPMG LLP study", Journal of the American Veterinary Medical Association, Vol. 226 No. 7.

Lincoln, A., (2004) "Vetting Feminization Beyond Motives: Structural and Economic Influences on Applications to American Veterinary Medical Colleges, 1976-1988", Paper presented at the annual meeting of the American Sociological Association, Hilton San Francisco & Renaissance Parc 55 Hotel, San Francisco, CA, Online Last accessed: 19th January 2011 via:
http://www.allacademic.com/meta/p110046_index.html

Lincoln A. E. (2010) The shifting supply of men and women to occupations: feminization in veterinary education. Social Forces 88, 1969–1998. doi: 10.1353/sof.2010.0043

Lofstedt, J. (2003), "Gender and veterinary medicine", Canadian Veterinary Journal, Vol. 44 No. 7, pp. 533-5.

Lowe, P. (2009), Unlocking Potential – A Report on Veterinary Expertise in Food Animal Production, Department for Environment and Food Rural Affairs (DEFRA), London.

McElwee, G. and Bosworth, G. (2010). "Exploring the strategic skills of farmers across a typology of farm diversification approaches," Journal of Farm Management, 13 (12), pp. 819-838.

McNair, S. (2003), "Employability in Higher Education," LTSN Generic Centre, University of Surrey.

QAA – Quality Assurance Agency. (2002), "Veterinary Science – Subject Benchmark Statements," Quality Assurance for Higher Education, Gloucester.

RCVS – Royal College of Veterinary Surgeons. (2006). "The UK Veterinary Profession in 2006: The findings of a survey of the profession, conducted by the Royal College of Veterinary Surgeons", London: Royal College of Veterinary Surgeons. Available at: http://www.rcvs.org.uk/shared_asp_files/uploadedfiles/97d3daf0-9567-4b2f-9972-b0a86cfb13c7_surveyprofession2006.pdf (last accessed: 8th January, 2010).

RCVS. (2010), "The 2010 RCVS Survey of the UK Veterinary and Veterinary Nursing Profession", London: Royal College of Veterinary Surgeons. Available at: http://www.rcvs.org.uk/Templates/SinglePublication.asp?NodeID=7828174 (last accessed: 4 November 2010).

Reskin, B. & Roos, P. Job queues, gender queues. Explaining women's inroads into male occupations. Philadelphia: Temple University Press, 1990

Rosa, P. and Dawson, A. (2006), "Gender and the commercialization of university science: Academic founders of spinout companies," Entrepreneurship and Regional Development, July, pp.341-366.

Rubin, H. E. (2001). "Generation and gender – a critical mix," JAVMA, 218(11), pp.1753-1754.

Rudmann, C. (Ed) (2008), "Entrepreneurial skills and their role in enhancing the relative independence of farmers", Research Institute of Organic Agriculture FiBL, Ackerstrasse, available from: www.fibl.org

Rushton, J. & McLeod, A. (2006). "Animal health economics – UK veterinary services and practices", presentation to Defra.

Slater, R.S. & Slater, M.S. (2000). "Women in veterinary medicine" Journal of the American Veterinary Medical Association, 217(4), pp. 472-476.

Smith, C.A. (2002) "Gender and Work: What veterinarians can learn from research about women, men and work", JAVMA, Vol 220, No. 9, pp. 1304 – 1311.

Tuchman, G. (1989). "Edging women out: Victorian novelists, publishers and social change", New Haven, CT: Yale University Press.

Zhao, Yilu. "Women Soon to be Majority of Veterinarians." New York Times 9 June 2002. Melissa Kaplan's Herp Care Collection. 2 Mar. 2009 <http://www.anapsid.org/vets/vetdermos.html

3

Artificial Insemination in Veterinary Science

Annett Heise
Faculty of Veterinary Science
University of Pretoria
South Africa

1. Introduction

Artificial insemination (AI) is widely used by veterinarians and veterinary specialists in most domestic as well as wild animal species. Reasons for use of AI instead of natural matings are diverse and different for individual species. As in humans, AI can be used as a tool to increase conception rate in animals that have fertility problems. This is usually performed in companion animals, like horses and dogs, where individuals are important as breeding animals. In these cases, breeding animals are mostly chosen for performance and pedigree instead of breeding soundness. Breeders go through a lot of effort to produce offspring of a specific female or male animal irrespective of potential reproductive problems.

In production animals, AI is a way to increase reproductive efficiency and production. AI has proven to be a very effective reproductive technology that selectively increases genetic gain through increased selection pressure on males. In Holstein cattle, for example, AI supported selection for the milk production trait and within 40 years milk production has nearly doubled. Farm animals, males as well as females, are usually chosen for breeding programs based on breeding soundness examinations (BSEs). These BSEs determine suitability and likelihood of females or males to participate successfully in breeding programs. Animals that do not fulfill certain criteria are identified. These "problem" animals are excluded from insemination programs. Estrus cycles of females can be manipulated to institute efficient insemination programs. With the use of these estrus synchronization programs, large groups of females can be inseminated at the same time. This does not only have the advantage of concentrating work on specific days during breeding, but will ultimately also simplify the herd management before and after the offspring are born. Group feeding of pregnant animals, partus observation, vaccination programs for calves and tail docking of lambs are just a few examples of improved herd management areas through the group effect achieved through AI.

Another reason for AI is to ensure effective use of semen. An increased number of offspring from a superior sire can be produced when AI is employed. For example, a stallion's ejaculate can be sufficient to inseminate 5-10 mares at the same time when split into doses instead of one live cover on a mare. Ram ejaculates can also be split into up to 15 fresh AI doses. Freezing bull semen can provide up to 200 straws of frozen semen from one ejaculate, equaling 200 AI doses. Overuse of males is prevented and commercial distribution facilitated. Other important aspects are the prevention of venereal disease transmission that plays a major role in the economic system of offspring production, and increased safety for valuable breeding animals as mating related injuries are avoided.

Venereal diseases that play a major economic role in cattle production are for example Trichomonosis and Campylobacteriosis both of which decrease reproductive efficiency through decreased pregnancy rates, high return rates to estrus and increased pregnancy losses. In general, shipping fresh and frozen semen nationally and internationally involves fewer health risks and welfare implications than transporting live animals.

Import and export of frozen semen is a huge economic market. Semen of a specific bloodline, a specific individual male or breed is imported. This is especially important in countries where breeds were introduced and are somewhat isolated with a small genetic pool. To eventually prevent breeding setbacks due to inbreeding and to expand the genetic pool, imported semen is used. Furthermore, AI can be used for frozen semen from males that have died or are not physically available for matings due to distance or physical inability. A great advantage of frozen semen in general is that it can be stored indefinitely and has the potential to outlive the male donor animal by years.

2. First developments and milestones in the field of veterinary Artificial Insemination

Artificial insemination (AI) was the first assisted reproductive technique applied to control and improve reproduction as well as genetics. The first successful insemination was performed by the Italian physiologist and priest Abbe Lazzaro Spallanzani (1784) in a dog which whelped three pups 62 days later (Foote, 2002). The establishment of AI as a practical procedure was initiated in Russia in 1899 by Ivanov who studied AI in domestic farm animals, dogs, foxes, rabbits and poultry. He also developed semen extenders. Milanov, another Russian scientist and successor of Ivanov, started large scale breeding programs for cattle and sheep, and designed and made artificial vaginas. Horse breeding programs and research was initiated at the same time in Japan even though translations of the original research only became available to the western world after 1958. Some AI work, especially in horses and cattle, had been done in Denmark in the early 1900s. It was Danish veterinarians who established the method of rectovaginal fixation of the cervix for insemination in cattle which enabled semen deposition deep into the cervix or into the uterine body (Foote, 2002). This technique is still used today. Another Danish invention was the straw for packaging semen. These straws have been further developed and modified by the French and are now used worldwide for processing and storage of frozen semen. Research on artificial insemination in Italy led to the development of an artificial vagina for dogs in 1914 and to the establishment of the "International Congress on AI and Animal Reproduction" in 1948. This congress is held every four years since (Foote, 2002). Rapid development of AI in dairy cattle occurred in the USA in the 1940s. One of the important milestones was the establishment of the "Dairy breeding research centre" on the campus of the Pennsylvania State University in 1949 to assist in the development of artificial insemination in dairy cattle. Interest in and development of frozen semen started with successful cryopreservation of gametes from a variety of animal species after discovery of the protective action of glycerol by scientists in Cambridge, England, in 1949 (Amann & Pickett, 1987). Early research focused on bull spermatozoa; methods successful to cryopreserve bull spermatozoa have been less successful for other species. Barker and Gandier reported the first pregnancy from frozen stallion semen in 1957 (Barker & GaPndier, 1957). Poor pregnancy results with the use of frozen-thawed stallion semen limited research funding for breeding trials in this species (Amann & Pickett, 1987). Only later the Chinese inseminated more than 110'000 mares with frozen-thawed stallion semen (between 1980 and 1985). The United States also did not have interest in developing improved procedures for freezing stallion spermatozoa in the seventies. Only in 1980 the Animal Reproduction Laboratory of Colorado State University began a long-range research program aimed at developing satisfactory procedures to freeze stallion semen. The acceptance of frozen semen as a method to produce registered foals by two of the largest breed associations, the American Quarter Horse and the American Paint Horse association in 2001 has furthermore stimulated new interest in the frozen semen technology (Loomis, 2001).

3. AI techniques in different species

Insemination techniques used depend on species, type of semen, breeding system, availability of equipment and expertise. Intravaginal (dogs), intracervical (sheep), transcervical intrauterine (cattle, horses, dogs, sheep), transcervical deep horn intrauterine (horses, cattle, pigs), laparoscopic (sheep), surgical intrauterine (dogs) insemination as well as endoscopic semen deposition at the uterotubal junction (horses) is available.

3.1 AI techniques in dogs

In dogs, fresh, chilled extended and frozen semen can be used. AI using fresh semen is usually performed if the animals will not or cannot copulate naturally. There are certain breeds, like English bulldogs and other brachycephalic breeds that almost always require AI due to their anatomical incompatibility to mate naturally. AI is also used if time constraints are an issue as fresh semen AI in the bitch is much quicker than a natural mating where the coital tie between male and female can last up to 40 minutes or more. AI can be used in bitches with congenital vaginal abnormalities like vaginal strictures or septae which might cause copulation failure. These cases often have ethical implications as well. Owners need to understand that even though AI can be performed easily these bitches might require Cesarian sections as the vaginal abnormalities might also impair natural delivery or that certain vaginal abnormalities are heritable and offspring with the same problem might be produced. AI is also used if the semen quality of the specific male is poor and addition of semen extender or pooling of more than one ejaculate is required for one insemination dose. Fresh semen is deposited into the cranial vagina of the bitch using an insemination pipette that is inserted through the vulva and directed into the vagina. Once the semen has been deposited, the hindquarters of the bitch are usually elevated for a few minutes to facilitate movement of the semen from the vagina through the cervix into the uterus. Vaginal contractions can be elicited for the same reason at the same time by either tickling the vaginal wall or massaging the clitoris. An insemination dose of at least 150×10^6 sperm is recommended and most commonly the whole ejaculate is used which may contain $250\text{-}2500 \times 10^6$ sperm (Johnston et al., 2001).

Pregnancy rates with the use of fresh semen for insemination is reported to vary between 65-84% on average depending on semen quality, timing of insemination and correct site of semen deposition (Johnston et al., 2001; Linde-Forsberg & Forsberg, 1989).

Chilled extended semen is usually used if the male and female are geographically separated. An extender is added to the collected semen before shipment in order to prolong the lifespan of sperm. For the same reason, the extended semen is slowly cooled down to 4 degrees Celsius. The entire ejaculate is usually used for the AI but an insemination dose of at least 150 x 10^6 sperm is recommended. Average pregnancy rate for chilled extended semen is 50% but can vary between 33-89% (Johnston et al., 2001). Extended semen can be used for up to 4 days after collection but should be inseminated as soon as possible. The insemination technique is the same as described above for fresh semen or transcervical intrauterine insemination can be used. Transcervical AI is performed using special catheters (e.g. Norwegian catheters) or endoscopes. The anatomy and location of the cervix in the bitch is such that it is difficult to penetrate the cervix and perform transcervical intrauterine inseminations due to a vaginal fold that is obscurring direct access to the cervix. Therefore, special equipment is needed for transcervical intrauterine AI. Norwegian catheters have been developed in the 1970s (Andersen, 1972, 1975) and are available in three different sizes to accommodate different sized bitches. For this technique, the cervix must be fixed through abdominal palpation and the catheter is moved slowly to find the cervical canal while the cervix is pulled downward. This method requires a lot of practice and there is a potential danger that inexperienced veterinarians might traumatize the cervix. Used by experienced clinicians this technique offers an inexpensive, fast way of inseminating non anesthetized bitches. Using a rigid endoscope for transcervical AI enables the operator to visualize the cervix, straighten the cervical canal and insert a catheter into the uterus to deposit the semen. The advantage of this technique is that it is not blind and the danger of trauma to the reproductive tract is minimal. Bitches do not usually have to be sedated for the procedure and AI can be repeated a few times if necessary.

For frozen semen, deposition of the semen into the uterine lumen is recommended in order to achieve good pregnancy rates (Thomasse et al., 2001; Thomassen et al., 2006). Even though the first report of successful AI with frozen semen in dogs was a result of intravaginal deposition of the semen (Seager, 1969) it has been shown that success rates with intrauterine inseminations are far superior (Thomassen et al., 2001; Thomassen et al., 2006). Intrauterine insemination can be performed by transcervical intrauterine AI as described above or surgical AI via laparotomy. In cases where transcervical intrauterine AI is unsuccessful or the equipment is not readily available, surgical intrauterine AI is performed. It is usually a quick procedure that requires general anesthesia for about 20 minutes. A small abdominal incision is made, the uterus exteriorized and the semen injected directly into the uterine lumen through the uterine wall. Disadvantages of this procedure are the relatively high costs as well as the anesthetic and surgical risk. Surgical insemination is considered an unethical procedure in some countries (Linde-Forsberg, 1991). Insemination doses are usually composed of 100-150 x 10^6 motile spermatozoa. Whelping rates for frozen semen AI are reported to be as high as 70-75% if the timing of insemination is accurate, good quality frozen-thawed semen is used and the semen deposition is correct (Thomassen et al., 2001; Thomassen et al., 2006).

3.2 AI techniques in horses

AI is a widely practiced breeding method in most sport horse breeds worldwide. Fresh, chilled extended and frozen-thawed semen can be used in horses. Common reasons for the use of insemination for fresh semen instead of natural mating are the reduced risk of injury to the often very valuable stallion by avoiding live coverings, insemination of mares that do not want to allow a mating or splitting of an ejaculate into several insemination doses if more than one mare is to be inseminated at the same time. Generally accepted insemination doses for fresh semen as supported by the World Breeding Federation of Sport Horses (WBFSH) are 300×10^6 straight forward swimming (progressively motile) spermatozoa (Katila, 2005) which is slightly lower than the originally recommended fresh semen AI dose of 500×10^6 progressively motile spermatozoa (PMS) (Pickett & Voss, 1975). First cycle pregnancy rate for fresh semen AI is approximately 60%. Chilled extended semen is usually used if the mare and the stallion are in distant places. Semen is collected, extended with a suitable semen extender to provide buffers, nutrients, antibiotics etc. in order to prolong lifespan of the spermatozoa and slowly cooled down to 4 degrees Celsius. Usually, special transport containers that form cooling units (e.g. Equitainer®, Hamilton Thorne) are used and the semen of most stallions is viable for at least 48 hours. Most insemination centres try to inseminate mares with chilled extended semen within 24 hours of collection. One billion spermatozoa or 600×10^6 progressively motile spermatozoa (according to WBFSH (Katila, 2005)) form one insemination dose and pregnancy rates of about 60 % (Sieme et al., 2003) can be expected depending on timing of insemination relative to ovulation, AI dose and semen quality after chilling. Some stallions' semen is not suitable for chilling and the semen quality deteriorates very rapidly. It is therefore recommended to perform a trial cooling of equine semen before a shipping is done and to evaluate semen quality parameters over time to assess longevity.

The insemination technique for fresh and chilled extended semen is similar in the horse. A transcervical intrauterine insemination is performed where the semen is deposited into the uterine body. A commercially available insemination pipette is inserted manually into the vagina, the external opening of the cervix is located using the index finger and the pipette is guided through the cervical canal into the uterus. The penetration of the cervix is generally very easy as the cervical tissue is smooth muscle that relaxes under estrogen influence. That allows easy access to the equine uterus at the time of insemination. Frozen-thawed semen has first been used to inseminate mares in 1957 (Barker & Gandier, 1957) even though it only gained increasing popularity over the last 15-20 years. Using frozen semen has a lot of benefits: accessibility to semen from stallions in competition or stallions that become ill, injured or overbooked during the breeding season. Using frozen semen eliminates the need to organize stallion availability at the optimum time for breeding of the mare and disease transmission. Chances for injury are decreased as direct mare-stallion contact is avoided. Pregnancy rate per cycle for frozen semen varies between 30-50% on average (Leipold et al., 1998; Metcalf, 2007; Sieme et al., 2003; Vidament, 2005; Vidament et al., 1997). There are, however, some disadvantages regarding frozen semen. The management of mares during estrus is more intense which increases the costs involved for frozen semen inseminations. This is necessary as inseminations with frozen semen should be done as close to ovulation as possible since frozen-thawed spermatozoa have a shortened lifespan. Frozen-thawed spermatozoa survive for about 12 hours in the reproductive tract of mares whereas fresh semen can survive for 48-72 hours. Frozen-thawed equine semen can be inseminated into the uterine body as described for fresh and chilled distended semen if an insemination dose of 250×10^6 progressively motile spermatozoa is available (Katila, 2005). If the insemination dose is lower or a very small volume is to be inseminated (0.25-0.5ml), the semen can be deposited deeply into the uterine horn ipsilateral to the ovary where ovulation will take place or has taken place (Katila, 2005). Other possibilities for low dose ($5\text{-}25 \times 10^6$

progressively motile sperm) or very low volume (0.02-0.2 ml) inseminations (Katila, 2005) are endoscopic deposition of semen at the utero-tubal junction right in the tip of the uterine horn ipsilateral to the ovary where ovulation will take place (Lindsey et al. , 2001; Lindsey et al. , 2002; L. H. A. Morris, 2004), and surgical deposition of spermatozoa directly into the oviduct (McCue et al. , 2000).

3.3 AI techniques in dairy cattle

In Britain, AI in dairy cattle began to be available in 1942, and by 1950 20% of dairy cattle were being inseminated. By 1960, more than 2 million cows were inseminated yearly, which was about 80% of the maximum level that AI would reach (Brassley, 2007). The established procedure for AI in cattle since the 1960s is transcervical deposition of semen into the uterine body. This technique replaced the original vaginal or shallow cervical insemination performed in the 1940s as the intrauterine method proved to be more efficient and resulted in higher fertility (Lopez-Gatius, 2000). Transcervical intrauterine AI involves the technique of cervical fixation per rectum to facilitate easier penetration of the cervical rings with a stainless steel Cassou device (AI pistolette) (Noakes et al. , 2001). Other techniques like unicornual or bicornual insemination where semen is deposited into one or both uterine horns, and intraperitoneal insemination have been investigated (Lopez-Gatius, 2000) but could not replace the transcervical intrauterine AI with semen deposition into the uterine body. For commercial AI in cattle, frozen-thawed semen is routinely used and a generally accepted insemination dose contains 10-20 x 10^6 spermatozoa. Deep horn AI close to the uterotubal junction has been investigated and facilitates AI with a conventional number of spermatozoa reduced x 100 or if very small volumes of semen (0.1-0.25 ml) are to be used (Hunter, 2003). Potential advantages of deep horn AI include: raising fertility of genetically valuable bulls whose non-return rates to estrus are sub-optimal, reducing the number of sperm per AI dose, facilitating the use of limited numbers of sex selected sperm cells available from flow cytometry, and breeding from valuable but oligospermic (too few sperm in ejaculate) bulls (Hunter, 2003).

3.4 AI techniques in pigs

Even though AI in pigs has been used since the 1930s, wider commercial application only started in the 1980s, with a dramatic increase in the use of AI in pork production in the last 20 years. International comparison shows that in 1990, 80% of pigs in former Eastern Germany were bred by AI, compared to only 23% in West Germany, while the figures for Norway were 71% and for the Netherlands 51%. France and the UK were about the same with 10% and the USA was only 7% (Brassley, 2007). By the end of the 1990s, close to 50% of the worldwide gilts and sows were inseminated (Roca et al., 2006). Nowadays, AI is used routinely in pig companies. In some European countries, like Belgium, Italy, the Netherlands, Norway and Spain, more than 80% of females are bred by AI and in North America and Brazil the percentage has reached 75% (Roca et al., 2006). One reason for the slow take-off for AI in pigs were initial conception rates which were as low as 18.1% in 1955 rising to 62% in 1961 while natural conception rates were expected to be close to 90% (Brassley, 2007). Conception rates could be increased to about 80% by the mid 1970s. Consistent 80-90% fertility rates with the use of liquid extended semen are common on many farms by now with an overall fertility success (measured as farrowing rates and litter sizes) similar to or better than those resulting from natural matings (Roca et al., 2006). Apart from good conception rates, there are other reasons for the dramatic increase in AI utilization for pig breeding systems. On one hand there was the change of breeding and farrowing units that became larger and more specialized, and that the application of AI mating technologies became more feasible and cost effective on the other hand (Singleton, 2001). At the same time, the pork industry initiated payment programs based on actual carcass value instead of live weight basis. Genetic evaluation programs were used to implement genetic improvement programs through the use of AI to produce higher quality pork carcasses. For most commercial breeders it was the prospect of genetic improvement that was the major incentive to engage in AI (Brassley, 2007). Semen processing centres (boar studs) or on-farm collection facilities provide boar semen used for AI programs. More than 99% of AIs are performed with semen extended in a liquid state that can be stored at 15-20°C for up to 3 days (cooled semen)(Roca et al., 2006). The number of viable sperm per dose ranges between 2.5- 4 billion motile spermatozoa. Dose volumes range from 80-100ml for fresh liquid semen. The insemination procedure, called intra-cervical insemination (intra-CAI), involves the deposition of spermatozoa into the posterior part of the cervix using a catheter that engages with the folds of the cervix, stimulating the corkscrew tie of the boar's penis (Roca et al., 2006). This easy and quick procedure has been developed in the mid 1950s, standardized in the 1970s and is still used worldwide today (Roca et al., 2006). The remaining 1% of AIs utilizes frozen-thawed semen at doses of $5\text{-}6 \times 10^9$ spermatozoa. Even though large sperm numbers are used, fertility is substantially lower than that obtained with cooled semen. Due to the lowered reproductive performance, frozen-thawed boar semen is mostly limited to specialized breeding programs, research and for export puposes (Singleton, 2001; Wongtawan et al. , 2006). There are two insemination procedures available that allow insemination with low numbers of spermatozoa: post-cervical insemination (post-CAI) and deep uterine insemination (DUI). Both techniques facilitate deposition of semen into the uterus. Using post-CAI, semen is placed into the uterine body while DUI facilitates placement of semen in the proximal 1/3 of one uterine horn (Martinez et al., 2005). Similar fertility results can be expected for DUI using 600×10^6 spermatozoa and $1\text{-}1.5 \times 10^9$ spermatozoa for post-CAI as compared to intra-CAI using 3000×10^9 sperm per dose (Roca et al., 2006). Or in other words, a threefold reduction of fresh sperm numbers using post-cervical AI, and for DUI a 20-fold reduction for fresh and sixfold reduction for frozen semen can achieve acceptable pregnancy rates (J. M. Vazquez et al., 2008). Other possibilities for inseminations with low sperm numbers are surgical intrauterine inseminations where high pregnancy rates (89%) can be obtained with as few as 10×10^6 cooled stored spermatozoa that are placed on the uterotubal junction (Krueger & Rath, 2000; Krueger et al. , 1999). A further reduction in sperm numbers to 5×10^6 can be achieved if spermatozoa are placed close to the uterotubal junction by laparoscopy (Fantinati et al., 2005). A new procedure where semen is placed into the oviduct via laparoscopy also displays an opportunity for the use of diluted and sex sorted spermatozoa (Vazquez et al., 2008). Other insemination techniques like intraperitoneal insemination, where semen was deposited directly into the abdominal cavity, have been used to investigate insemination possibilities other than intra-CAI (Hunter, 1978). This technique, however, has never come to use in the AI industry due to ineffective sperm transport to the oviducts, reduced fertility and difficulty of the procedure when compared to intra-CAI. It has also been shown that specific boar stimuli (such as olfactory and tactile stimuli) at or around the time of AI positively influence reproductive performance through an effect on reproductive processes like sperm transport and ovulation (Soede, 1993).

3.5 AI in sheep (Youngquist & Threlfall, 2007)

Fresh, chilled and frozen semen is utilized for AI in sheep. Methods used are vaginal, cervical, laparoscopic intrauterine and transcervical intrauterine insemination. Vaginal insemination can be used for fresh and chilled semen and is also referred to as the "shot in the dark", or SID, method as the semen is blindly deposited into the cranial vagina. Pregnancy rates performing vaginal AI for fresh and chilled semen are acceptable while they are not for frozen semen. The technique is very fast but the use of semen is inefficient as AI doses have to contain large numbers of sperm. For cervical insemination, the hindquarters are elevated while the ewe is restrained "over the rail". The cervix is visualized using a speculum and a light source. Semen is deposited into the cervix with an angled tip insemination gun.

In contrast to horses and cattle, a successful method for transcervical intrauterine insemination in sheep has not been well established due to the specific anatomy of the ovine cervix (Halbert et al. , 1990). The cervical canal is approximately 7 cm long with a series of 6-8 rearward facing, offset rings that make transcervical insemination difficult to impossible. The Guelph system for transcervical AI (GST-AI) has been developed which requires special positioning of the ewe, cervical retraction and stabilization, and the use of specially designed instruments. Trained, experienced inseminators may penetrate the cervix in as much as 75-85% of ewes. Cervical injury, abscesses, infections and poor pregnancy rates are associated with this technique. Surgical AIs (i.e. via midventral laparotomy) are effective, but they are costly, time consuming, require technical proficiency, limit the number of times ewes can be used and require anesthesia (Evans & Maxwell, 1987). Laparoscopic intrauterine AI is used for frozen semen, and requires laparoscopic equipment as well as technical expertise. Animals are usually sedated and restrained in a laparoscopic cradle in dorsal recumbency. The laparoscope is used to identify the uterus and a loaded insemination pipette directed to the uterus to facilitate intrauterine deposition of the semen. Three hundred or more ewes can be inseminated per day using this technique if an experienced team works in a well-equipped and organized operation. Insemination doses for fresh as well as frozen-thawed semen are 400×10^6, 200×10^6, 20×10^6, 100×10^6 progressively motile spermatozoa for vaginal, cervical, laparoscopic and transcervical AI, respectively. Expected lambing rates for fresh semen are 20-60%, 40-80%, 70-100%, 40-80%, and 5-20%, 25-60%, 40-80%, 30-70% for frozen semen for vaginal, cervical, laparoscopic and transcervical AI, respectively.

3.6 AI in other species

Since the 1920s, AI has been a reproductive tool in commercial rabbitries that permits more controlled management and better planning (e.g. in batch parturition and weaning) than natural mating (Morrell, 1995). Conception rates after AI can be equivalent to or better than that achieved with natural breeding (Morrell, 1995). Natural matings in healthy individuals can result in conception rates of 85%. A single ejaculate can be split into 20-50 insemination doses and used for AI (Lavara et al. , 2005). For the AI procedure, the female is placed into a restraining box, the tail is lifted and an insemination pipette with a bend approximately 8cm from the end is inserted into the vagina at an angle of 45° in order progress beyond the pelvic rim (Morrell, 1995). Semen is deposited intravaginally. Due to the fact that rabbits have two separate uterine horns and cervices, intracervical AI is not performed as it would be required to release semen into both cervices. Other peculiarities regarding AI in rabbits are that females should be kept separate from males for about 19 days before breeding to exclude pseudopregnancy, that timing of AI is based on general behaviour and vulva colour of the doe, and that rabbits are induced ovulators that always require induction of ovulation when AI is used. Three methods for induction of ovulation are available: 1) mating with a vasectomized buck, 2) administration of human chorionic gonadotropin (hCG) or 3) administration of gonadotropin releasing hormone (GnRH) analogues (Morrell, 1995).

AI in non-human primates is based on captive colony management and propagation of endangered or valuable founder animals. Its application, (although limited due to high costs, substantial technical requirements and limited available captive populations), has found use in Great Apes as well as Old World and New World Macaques (Wolf, 2009). Initially, intravaginal AI was performed while intrauterine insemination is the technique of choice today.

Application of AI in South American camelids has been challenging due to the inconsistent success in collecting semen from males. Llamas as well as alpacas copulate for extended periods of time (10-60 min), display a recumbent mating posture, deposit semen into the uterus, and the semen is very viscous (Adams et al., 2009). Camelids are not as easily trained to mount an AV as rams, bulls or stallions. It is necessary to maintain a stable AV temperature during prolonged copulation. Other semen collection attempts using condoms or intravaginal sacs, vaginal sponges, electro-ejaculation, post-coital vaginal aspiration, and fistulation of the penile urethra were associated with recovery of poor semen samples and contamination of semen samples with blood (Adams et al., 2009). For AI, semen is deposited into the uterus transcervically or via laparoscopy. Reported pregnancy rates after AI vary widely between 2-68% (Adams et al., 2009).

4. Use of epididymal spermatozoa for AI

Another interesting field for application of AI is the use of epididymal spermatozoa. Harvesting of epididymal sperm enables storage and usage of valuable genetic material of males after death or shortly before death if unexpected accidents or health problems occur. The epididymis is part of the male reproductive tract, is connected to the testis and forms a site for sperm maturation and storage. The epididymis can be dissected free from the testis after castration and epididymal spermatozoa can be harvested by flushing or slice-and-dice techniques (Bruemmer, 2006). Aspiration of spermatozoa from the epididymis has also been performed. Interestingly, the first reported pregnancy in a mare after AI was achieved with frozen-thawed epididymal stallion spermatozoa in 1957 (Barker & Gandier, 1957).

Epididymal spermatozoa have been harvested from a variety of species like cats (Filliers et al., 2008; Hermansson & AxnÈr, 2007), dogs (Garcia-Macias et al., 2006; Hewitt et al., 2001; ☼Nothling et al., 2007; Ponglowhapan et al., 2006), rats (Yamashiro et al., 2007), horses (Braun et al., 1994; Bruemmer, 2006; Heise et al., 2011; Johnson & Coutinho da Silva, 2008; Melo et al., 2008), cattle (Goovaerts et al., 2006; Martins, Rumpf, Pereira, & Dode, 2007), pigs (Ikeda et al., 2002), sheep (Garcia-Macias et al., 2006), goats (Blash, Melican, & Gavin, 2000), red deer (Fernandez-Santos et al., 2006; Garcia-Macias et al., 2006; Martìnez-Pastor et al.,

2006), Spanish Ibex (Santiago-Moreno et al., 2006), African buffalo (Herold et al., 2006), North American buffalo (Lessard at al., 2009) and monkeys (Goff et al., 2009; Ng et al., 2002). Pregnancies and offspring after AI with epididymal spermatozoa have been produced amongst others in horses (Barker & Gandier, 1957; Heise et al., 2010; Morris et al., 2002; Papa et al., 2008), dogs (Hori, Hagiuda, Kawakami, & Tsutsui, 2005) and Spanish Ibex (Santiago-Moreno et al., 2006). Application of AI for epididymal spermatozoa holds tremendous potential for future use of valuable genetics not only in domestic but also especially in wild animal species.

5. Use of sexed semen for AI

Another aspect of artificial insemination in animals is the use of sex sorted spermatozoa. Separation of the X and Y bearing sperm is desirable in animals as one sex has significantly more value than the other in certain species. For dairy cattle for example, cows as the "milk producers" are the main source of income for the industry while bull calves are of less value as lactation is limited to females. For other food producing animals a higher percentage of male offspring might be beneficial as they grow faster and produce more meat. In many large, long-lived species like elephants, rhinoceroses, dolphins that are kept in captivity, sex selection could ease and avoid housing problems with males of these species (Durrant, 2009).

It has first been established for human spermatids in 1979 that there is a difference in DNA content between the mammalian X-chromosome-bearing spermatozoa and the Y-chromosome (Otto et al., 1979). Since then, DNA content measurements have been used to identify the sex-chromosome bearing sperm populations with good accuracy in semen from at least 23 mammalian species (Garner, 2006; Garner et al., 1983; Lu et al., 2010; Pinkel et al., 1982), and offspring have been produced from sexed sperm of at least seven species, including rabbits (Johnson et al., 1989), humans (Levinson et al., 1995), cattle (Cran et al., 1993), horses (Buchanan et al., 2000), sheep (Catt et al., 1996), dogs (Meyers et al., 2008), cats (Pope et al., 2008), elk (Schenk & DeGrofft, 2003), buffalo (Presicce et al., 2005) and dolphins (O'Brien & Robeck, 2006). The first offspring born with flow cytometrically sex sorted spermatozoa was in rabbits after surgical AI into the oviduct (Johnson et al., 1989).

The Beltsville Sperm Sexing technology (Garner, 2006) uses the difference in DNA content of the X- and Y-chromosome to sort the sex-determining gametes. The procedure is called fluorescence-activated cell separation (FACS) where ejaculated spermatozoa are treated with a DNA stain (called a flourochrome) and due to the fact that X-chromosomes contain more DNA, the stain take-up will be higher for the X-chromosome bearing spermatozoa than the Y-chromosome bearing spermatozoa. This difference in stain absorption is used in a flow cytometer chamber where the fluorescent stain in the spermatozoa is excited by a laser. Each live sperm produces an emission with an intensity that is directly related to the quantity of DNA within the sperm head. The X bearing spermatozoa emit more intense light than the Y bearing spermatozoa. A high speed computer is used to analyze the relative fluorescence of the X- and Y-sperm populations as they flow through a cytometer chamber. Spermatozoa are then assigned either a negative or positive charge depending on the DNA content while passing by charged plates. An electromagnetic field separates the X- and Y-chromosome bearing spermatozoa (Senger, 2003). This separation technology has a 85-95% success rate (Garner, 2006).

Not all mammalian sperm are equally suitable for sex sorting of spermatozoa. Apart from the DNA content difference of the X- and Y-bearing spermatozoa, the head shape of the spermatozoa plays a role as well. Flattened, oval shaped sperm heads (e.g. bull, boar, ram spermatozoa) are more readily oriented in a sperm sorter using hydrodynamics than those gametes with more round or angular head shapes (rodent spermatozoa) (Garner, 2006). The area of the flat profile of the sperm head can be multiplied times the difference in DNA content of the X-and Y-chromosome bearing sperm to give the sorting index. This index suggests that bull and boar sperm are well suited for separation in a flow sorter.

Initially, the use of sex sorted spermatozoa was limited due to the slow separation process where only a few hundred thousand sperm per hour could be sorted. Newer sperm sorter systems are able to sort 20,000 sperm/s resulting in up to 6000 or more sperm/s each of X- and Y-sperm at 90% accuracy (Garner & Seidel Jr, 2008). Due to low sperm numbers acquired with sex sorting, initial efforts to predetermine the sex required surgical insemination. Later, with improvement of the equipment, quantities were sufficient for in vitro fertilization (IVF). Today, sexed sperm are commercially available for cattle where the standard insemination doses of 2×10^6 sexed sperm achieve 70-80% of the pregnancy rates achieved with non-sorted sperm in doses of $10\text{-}20 \times 10^6$ (Bodmer et al., 2005; Garner, 2006). In pigs, low dose (70×10^6 spermatozoa) AI with flow cytometrically sorted sperm deep into the uterine horn resulted in pregnancy rates of 35-45.6% (Vazquez et al., 2003). In horses, hysteroscopic insemination into the uterine horn (Lindsey et al., 2002; Morris & Allen, 2002) and ultrasound guided deep uterine AI were performed using sex sorted spermatozoa in low concentrations (5×10^6 sperm cells/ dose).

6. Conclusion

AI has been and still is the most used reproductive technique in animals. A lot of research has been done over the last few decades, constantly improving techniques, methods and applications of AI. Routine AI procedures as well as specialized techniques like low-dose inseminations or use of sexed semen offer a wide variety for application of AI in domestic as well as wild and endangered animal species.

7. References

Adams, G. P., Ratto, M. H., Collins, C. W., & Bergfelt, D. R. (2009). Artificial insemination in South American camelids and wild equids. *Theriogenology, 71*(1), 166-175.

Amann, R. P., & Pickett, B. W. (1987). Principles of cryopreservation and a review of cryopreservation of stallion spermatozoa. *Journal of Equine Veterinary Science, 7*(3), 145-173.

Andersen, K. (1972). Fertility of frozen dog semen. *Acta Veterinaria Scandinavia, 13*, 128-130.

Andersen, K. (1975). Insemination with frozen dog semen based on a new insemination technique. *Zuchthygiene, 10*, 1-4.

Barker, C. A. V., & Gandier, J. C. C. (1957). Pregnancy in a mare resulted from frozen epididymal spermatozoa. *Canadian Journal of Comparative Veterinary Medical Science, 21*, 47-51.

Blash, S., Melican, D., & Gavin, W. (2000). Cryopreservation of epididymal sperm obtained at necropsy from goats. *Theriogenology, 54*(6), 899-905.

Bodmer, M., Janett, F., Hoessig, M., Daas, N. d., Reichert, P., & Thun, R. (2005). Fertility in heifers and cows after low dose insemination with sex-sorted and non-sorted sperm under field conditions. *Theriogenology, 64*(7), 1647-1655.

Brassley, P. (2007). Cutting across nature? The history of artificial insemination in pigs in the United Kingdom. *Studies in History and Philosophy of Science Part C: Studies in History and Philosophy of Biological and Biomedical Sciences, 38*(2), 442-461.

Braun, J., Sakai, M., Hochi, S., & Oguri, N. (1994). Preservation of ejaculated and epididymal stallion spermatozoa by cooling and freezing. *Theriogenology, 41*(4), 809-818.

Bruemmer, J. E. (2006). Collection and Freezing of Epididymal Stallion Sperm. *Veterinary Clinics of North America: Equine Practice, 22*(3), 677-682.

Buchanan, B. R., Seidel, G. E., McCue, P. M., Schenk, J. L., Herickhoff, L. A., & Squires, E. L. (2000). Inseminations of mares with low numbers of either unsexed or sexed spermatozoa. *Theriogenology, 53*, 1333-1344.

Catt, S. L., Catt, J. W., Gomez, M. C., Maxwell, W. M. C., & Evans, G. (1996). Birth of a male lamb derived from an in vitro matured oocyte fertilised by intracytoplasmic injection of a single presumptive male sperm. *Veterinary Record, 139*, 494-495.

Cran, D. G., Johnson , L. A., Miller, N. G. A., Cochrane, D., & Polge, C. (1993). Production of bovine calves following separation of X-chromosome and Y-chromosome bearing sperm and *in vitro* fertilization. *Veterinary Record, 132*, 40-41.

Durrant, B. S. (2009). The importance and potential of artificial insemination in CANDES (companion animals, non-domestic, endangered species). *Theriogenology, 71*(1), 113-122.

Evans, G., & Maxwell, W. M. C. (1987). *Salamon's artificial insemination of sheep and goats.* Sydney: Butterworths.

Fantinati, P., Zannoni, A., Bernardini, C., Webster, N., Lavitrano, M., Forni, M., et al. (2005). Laparoscopic insemination technique with low numbers of spermatozoa in superovulated prepuberal gilts for biotechnological application. *Theriogenology, 63*(3), 806-817.

Fernandez-Santos, M. R., Esteso, M. C., Montoro, V., Soler, A. J., & Garde, J. J. (2006). Cryopreservation of Iberian red deer (Cervus elaphus hispanicus) epididymal spermatozoa: Effects of egg yolk, glycerol and cooling rate. *Theriogenology, 66*(8), 1931-1942.

Filliers, M., Rijsselaere, T., Bossaert, P., De Causmaecker, V., Dewulf, J., Pope, C. E., et al. (2008). Computer-assisted sperm analysis of fresh epididymal cat spermatozoa and the impact of cool storage (4°C) on sperm quality. *Theriogenology, 70*(9), 1550-1559.

Foote, R. H. (2002). The history of artificial insemination: Selected notes and notables. *Journal of Animal Science, 80*, 1-10.

Garcia-Macias, V., Martinez-Pastor, F., Alvarez, M., Garde, J. J., Anel, E., Anel, L., et al. (2006). Assessment of chromatin status (SCSAÆ) in epididymal and ejaculated sperm in Iberian red deer, ram and domestic dog. *Theriogenology, 66*(8), 1921-1930.

Garner, D. L. (2006). Flow cytometric sexing of mammalian sperm. *Theriogenology, 65*(5), 943-957.

Garner, D. L., Gledhill, B. L., Pinkel, D., Lake, S., Stephenson, D., & Van Dilla, M. A. (1983). Quantification of the X- and Y-chromosome bearing spermatozoa of domestic animals by flow cytometry. *Biology of Reproduction, 28*, 312-321.

Garner, D. L., & Seidel Jr, G. E. (2008). History of commercializing sexed semen for cattle. *Theriogenology, 69*(7), 886-895.

Goff, K., Liukkonen, J., & Kubisch, H. M. (2009). Postmortem recovery and cryopreservation of spermatozoa from the vas deferens of rhesus macaques (Macaca mulatta). *Theriogenology, 72*(6), 834-840.

Goovaerts, I. G. F., Hoflack, G. G., Van Soom, A., Dewulf, J., Nichi, M., de Kruif, A., et al. (2006). Evaluation of epididymal semen quality using the Hamilton-Thorne analyser indicates variation between the two caudae epididymides of the same bull. *Theriogenology, 66*(2), 323-330.

Halbert, G. W., Dobson, H., Walton, J. S., & Buckrell, B. C. (1990). The structure of the cervical canal of the ewe. *Theriogenology, 33*, 977-992.

Heise, A., K‰hn, W., Volkmann, D. H., Thompson, P. N., & Gerber, D. (2010). Influence of seminal plasma on fertility of fresh and frozen-thawed stallion epididymal spermatozoa. *Animal Reproduction Science, 118*(1), 48-53.

Heise, A., Thompson, P. N., & Gerber, D. (2011). Influence of seminal plasma on fresh and post-thaw parameters of stallion epididymal spermatozoa. *Animal Reproduction Science, 123*(3-4), 192-201.

Hermansson, U., & AxnÈr, E. (2007). Epididymal and ejaculated cat spermatozoa are resistant to cold shock but egg yolk promotes sperm longevity during cold storage at 4°C. *Theriogenology, 67*(7), 1239-1248.

Herold, F. C., de Haas, K., Colenbrander, B., & Gerber, D. (2006). Comparison of equilibration times when freezing epididymal sperm from African buffalo (Syncerus caffer) using Triladyl(TM) or AndroMed®. *Theriogenology, 66*(5), 1123-1130.

Hewitt, D. A., Leahy, R., Sheldon, I. M., & England, G. C. W. (2001). Cryopreservation of epididymal dog sperm. *Animal Reproduction Science, 67*(1-2), 101-111.

Hori, T., Hagiuda, K., Kawakami, E., & Tsutsui, T. (2005). Unilateral intrauterine insemination with prostatic fluid-sensitized frozen caudal epididymal sperm in beagle dogs. *Theriogenology, 63*(6), 1573-1583.

Hunter, R. H. F. (1978). Intraperitoneal insemination, sperm transport and capacitation in the pig. *Animal Reproduction Science, 1*(2), 167-179.

Hunter, R. H. F. (2003). Advances in deep uterine insemination: a fruitful way forward to exploit new sperm technologies in cattle. *Animal Reproduction Science, 79*(3-4), 157-170.

Ikeda, H., Kikuchi, K., Noguchi, J., Takeda, H., Shimada, A., Mizokami, T., et al. (2002). Effect of preincubation of cryopreserved porcine epididymal sperm. *Theriogenology, 57*(4), 1309-1318.

Johnson, A. E. M., & Coutinho da Silva, M. A. (2008). Effects of recovery technique, freezing extender and antioxidants on motility parameters of cryopreserved stallion epididymal sperm. *Theriogenology, 70*(3), 579-580.

Johnson, L. A., Flook, J. P., & Hawk, H. W. (1989). Sex pre-selection in rabbits: live birth from X and Y sperm separated by DNA and cell sorting. *Biology of Reproduction, 41*, 199-203.

Johnston, S. D., Root Kustritz, M. V., & Olson, P. N. S. (2001). *Canine and Feline Theriogenology*: W. B. Saunders Company.

Katila, T. (2005). Effect of the inseminate and the site of insemination on the uterus and pregnancy rates of mares. *Animal Reproduction Science, 89*(1-4), 31-38.

Krueger, C., & Rath, D. (2000). Intrauterine insemination in sows with reduced sperm number. *Reproduction, Fertility and Development, 12*, 113-117.

Krueger, C., Rath, D., & Johnson, L. A. (1999). Low dose insemination in synchronized gilts. *Theriogenology, 52*, 1363-1373.

Lavara, R., Mocé, E., Lavara, F., de Castro, M. P. V., & Vicente, J. S. (2005). Do parameters of seminal quality correlate with the results of on-farm inseminations in rabbits? *Theriogenology, 64*, 1130-1141.

Leipold, S. D., Graham, J. K., Squires, E. L., McCue, P. M., Brinsko, S. P., & Vanderwall, D. K. (1998). Effect of spermatozoal concentration and number on fertility of frozen equine semen. *Theriogenology, 49*(8), 1537-1543.

Lessard, C., Danielson, J., Rajapaksha, K., Adams, G. P., & McCorkell, R. (2009). Banking North American buffalo semen. *Theriogenology, 71*(7), 1112-1119.

Levinson, G., Keyvanfar, K., Wu, J. C., Fugger, E. F., Fields, R. A., & Harton, G. L. (1995). DNA-based X-enriched sperm separation as an adjunct to preimplantation genetic testing for the prevention of X-linked disease. *Human Reproduction, 10*, 797-782.

Linde-Forsberg, C. (1991). Achieving canine pregnancy by using frozen or chilled extended semen. *Veterinary Clinics of North America, 21*, 467-485.

Linde-Forsberg, C., & Forsberg, M. (1989). Fertility in dogs in relation to semen quality and the time and site of insemination with fresh and frozen semen. *Journal of Reproduction and Fertility Supplement, 39*, 299-310.

Lindsey, A. C., Bruemmer, J. E., & Squires, E. L. (2001). Low dose insemination of mares using non-sorted and sex-sorted sperm. *Animal Reproduction Science, 68*(3-4), 279-289.

Lindsey, A. C., Schenk, J. L., Graham, J. K., Bruemmer, J. E., & Squires, E. L. (2002). Hysteroscopic insemination of low numbers of non sorted or flow-sorted spermatozoa. *Equine Veterinary Journal, 34*, 128-132.

Loomis, P. R. (2001). The equine frozen semen industry. *Animal Reproduction Science, 68*(3/4), 191-200.

Lopez-Gatius, F. (2000). Site of semen deposition in cattle: A review. *Theriogenology, 53*(7), 1407-1414.

Lu, Y., Zhang, M., Lu, S., Xu, D., Huang, W., Meng, B., et al. (2010). Sex-preselected buffalo (Bubalus bubalis) calves derived from artificial insemination with sexed sperm. *Animal Reproduction Science, 119*(3-4), 169-171.

Martinez, E. A., Vazquez, J. M., Roca, J., Cuello, C., Gil, M. A., Parrilla, I., et al. (2005). An update on reproductive technologies with potential short-term application in pig production. *Reproduction in Domestic Animals, 40*, 300-309.

Martìnez-Pastor, F., Anel, L., Guerra, C., ¡lvarez, M., Soler, A. J., Garde, J. J. n., et al. (2006). Seminal plasma improves cryopreservation of Iberian red deer epididymal sperm. *Theriogenology, 66*(8), 1847-1856.

Martins, C. F., Rumpf, R., Pereira, D. C., & Dode, M. N. (2007). Cryopreservation of epididymal bovine spermatozoa from dead animals and its uses in vitro embryo production. *Animal Reproduction Science, 101*(3-4), 326-331.

McCue, P. M., Fleury, J. J., & Denniston, D. J. (2000). Oviductal insemination of mares. *Journal of Reproduction and Fertility Supplement, 56*, 499-502.

Melo, C. M., Papa, F. O., Fioratti, E. G., Villaverde, A. I. S. B., Avanzi, B. R., Monteiro, G., et al. (2008). Comparison of three different extenders for freezing epididymal stallion sperm. *Animal Reproduction Science, 107*(3-4), 331-331.

Metcalf, E. S. (2007). The efficient use of equine cryopreserved semen. *Theriogenology, 68*(3), 423-428.

Meyers, M. A., Burns, G., Arn, D., & Schenk, J. L. (2008). Birth of canine offspring following insemination of a bitch with flow-sorted spermatozoa. [Abstract]. *Reproduction, Fertility and Development, 20,* 213.

Morrell, J. M. (1995). Artificial insemination in rabbits. *British Veterinary Journal, 151*(5), 477-488.

Morris, L. H., & Allen, W. R. (2002). An overview of low dose insemination in the mare. *Reproduction in Domestic Animals, 37,* 206-210.

Morris, L. H. A. (2004). Low dose insemination in the mare: an update. *Animal Reproduction Science, 82-83,* 625-632.

Morris, L. H. A., Tiplady, C., & Allen, W. R. (2002). The in vivo fertility of cauda epididymal spermatozoa in the horse. *Theriogenology, 58,* 643-646.

Ng, S. C., Martelli, P., Liow, S. L., Herbert, S., & Oh, S. H. (2002). Intracytoplasmic injection of frozen-thawed epididymal spermatozoa in a nonhuman primate model, the cynomolgus monkey (Macaca fascicularis). *Theriogenology, 58*(7), 1385-1397.

Noakes, D. E., Parkinson, T. J., & England, G. C. W. (2001). *Veterinary reproduction and obstetrics* (8th ed.): W. B. Saunders.

Nothling, J. O., Gerber, D., Colenbrander, B., Dijkstra, M., Bakker, T., & De Cramer, K. (2007). The effect of homologous prostatic fluid on motility and morphology of dog epididymal spermatozoa extended and frozen in Biladyl with Equex STM paste or Andromed. *Theriogenology, 67*(2), 264-275.

O'Brien, J. K., & Robeck, T. R. (2006). Development of sperm sexing and associated reproductive technology for sex preselection of captive bottlenose dolphins (Tursiops truncatus). *Reproduction, Fertility and Development, 18,* 319-329.

Otto, F. J., Hacker, U., Zante, J., Schumann, J., Göhde, W., & Meistrich, M. L. (1979). Flow cytometry of human sperm. *Histochemistry, 62,* 249-254.

Papa, F. O., Melo, C. M., Fioratti, E. G., Dell'Aqua Jr, J. A., Zahn, F. S., & Alvarenga, M. A. (2008). Freezing of stallion epididymal sperm. *Animal Reproduction Science, 107*(3-4), 293-301.

Pickett, B. W., & Voss, J. L. (1975). The effect of semen extenders and sperm numbers on mare fertility. *Journal of Reproduction and Fertility Supplement, 23,* 95-98.

Pinkel, D., Lake, S., Gledhill, B. L., Van Dilla, M. A., Stephenson, D., & Watchmaker, G. (1982). High resolution DNA content measurements of mammalian sperm. *Cytometry, 3,* 1-9.

Ponglowhapan, S., Chatdarong, K., Sirivaidyapong, S., & Lohachit, C. (2006). Freezing of epididymal spermatozoa from dogs after cool storage for 2 or 4 days. *Theriogenology, 66*(6-7), 1633-1636.

Pope, C. E., Crichton, E. B., Gomez, M. C., Dumas, C., & Dresser, B. (2008). Birth of domestic cat kittens of predetermined sex after transfer of embryos produced by in vitro fertilization of oocytes with flow-sorted spermatozoa. [Abstract]. *Reproduction, Fertility and Development, 20,* 213-214.

Presicce, G. A., Rath, D., Klinc, P., Senatore, E. M., & Pascale, M. (2005). Buffalo calves born following AI with sexed semen. [Abstract]. *Reproduction in Domestic Animals, 40,* 349.

Roca, J., Vaszques, J. M., Gil, M. A., Cuello, C., Parrilla, I., & Martinez, E. A. (2006). Challenges in Pig Artificial Insemination. *Reproduction in Domestic Animals, 41*(2), 43-53.

Santiago-Moreno, J. n., Toledano-Dìaz, A., Pulido-Pastor, A., Dorado, J. s., Gûmez-Brunet, A., & Lûpez-Sebasti n, A. (2006). Effect of egg yolk concentration on cryopreserving

Spanish ibex (Capra pyrenaica) epididymal spermatozoa. *Theriogenology, 66*(5), 1219-1226.

Santiago-Moreno, J. n., Toledano-Dìaz, A., Pulido-Pastor, A., GÛmez-Brunet, A., & LÛpez-Sebasti n, A. (2006). Birth of live Spanish ibex (Capra pyrenaica hispanica) derived from artificial insemination with epididymal spermatozoa retrieved after death. . *Theriogenology, 66*(2), 283-291.

Schenk, J. L., & DeGrofft, D. L. (2003). Insemination of cow elk with sexed frozen semen. [Abstract]. *Theriogenology, 59*, 514.

Seager, S. W. J. (1969). Successful pregnancies utilizing frozen dog semen. *AI Digest, 17*, 6-16.

Senger, P. L. (2003). *Pathways to Pregnancy and Parturition* (Second ed.): Current Conceptions,Inc.

Sieme, H., Sch‰fer, T., Stout, T. A. E., Klug, E., & Waberski, D. (2003). The effects of different insemination regimes on fertility in mares. *Theriogenology, 60*(6), 1153-1164.

Singleton, W. L. (2001). State of the art in artificial insemination of pigs in the United States. *Theriogenology, 56*(8), 1305-1310.

Soede, N. M. (1993). Boar stimuli around insemination affect reproductive processes in pigs: A review. *Animal Reproduction Science, 32*(1-2), 107-125.

Thomassen, R., Farstad, W., Krogenaes, A., Fougner, J. A., & Andersen Berg, K. (2001). Artificial insemination with frozen semen in dogs: a retrospective study. *Journal of Reproduction and Fertility Supplement, 57*, 341-346.

Thomassen, R., Sanson, G., Krogenes, A., Fougner, J. A., Berg, K. A., & Farstad, W. (2006). Artificial insemination with frozen semen in dogs: A retrospective study of 10 years using a non-surgical approach. *Theriogenology, 66*(6-7), 1645-1650.

Vazquez, J. M., Martinez, E. A., Parrilla, I., Roca, J., Gil, M. A., & Vazquez, J. L. (2003). Birth of piglets after deep intrauterine insemination with flow cytometrically sorted boar spermatozoa. *Theriogenology, 59*(7), 1605-1614.

Vazquez, J. M., Roca, J., Gil, M. A., Cuello, C., Parrilla, I., Vazquez, J. L., et al. (2008). New developments in low-dose insemination technology. *Theriogenology, 70*(8), 1216-1224.

Vidament, M. (2005). French field results (1985-2005) on factors affecting fertility of frozen stallion semen. *Animal Reproduction Science, 89*(1-4), 115-136.

Vidament, M., Dupere, A. M., Julienne, P., Evain, A., Noue, P., & Palmer, E. (1997). Equine frozen semen: Freezability and fertility field results. *Theriogenology, 48*(6), 907-917.

Wolf, D. P. (2009). Artificial insemination and the assisted reproductive technologies in non-human primates. *Theriogenology, 71*, 123-129.

Wongtawan, T., Saravia, F., Wallgren, M., Caballero, I., & RodrÌguez-MartÌnez, H. (2006). Fertility after deep intra-uterine artificial insemination of concentrated low-volume boar semen doses. *Theriogenology, 65*(4), 773-787.

Yamashiro, H., Han, Y.-J., Sugawara, A., Tomioka, I., Hoshino, Y., & Sato, E. (2007). Freezability of rat epididymal sperm induced by raffinose in modified Krebs-Ringer bicarbonate (mKRB) based extender solution. *Cryobiology, 55*(3), 285-294.

Youngquist, R. S., & Threlfall, W. R. (2007). *Current Therapy in Large Animal Theriogenology* (2nd ed.): Saunders Elsevier.

4

Veterinary Dysmorphology

Enio Moura[1] and Cláudia T. Pimpão[2]
[1]Service of Medical Genetics,
[2]Laboratory of Pharmacology and Toxicology,
Faculty of Veterinary Medicine, Campus São José,
Agricultural and Environmental Sciences Center,
Pontifícia Universidade Católica do Paraná, Curitiba
Brazil

1. Introduction

Dysmorphology is a branch of clinical genetics that deals with birth defects on a multidisciplinary basis. It involves knowledge of genetics, embryology, pathology, pediatrics and clinical medicine in order to diagnose birth defects and treat patients. Literally, dysmorphology means "the study of abnormal form". It is a word of Greek origin: *dys*, defect, disorder; *morphé*, form; and *lógos*, word, study. The term was coined by David Smith[1] in the 1960s (Aase, 1990), emphasizing its multidisciplinary aspects to differentiate it from traditional teratology. Due to its multidisciplinary nature, a specialist in dysmorphology works alongside cardiologists, ophthalmologists, neurologists, urologists, orthopedists, imaginologists, pathologists, biochemists and other specialists. It is a field that requires not only medical and biological knowledge but also high level of humanitarian feeling and respect for life, with dedication and perception to reduce the suffering of others. This chapter introduces the fundamentals of dysmorphology and offers an overview of this science in the context of veterinary medicine, with significant examples and emphasis on nosological, pathological, embryological, genetic and clinical aspects. The purpose of this is to provide veterinarians with an approach to congenital defects rather than the usual approach, emphasizing that much can be done instead of simply submitting affected animals to euthanasia. Therapeutic methods and surgical procedures will not be discussed, as each condition requires its own procedures, and these can easily be found in textbooks on medical therapy or surgery and also in scientific journals on veterinarian or human medicine.

---

[1] David Weyhe Smith (Oakland, 1926 – Seattle, 1981) was an American pediatrician and professor who dedicated his life to children affected by congenital defects, also providing guidance and support to their parents. He was a pioneer of dysmorphology, publishing a large number of articles on this science, of which he was the grand master. One of his books, *Recognizable Patterns of Human Malformation*, became a worldwide classic in the field of human dysmorphology (Wiedemann, 1991), and is now in its sixth edition, updated by Jones (2006). Aase (1990), in a posthumous homage, referred to David W. Smith as "the best and finest man I ever knew".

2. Dysmorphology in veterinary medicine

In veterinary medicine, dysmorphology is still a neglected field of knowledge, but has begun to take shape in line with the advances in veterinary medical genetics. Its basis is derived from human dysmorphology due to current knowledge of the genomic similarities between man and other vertebrates, especially mammals, showing that morphogenesis is evolutionarily conserved throughout the zoological scale. The inductive molecular mechanisms that form the embryonic pattern are identical in all vertebrates (Opitz et al., 2002). Furthermore, veterinary medicine and human medicine share most of the same methods and techniques, both in terms of diagnosis and therapy. However, in the current stage of the development of veterinary dysmorphology, some minute criteria used in human dysmorphology, especially those concerning the extension of concepts, could not always be adopted here.

2.1 Importance

The meaning of dysmorphology in veterinary medicine becomes clear when one considers that congenital defects in animals cause different types of impact: 1) the obvious suffering of the affected individual; 2) the psychological stress for the owners, who are more affectionate towards animals; 3) the abandonment of affected animals by many owners; and 4) the economic loss suffered by breeders, both of companion and production animals. All of these situations are directly linked to the professional work of the veterinarian, meaning different goals in terms of intervention.

2.2 Objectives

The main objectives of veterinary dysmorphology are humanitarian, professional, scientific, preventive and educational. The goal in humanitarian terms is to strive to minimize the suffering of affected individuals and have to do with the perception that animals are sentient beings, i.e., they can feel pain, discomfort, a number of difficulties and other feelings when they are affected by a defect or illness and, consequently, they suffer. The professional goals are to offer qualified assistance to clients who seek guidance and a solution to the congenital health problems of their animals. With these aims in mind more and more people are seeking veterinary clinics and hospitals, especially those dedicated to small animals. The scientific goals have to do with producing knowledge that will result in benefits for the animals themselves and also human beings. The study of spontaneous animal models of human diseases generates knowledge that could not be obtained from human patients for legal and ethical reasons. There are a great number of these animal models recognized today. New medical and molecular biology technology greatly facilitate these studies. The preventive goals are to attempt to advise owners and breeders of animals to help them make decisions and prevent the birth of new individuals with congenital defects. Scientifically based advice is an important step to avoiding the perpetuation of abnormalities, be they of a genetic nature or caused by environmental factors. The educational objectives include raising awareness that veterinarians, like any other professional, should contribute to the development of a better society in every way possible, encouraging ethical values and respect for human beings, animals, nature and life in general.

3. Dysmorphisms: Concept and classification

3.1 Concept

Dysmorphism[2] is the generic name for abnormalities of the form and structure of an animal's body, being used especially for congenital abnormalities, thus constituting an *inborn error of development*. It is important to remember that the adjective "congenital" means born with the individual, independent of the cause. However, it is not synonymous with either "genetic" or "hereditary". Therefore, there are congenital defects that have a genetic cause (the majority) while others have an environmental cause. The word dysmorphism has a broad meaning and can also refer to alterations that are expressed in deviations of size, position, number and even the coloring of one or more parts of the body. Thus, all of the following examples are dysmorphisms: cleft lip and palate (*cheilopalatoschisis*); absence of the cranial vault and cerebral hemispheres (*anencephaly*); very small jaw (*micrognathia*); heart with the apex to the right-hand side (*dextrocardia*); an out of place kidney (*renal ectopia*); one or two missing eyes (*anophthalmia*); extra toes (*polydactyly*); two heads (*dicephaly*); a simple and hyperplasic congenital stain on the skin (*congenital nevus*). Some are extremely serious and lead to death in early life, such as anencephaly; others cause little or no harm to the animal, such as polydactyly (Fig.1).

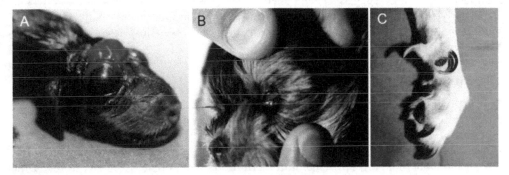

Fig. 1. Examples of dysmorphisms in dogs: A) Anencephaly; B) Anophthalmia; C) Polydactyly.

3.2 Classification

According to the nature of the alteration that causes the dysmorphism and the stage at which it manifests, the phenomenon can be divided into three categories: *malformation, disruption and deformation*. Malformations begin earlier, during the embryonic period, while disruptions appear later. Most deformations begin during the fetal stage, which is when the conceptus grows more rapidly (Kumar & Burton, 2008). If subjacent histological alterations are also considered, a fourth category can be added: *dysplasia*.

---

[2] Dysmorphism should not be confused with dimorphism, which means the existence of "two different and normal forms" of a given characteristic (from the Greek *di*, two; *morphé*, form), commonly used in the expression "sexual dimorphism" to indicate the natural differences between male and female in a given species.

3.2.1 Malformation

This is a morphological defect of an organ, part of an organ, or a larger region of the body, resulting from an intrinsically abnormal developmental process (Spranger, 1982)[3]. This definition highlights that malformations are disorders in the formation of organs and manifest early, i.e., they are *abnormal processes since the time of their origin*. The affected organ can show varying degrees of imperfection or simply not exist. Malformations arise during blastogenesis or organogenesis and are causally heterogeneous and those that appear earlier (blastogenesis) tend to affect more than one region of the body (Opitz et al., 2002). Although they can be induced by environmental factors, they are commonly caused by gene mutations, chromosomal aberrations or a combination of genetic and environmental factors (Kumar & Burton, 2008). Examples: 1) A nonsyndromic cleft lip and palate can be caused by a recessive autosomal mutation in Brittany spaniels (Richtsmeier et al., 1994), Pyrenees shepherds (Kemp et al., 2009) and boxers (Moura et al., 2011); 2) In Rocky Mountain horses ciliary body cysts, iridal hypoplasia, iridocorneal adhesions and megalocornea are caused by codominant autosomal mutation, with cysts expressed in the heterozygotes and multiple ocular anomalies expressed in the homozygotes (Ewart et al., 2000), whose locus was mapped to the long arm of chromosome 6 (Andersson et al. 2008); 3) The trisomy 18 in cattle causes brachygnathia and is lethal (Herzog, 1974); 4) Cardiac malformations usually have a multifactorial etiology, such as a patent ductus arteriosus in poodles (Buchanan & Patterson, 2003); 5) Neural tube closure defects, such as spina bifida and anencephaly, also have a multifactorial etiology, including mutations in genes involved in folate metabolism (De Marco et al., 2011).

3.2.2 Disruption

A disruption is a morphological defect of an organ, part of an organ or a larger region of the body, resulting from a disturbance in an originally normal developmental process (Spranger, 1982)[4]. This definition highlights that the *formation process of the organs was initially normal, but suffered negative interference during its development*, having affected the organ during the embryonic or fetal stage. In a disruption there is damage to structures of the conceptus because of interference in the blood supply, anoxia, infection or mechanical force (Epstein, 2004), affecting several different tissues and the defect does not respect the boundaries imposed by embryonic developmental process (Aase, 1990). In general, disruptions are caused by environmental factors, but genetic factors can predispose to the development of a disruption (Kumar & Burton, 2008). Examples: 1) A number of therapeutic drugs can cause damage to the embryo when used during pregnancy, especially drugs for continuous use, such as the anticonvulsant valproic acid (Jentink et al., 2010); 2) The feline panleukopenia virus has long been known to cause cerebellar hypoplasia and eventually

---

[3] In the early 1980s, due to divergences and mistaken nomenclature at that time, specialists in congenital defects formed an International Work Group (IWG) to classify and define terms and expressions for morphogenesis disorders. Their recommendations were published in 1982 (Spranger et al., 1982) and adopted by most dysmorphologists and are still in use today, with very few modifications.
[4] The definitions of malformation and disruption used here correspond, respectively, to the *primary malformation* and *secondary malformation* that were previously in use in dysmorphology. In 1982, the IWG restricted the use of malformation to intrinsically abnormal or primary defects (Opitz, 1984).

hydranencephaly in cats (Résibois et al., 2007); 3) The intrauterine infection caused by the blue tongue virus (BTV serotype 8) causes hydranencephaly in cattle (Wouda et al., 2009); 4) A well known cause of disruption in human beings and which has also been found in the rhesus monkey (Tarantal & Hendrickx, 1987), are amniotic bands that can cause constriction of body structures, leading to facial clefts, amputation of fingers and toes or limbs and other abnormalities.

3.2.3 Deformation

This is a defect of the shape or position of part of the body caused by mechanical forces (Spranger, 1982). These forces may be of internal or external origin and are most evident in the bones, cartilage and joints, as soft tissues tend to return to their original form as soon as the force ceases. Deformations set in during the fetal stage and are normally caused by forces that act late in pregnancy (Epstein, 2004). A large number of deformations have a spontaneous resolution after birth, although this normally takes place slowly. Sometimes, however, treatment is necessary to correct a deformation (Aase, 1990). Like disruptions, although later on, deformations also cause damage to previously intact developed structures with no intrinsic tissue abnormality (Kumar & Burton, 2008). Examples: 1) Club foot as a result of too little space in the uterus and muscular hypotonia or joint laxity, impeding movement of the extremities. Among the factors that reduce uterine space are a very large fetus and a reduction in amniotic fluid, a condition known as oligohydramnios; 2) Increased cephalic perimeter in the hydrocephaly[5] due to pressure from the accumulation of cerebrospinal fluid. The first example is caused by an external force (pressure from the uterus) whereas the second one is caused by an internal force (pressure from the cerebrospinal fluid). It is worth bearing in mind, however, that not all deformations are congenital. They can also develop in postnatal life. For example, bones can be bent because of a lack of calcium or the joints can lose alignment because of the laxity of the joints or lack of calcium. These structures become deformed because of the weight of the body.

3.2.4 Dysplasia

Dysplasia is a morphological defect that results from a disorganization of cells (Spranger, 1982) and other components of a tissue, which, in turn, does not have normal architecture. Therefore, dysplasias are disorders of histogenesis and the alterations occur on a microscopic level and are reflected in the imperfect appearance of the organ or other affected regions of the body. Examples: 1) Congenital alopecia and dental abnormalities in dogs with X-linked hypohidrotic ectodermal dysplasia. There is also absence of piloglandular units in the areas of alopecia (Moura & Cirio, 2004). 2) Thoracic and pelvic limbs are short and bent in dogs affected by chondrodysplasia as can be seen in Great Pyrenees dogs (Bingel & Sande, 1994) or in Labrador retrievers (Smit et al., 2011). Figure 2 shows a visual comparison between normal development and the four types of inborn errors of development (malformation, disruption, deformation and dysplasia).

---

[5] The cause of hydrocephaly is a malformation or disruption that blocks the drainage of cerebrospinal fluid which, in turn, dilates the cerebral ventricles and separates the cranial bones, *deforming* the head.

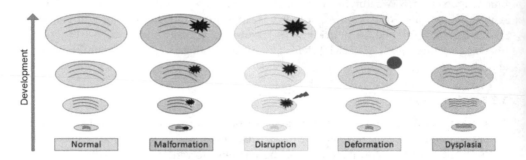

Fig. 2. Types of dysmorphisms compared with normal development.

3.3 Further considerations

Dysmorphisms can also be classified based on criteria other than those presented above. When the medical consequences are considered, they are divided into major and minor dysmorphisms. The former have a significant effect on the quality of life of the affected individual, such as oral clefts, or even impede survival (lethal dysmorphisms), such as anencephaly. The latter have little or no effect on the quality of life of the affected individual and do not require treatment or can be easily treated, such as polydactyly. Dysmorphisms can occur due to increased size or number of body parts and are known as excess dysmorphisms, e.g., extra fingers and toes (polydactyly), duplication of the face (diprosopia) and two heads (dicephaly); or missing body parts, known as reduction dysmorphisms, such as unilateral or bilateral absence of the radius (radial agenesis), missing pinna (anotia) and missing tail (anury). Figure 3 shows some of these defects.

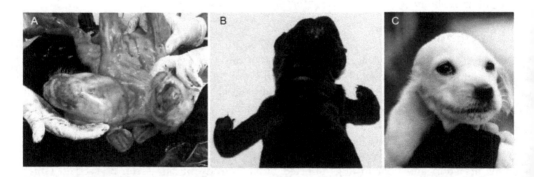

Fig. 3. A) Dicephaly (excess dysmorphism) in extreme premature calf); B) Bilateral radial agenesis in a dog (reduction dysmorphism); C) Anotia in a dog (reduction dysmorphism). Photograph **A** courtesy of Dr. Antonia M. R. B. do Prado and Dr. Joséli Maria Büchele, Laboratory of Anatomy, Faculty of Veterinary Medicine, Pontifícia Universidade Católica do Paraná

4. Epidemiological aspects of dysmorphisms

On its own, a certain type of congenital defect may be rare, but congenital defects as a whole are relatively common in all domestic species and their different breeds and are a significant cause of neonatal and infant mortality and morbidity. Preliminary data suggest that the frequency of dysmorphisms is greater in pigs, followed in descending order by dogs, horses, cattle and cats[6] (Hámori, 1983).

4.1 Frequency, mortality and morbidity

The *frequency* of major dysmorphisms in humans is estimated at 3% of live births (Marden et al, 1964). This number practically doubles by the end of the first year of life, with the identification of defects that manifest later (Kumar & Burton, 2008). In domestic animals, these numbers must be similar or even higher because inbreeding is common in selective breeding both for companion animals and for farm animals, increasing the coefficient of consanguinity. One study (Priester et al, 1970), which included all domestic species, analyzed almost 138,000 individuals and found a rate of 4.68%. However, minor dysmorphisms are not always identified and are seldom included in statistics. The same may occur in the case of major dysmorphisms when they affect internal structures and cause intrauterine or neonatal death and are not always reported. Rates of occurrence vary according to each abnormality and can also vary according to species, breed and geographical location. *Mortality* varies a great deal from one dysmorphism to another. Some are so serious that they cause intrauterine or perinatal death, such as combined heart-lung defects; others are incompatible with life and the affected individual dies soon after birth, as is the case with anencephaly. However, a large number of major dysmorphisms can be corrected surgically or be given some form of treatment, making life viable. Furthermore, minor dysmorphisms have no meaning in terms of mortality. Like mortality, *morbidity* also varies according to the dysmorphism. In many cases, treatment definitively cures the defect and the individual goes on to live a normal life; in other cases, treatment can improve the quality of life, but the individual will have chronic difficulties until the end of his days.

4.2 Risk factors

The artificial selection in breeding to obtain animals with a new or better appearance or for financial gain often means consanguineous unions, increasing the risk of the recurrence of a given defect in future generations. The environment also poses many risk factors during pregnancy, such as: 1) residue from pesticides in water, pasture and other foods; 2) certain toxic plants[7] in the pasture; 3) inadequate conservation of animal feed and other foodstuff

---

[6] Cats are generally under-represented in samples involving several species. However, veterinarians of small animals often come across congenital defects in purebred cats, which are suggestive of a relatively high rate of dysmorphisms in this species, which is not always reported in journals. They have seen conjoined twins, poliotia, radial agenesis, frontonasal dysplasia, cyclopia, diprosopia, meningocele, anencephaly, spina bifida, hydrocephaly, polydactyly, syndactyly, anal atresia, hypospadias, true hermaphroditism, pseudohermaphroditism and others.

[7] Examples include certain species of the genus *Lupinus* (lupines) that contain teratogenic alkaloids (anagyrine, ammodendrine) that cause a form of congenital arthrogryposis in calves, known as "crooked calf disease". This disease occurs when pregnant cows ingest the plants between the fortieth

which results in mycotoxins; 4) excessive levels of nitrogen-containing food preservatives[8] in low quality animal feed; 5) medicine[9] in the early stages of pregnancy; 6) medicines for continuous use during pregnancy, such as some anticonvulsants; 7) occurrence of certain infectious or metabolic diseases during pregnancy.

5. Etiopathogenesis of dysmorphisms

5.1 Etiology

The *etiological agents* of dysmorphisms can be divided into three large groups: *genetic, environmental and multifactorial*. Although, presumably, any cause of congenital defect is included in one of these groups, a large number of dysmorphsisms have no identified cause and are provisionally separated as a group of *unknown etiology*.

5.1.1 Genetic etiology

In humans, genetic factors are responsible for most dysmorphisms with a known cause (Kumar & Burton, 2008). Considering that mammals in general share most of their genes with humans and that the genes responsible for morphogenesis are highly conserved, the genetic factors must be equally responsible for most of the congenital defects of domestic mammals. These factors are: 1) *dominant autosomal mutations*, such as the fibrillin-1 gene (*FBN 1*), which causes Marfan syndrome in cattle (Singleton et al., 2005). The affected animals have long, thin limbs, laxity of the joints, lens abnormalities, aortic dilation, etc. (Besser et al., 1990); 2) *recessive autosomal mutations*, such as the one that causes anotia, cleft palate and bifid tongue in St. Bernard dogs (Villagómez & Alonso, 1998); 3) *recessive X-linked mutations*, such as the one that occurs in the ectodysplasin A1 and A2 gene isoforms (*EDA-A1* and *EDA-A2*) and causes X-linked hypohidrotic ectodermal dysplasia in dogs (Casal et al. 2005). Affected individuals have imperfect teeth, oligodontia and cutaneous areas with no piloglandular units, as shown in Figure 4 (Moura & Cirio, 2004); 4) *deletions of Y chromosome genes*, such as the one of the sex-determining region Y gene (*SRY*), which determines sex reversal in horses, i.e., it leaves individuals with an male XY karyotype with a female phenotype and ovaries (Raudsepp et al., 2010); 5) *chromosomal aberrations*, such as trysomy of chromosome 30 in horses, which makes them smaller than normal, with a

---

and hundredth day of pregnancy. The affected calves characteristically have bent extremities and can also have scoliosis, torticollis and cleft palate. Ingestion of toxic plants by farm animals can have a serious economic impact on livestock producers in given geographical areas through death losses, abortions, and birth defects (Lee et al., 2008).

[8] It has not been completely established that N-nitroso compounds, such as nitrosamine and its precursors (nitrites and nitrates) naturally cause congenital diseases. Studies in animals indicate that they are highly carcinogenic and at higher levels can be teratogenic, but there is a need for further studies (Griesenbeck et al. 2010). Likewise, mycotoxins should also be considered. Fumonisins (frequent contaminants of corn) and ochratoxin-A (often found in stored grains) experimentally cause craniofacial and neural tube defects in mice (Marasas et al., 2004; Ueta et al. 2010).

[9] An example of routine use in veterinary medicine is griseofulvin, an antifungal drug for animals with dermatomycosis. Scott et al. (1975) observed multiple congenital defects in newborn cats whose mothers orally received high doses of griseofulvin (500-1000 mg, at weekly intervals). There were cerebral defects, skeletal defects, cleft palate, anophthalmia with absence of optic nerves, anal atresia, lack of atrioventricular valves and other defects.

serious angular deviation of the thoracic limbs and polydactyly (Bowling & Millon, 1990); 6) *structural chromosomal aberrations*, such as the translocation between the X chromosome and an autosome described by Schelling et al., (2001) in an intersex Yorkshire terrier.

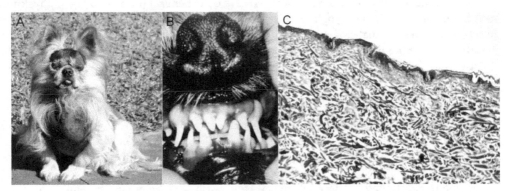

Fig. 4. X-linked hypohidrotic ectodermal dysplasia: A) Congenital absence of hair (congenital alopecia); B) Dental defects (conical teeth and oligodontia); C) Microphotograph of the skin (from an alopecic area) showing absence of hair follicles, sebaceous glands and sweat glands. Shorr stain, X10 objective. Photograph **C** courtesy of Dr. Silvana M. Cirio, Laboratory of Pathology, Faculty of Veterinary Medicine, FEPAR.

5.1.2 Environmental etiology

The environment can be a source of numerous potential teratogens, an important cause of congenital defects in both humans and animals because their presence is not always obvious or the harmful effect of certain products is unknown to the public at large, which increases the risk of maternal exposure to them. *Environmental teratogens* are agents in the *environment* that can negatively impact embryonic development, causing congenital defects. Many chemical products and medicines have been considered potentially teratogenic for decades. Some have been confirmed as such and others have been refused, while the potential of others is doubtful or has been mistakenly confirmed (Koren & Nickel, 2010; 2011). In principle, the risk of a defect is related to the frequency and degree of maternal exposure (Holmes, 2011). Agents that are commonly considered as potentially teratogenic can be separated into four groups: 1) *environmental contaminants*, such as mercury[10], lead, polychlorinated biphenyls, organochlorines and dioxins. There is also considerable doubt

---

[10] Mercury does not cause gross birth defects, but rather lesions in the central nervous system which cause psychomotor retard, convulsions and other neurological signs (Lancaster, 2011). The sad history of *Minamata disease* was first reported in 1953, but its cause was identified only three years later: a chemical plant discharged water containing inorganic mercury into Minamata Bay in Japan, and this was transformed into organic mercury (methylmercury) by marine microorganisms. Contaminated fish and clams with mythylmercury were consumed as food by the inhabitants of the town of Minamata and this was the source of poisoning which, in the case of pregnant women, affected the fetus, causing *congenital Mimata disease* (Moura, 1993). The number of people affected by the disease was officially established as 2,252, of whom 1,043 had already died 36 years later (Harada, 1995).

concerning their real effect on teratogenic processes. For example, dioxins have been held responsible for a variety of defects. However, that scientific data have so far only confirmed a link to spina bifida (Ngo, 2010); 2) *medicines*[11] such as phenytoin, valproic acid, coumarins and antibiotics; 3) *physical agents* such as heat and radiation[12]; 4) *infectious agents* such as viruses, bacteria and protozoa. Thus, teratogens are of a chemical (dioxins, drugs), physical (heat, radiation) and biological nature (microbes). Non-infectious maternal diseases can also cause dysmorphisms: diabetes mellitus, iodine deficiency, uterine myomas, autoimmune diseases, etc. Uterine dysmorphisms and abnormalities in the extra-embryonic membranes can also cause fetus defects.

5.1.3 Multifactorial etiology

The joint action of several genes (polygenic inheritance) can also play a significant role in the occurrence of dysmorphisms. Deleterious alleles of the different genes play an additive effect until they reach a threshold at which the defect occurs. Environmental factors usually add to this mechanism. Thus, an individual with a given genotype becomes more susceptible to developing a defect, which can be unleashed when environmental forces are at play (multifactorial inheritance). Neural tube closure defects (anencephaly, spina bifida) and conotruncal defects (truncus arteriosus, tetralogy of Fallot) generally have a multifactorial etiology.

5.2 Pathogenesis

The process that gives rise to an abnormal form is a *morphogenetic disturbance* and is known as dysmorphogenesis. The mechanisms involved in dysmorphogenesis are complex, compromising a number of the embryonic developmental phenomena (division of cells, cellular migration, cell adhesion, differentiation, etc.), including cell signaling pathways, e.g., the Sonic hedgehog pathway. They can also include hypoxia resulting from blocked

---

[11] The tragic history of thalidomide is a warning that the use of medicine during pregnancy should be strictly limited to what is absolutely necessary and should be taken only with medical advice. Thalidomide was launched in 1956, initially as a sedative. By the early 1960s it had become a popular medicine to control morning sickness during pregnancy and could be purchased without a prescription. The following year, Australian obstetrician *William McBride* and German pediatrician *Widukind Lenz* independently saw the link between thalidomide in the early stages of pregnancy and *phocomelia*. The children born with this defect had short limbs close to their bodies and malformed fingers and toes. The abnormality could affect one limb, both arms or all four limbs and often affected internal organs such as the heart and duodenum, constituting a pattern of abnormalities that became known as *thalidomide embryopathy*. It is estimated that there were 8,000 to 10,000 cases worldwide (von Moos et al. 2003). However, thalidomide has been used successfully to treat diseases such as cancer, leprosy and auto-immune diseases.

[12] The *Chernobyl nuclear accident* (Ukraine), in 1986, is a blatant and relatively recent example of the catastrophic effect of *ionizing radiation* on living beings. A number of disorders, including a variety of *malformations*, were registered in animals, from fish to mammals, and even in invertebrates. Congenital defects of the mouth, anus, legs and head were reported in domestic animals. Until today, in animal populations of the contaminated region, there is *transgenerational genomic instability* and *gene mutation rates* are significantly high. In some areas of Europe, the radionuclide levels remain high in mammals, birds, amphibians and fish (Yablokov, 2009).

circulation or non-formation of blood vessels like that caused by antiangiogenic drugs, such as thalidomide and retinoids (Holaday & Berkowitz, 2009). They manifest at the histological level in different ways, such as aplasia, hypoplasia, dysplasia, atrophy, hypertrophy, etc. To follow, we present the fundamental concepts of the developmental field theory, the knowledge of which facilitates the understanding of dysmorphogenesis.

5.2.1 Developmental fields

Developmental field is, initially, the entire embryo in the early stages of its development and, later, it is a region or part of the body of the embryo which responds as a unit to embryonic induction and gives rise to multiple or complex anatomic structures (Spranger et al., 1982; Opitz et al., 2002). Developmental fields are systems that control the progressive differentiation of the structure and size, and also the temporal and spatial distribution of the complex organ components. To understand better the developmental field concept, it is important to remember the meaning of the terms *blastogenesis, organogenesis, morphogenesis, histogenesis* and *phenogenesis* in the context of dysmorphology. *Blastogenesis* is the set of events of embryonic development from fertilization to the end of gastrulation, i.e., it includes phenomena such as the formation of the morula, blastocyst, ectoderm, endoderm, mesoderm, neural tube and midline, in addition to cardioangiogenesis, mesonephrogenesis and curving of the embryo, which then takes the shape of a C (Opitz et al., 2002). At the end of the gastrulation, *organogenesis* begins. This is the set of events that lead to the formation of the organs and other parts of the body (*morphogenesis*) and includes the differentiation of the cells and tissues (*histogenesis*). On average, the duration of blastogenesis is similar in the majority of mammals, but the duration of the phenomena that follow varies from one species to another, especially the fetal period, which is reflected in the duration of pregnancy. The development that ranges from the fetal period and postnatal period to puberty is called *phenogenesis* (Opitz et al., 2002). During the fetal period, phenogenesis is characterized by growth and maturation, preparing the individual for birth. The *primary developmental field* is the field represented by the entire embryo in the early stages of blastogenesis. The initial phenomena of this period include pattern formation, generating components known as **progenitor fields**, which are the primordia of all final structures (Davidson, 1993; Martínez-Frías et al., 1998), as they give rise to the heart, central nervous system and limb buds (Opitz et al. 2002). When the components of a field remain contiguous, they constitute a *monotopic field*, in other words, a developmental field related to the formation of a single area of the body. However, there are fields in which the components separate from one another to give rise to distant final structures among themselves, which are known as *polytopic fields*. Thus, a polytopic field has to do with the formation of structures situated in different areas of the body (Opitz, 1982). *Secondary developmental fields* are the fields formed by the subdivision of progenitor fields, and each of them originates a determined final structure during organogenesis (Martínez-Frías et al., 1998).

5.2.2 Congenital defects and developmental fields

Malformations, disruptions and dysplasias are the result of disorders that occur in one of more developmental field. If they result from alterations that occur during blastogenesis, when the progenitor fields are formed, they are *primary field defects*; if they are the result of alterations that occur during organogenesis, after the formation of the progenitor fields, they are *secondary field defects*. Those that are localized, i.e., the affect only one structure or part of the body, which was differentiated during organogenesis, are *monotopic field defects*; those affecting structures situated in different parts of the body are *polytopic field defects* and originate in the early stages of blastogenesis (Martínez-Frías, 1998).

5.2.3 Heterogeneity, pleiotropy and sequence

Developmental fields are embryonic morphogenetic units and, thus, respond to an inductive stimulus as an epimorphically hierarchical self-organizing unit that is temporally synchronized and spatially coordinated (Opitz, 1982). Consequently, a given abnormal phenotype can originate as a response of a field to different causes. This becomes clearer if we remember that different fields can share parts of the same cell signaling pathway involved in embryonic development. For example, the *Sonic hedgehog cell signaling pathway* is composed of genes that codify proteins that act as intercellular signals in many development processes. Mutations in these genes can result in malformations such as holoprosencephaly, syndactyly, polydactyly, heart defects, kidney defects and anal atresia, or even in neoplasias such as meningioma and squamous cell carcinoma (Cohen Jr, 2004). A congenital defect can be the result of mutations in different genes, chromosomal aberrations or the action of mutagenic agents or teratogens, i.e., it is *causally heterogeneous*. Evidently, the meaning of this is that defects that are clinically the same can have a genetic or environmental cause (Fig. 5). A defect caused by an environmental factor, but which is the same as another caused genetically, is known as a *phenocopy*.

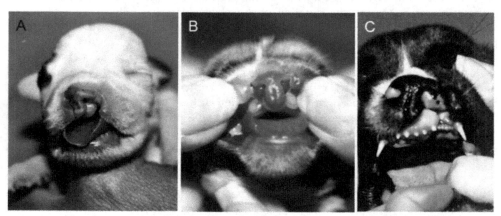

Fig. 5. Cleft lip and palate in dogs are phenotypically and etiologically heterogeneous. They can be unilateral (A) or bilateral (B). They can affect the entire extension of the palate or only the primary palate (C). They can have a multifactorial origin or a monogenic autosomal recessive origin, or be caused by environmental factors (phenocopy).

On the other hand, the same gene can give rise to a series of morphogenetic events that are necessary for the formation of different final structures. This genetic phenomenon in which a gene is responsible for several different phenotypic characteristics is known as *pleiotropy* and is also one of the phenomena that can occur in dysmorphogenesis. For example, a mutation in the gene that codifies ectodysplasin, a protein that regulates the initial epithelial-mesenchymal interaction necessary for the formation of ectodermal derivatives, causes X-linked hypohidrotic ectodermal dysplasia, which occurs in humans, cattle, mice and dogs, and is characterized by defects in the teeth and in the skin (absence of piloglandular units) and other ectodermal derivatives (Moura & Cirio, 2004). In addition to heterogeneity and pleiotropy, another phenomenon may be behind multiple abnormalities: they may be the consequence of only one initial defect that provokes the occurrence of new events in a chain reaction, characterizing a *dysmorphogenetic sequence*. For instance, micrognathia can unleash retroglossoptosis which, in turn, causes cleft palate and respiratory distress, a condition known as Pierre Robin sequence (Mackay, 2011).

5.2.4 More frequently affected systems and selected examples of abnormalities

Cardiovascular system: communication between the pulmonary trunk and the aorta artery (*patent ductus arteriosus*, Fig. 6-A); communication between the atria (*atrial septal defect*) or between the ventricles (*ventricular septal defect*); combination of pulmonary stenosis with a ventricular septal defect, hypertrophy of the right ventricle and an overriding aorta, i.e., the aorta is positioned directly over a ventricular septal defect (*tetratology of Fallot*); imperfect mitral valve and support structures (*mitral dysplasia*); imperfect tricuspid valve and support structures (*tricuspid dysplasia);* right or left atrium divided by a membrane, leaving it with two chambers (*cor triatriatum*); absence of communication between the right atrium and ventricle (*tricuspid atresia*); lack of differentiation of the origins of the pulmonary trunk, aorta and coronary arteries, forming a common arterial trunk (*truncus arteriosus*).

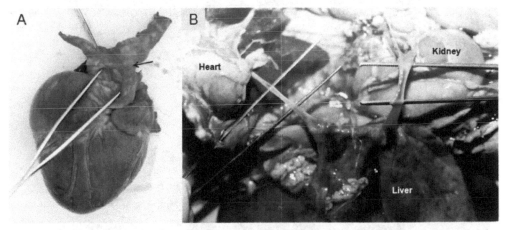

Fig. 6. Examples of abnormalities of the cardiovascular system: A) Patent ductus arteriosus (arrow); B) Abnormality of the caudal vena cava in a dachshund dog with Caroli disease. Note that this vein (raised by forceps) does not have normal morphology. Photograph **B** courtesy of Dr. Marconi R. de Farias, Companion Animal Veterinary Hospital, Faculty of Veterinary Medicine, Pontifícia Universidade Católica do Paraná.

Musculoskeletal system: missing jaw (*agnathia*); shorter-than-normal jaw (*brachygnathia*); abnormally small jaw (*micrognathia*); incompletely formed vertebra (*hemivertebra*, Fig. 7-A and B); missing vertebrae in the lumbar and sacral region (*lumbosacral agenesis*); absence of the radius (*radial agenesis, radial hemimelia*) which may be unilateral or bilateral; absence of one or more limbs (*amelia*); fused digits (*syndactyly*); missing digits and respective metacarpal bones (*ectrodactyly*, Fig. 7-C); existence of extra digits (*polydactyly*); presence of one or more supernumerary limbs (*polymelia*); shorter-than-normal bones due to deficient endochondral ossification (*chondrodysplasia*); incongruence of the elbow joint (*elbow dysplasia*); incongruence of the coxofemoral joint (*hip dysplasia*); congenital joint immobility (*arthrogryposis*); paraumbilical defect in the abdomen with evisceration (*gastroschisis*, Fig. 7-D); congenital umbilical hernia containing viscera (*omphalocele*); congenital cleft of the thoracic wall (*thoracoschisis*), with exteriorization of the heart (*ectopia cordis*).

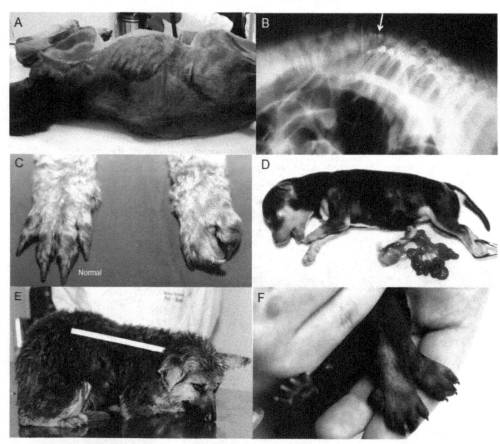

Fig. 7. Examples of abnormalities of the musculoskeletal system: A) Newborn foal with serious scoliosis as a result of spinal defects (hemivertebrae); B) Radiograph of the foal shown in A, revealing the hemivertebrae (arrow); C) Ectrodactyly in a poodle dog (left thoracic limb); D) Gastroschisis in a newborn Siberian husky; E) Pituitary dwarfism in a German shepherd at the age of 4 years; F) Duplication of the left hind paw of a newborn Rottweiler (polypodia). Photographs **A** and **B** courtesy of Dr. Pedro V. Michelloto Junior, Equine Veterinary Hospital, Faculty of Veterinary Medicine, Pontifícia Universidade Católica do Paraná.

Nervous system: absence of the upper parts of the brain and skull (*anencephaly*, Fig.1-A); retroflection of the head and partial or total absence of the cervical vertebrae associated with serious defects of the central nervous system (*iniencephaly*); stenosis of the aqueduct of Sylvius or another part of the brain's drainage system, leading to accumulated cerebrospinal fluid in the cerebral ventricles (*hydrocephaly*, Fig. 8-A); meningeal herniation, i.e., a protrusion of the meninges at some point of the spine (*meningocele*, Fig. 8-B); meningeal herniation containing a segment of the spinal cord (*meningomyelocele*); meningeal herniation containing part of the brain (*meningoencephalocele*); absence of the major connection between the two cerebral hemispheres (*agenesis of the corpus callosum*); failed development of the prosencephalon (forebrain), compromising the separation of the cerebral hemispheres and causing defects in the midline of the face (*holoprosencephaly*); absence of brain gyri (*lissencephaly*); presence of small and multiple brain gyri (*polymicrogiria*); enlargement of the brain gyri (*pachygiria*); lower than normal development of the cerebellum (*cerebellar hypoplasia*).

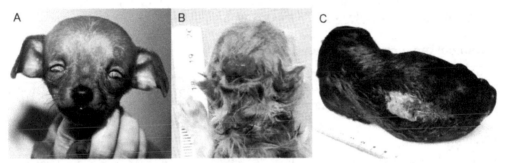

Fig. 8. Examples of abnormalities of the central nervous system: A) Hydrocephaly in a dachshund puppy ; B) Meningocele in a newborn Persian kitty; C) Spina bifida occulta with neural involvement in a newborn Rottweiler puppy.

Genitourinary System: missing kidney (*renal agenesis*) that can be unilateral or bilateral; disorganized renal tissue (*renal dysplasia*); cysts in the kidneys (*polycystic renal disease*); fusion of the kidneys by one of the poles, generally the lower, with a silhouette forming in the shape of a horseshoe (*horseshoe kidney*); proximal bifurcation of the renal pelvis (*bifid renal pelvis*); ureter flowing into an organ other than the bladder, commonly in the urethra or the vagina and even the uterus (*ureteral ectopia*); failure to close the urachus (*patent urachus*); urethral opening located on a point of the ventral side of the penis, scrotum or perineum (*hypospadias*, Fig. 9-A); urethra with a connection to the rectum (*urethrorectal fistula*); cystic tumors formed of tissue from different embryonic germ layers that are strangers to the affected organ (*teratoma*). They are more frequent in ovaries and testicles, but can occur in the prostate or in organs from other systems; absence of vagina (vaginal agenesis); larger-than-normal clitoris (*clitoromegaly*, Fig. 9-B); much smaller-than-normal penis (*micropenis*); testicle retained in the abdomen or inguinal canal (*cryptorchidism*), which can be unilateral or bilateral; presence of a membrane that totally or partially closes the vaginal opening (*persistent hymen*); presence of a fibrous ligament between the gland and the foreskin (*persistent penile frenulum*). In domestic mammals, unlike human beings where the hymen and the penile frenulum are characteristics found in adults, there is a regression of these structures during development.

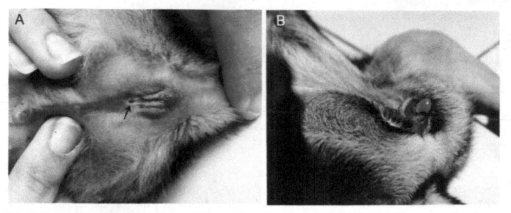

Fig. 9. Examples of abnormalities of the genitourinary system: A) Perineal hypospadias in a dog. Observe the urethral opening (arrow) located in the perineum, near the anus; B) Ambiguous genitalia in a dog with XX true hermaphroditism.

6. Clinical presentation of dysmorphisms

Dysmorphisms can affect an individual as a *single defect* (Fig. 10-A and B) or a set of defects (*multiple congenital anomalies*). The latter include syndromes, developmental field defects, associations and sequences. All arise from disorders in one of more developmental field.

6.1 Single defect

A *single defect* (*isolated defect*) affects only one specific part of an organ or a single organ or a local region of the body. Single defects include an eyelid coloboma, a cleft palate, a patent ductus arteriosus and a hypospadias. Most congenital defects are single and their etiology is often multifactorial. A given type of single defect may be viewed as part of certain syndromes, pointing out that different causes can affect the same developmental field, leading to the same result (Aase, 1990). Single defects are monotopic defects, which are the result of a disturbance in a single monotopic primary field or in a secondary field.

6.2 Multiple congenital anomalies

The occurrence of two or more defects in one or more parts of the body of the same individual is characterized as a *multiple congenital anomaly* (Fig. 10-C). However, the concomitant occurrence of anomalies does not define the etiology. A given pattern of defects may indeed have a specific etiology or may be caused by a variety of possible agents that affect the same developmental fields or a same monotopic or polytopic field.

6.2.1 Syndrome

A syndrome is a *set of defects* that occur simultaneously in the same individual and result from the *same cause*. Therefore, the pattern of defects must be repeated in all affected individuals. Syndromes are defined after several cases have been described, enabling one to determine which defects actually compose the syndrome and which are accidental. Strictly speaking, however, the cause is not always known, but it is presumed. Generally, syndromes are considered as having resulted from a disorder in more than one developmental field (Spranger, 1982). Examples: 1) Hurler Syndrome (mucopolysaccharidosis I), a recessive autosomal syndrome in which there is a deficiency of alpha-L-iduronidase. Affected dogs have corneal opacity, facial dysmorphism, joint abnormalities, aortic dilation and thickened heart valves (Traas et al., 2007); 2) Hunter Syndrome (mucopolysaccharidosis II), an X-linked recessive syndrome in which there is iduronate-sulfatase deficiency. Affected dogs have a course facial appearance, macrodactyly, corneal dystrophy and neurological alterations (Wilkerson, 1998).

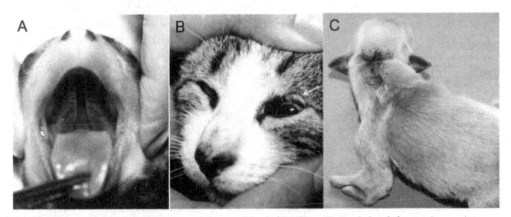

Fig. 10. Examples of single defect: A) Dog with cleft palate; B) Eyelid coloboma (arrow) in a cat; C) Example of a multiple congenital anomaly in a dog (meningocele and peromelia).

6.2.2 Developmental field defects

Developmental field defects are resulting from a *dysmorphogenetic response* of a developmental field (Hersch et al., 2002) and are causally heterogeneous. This means that the *same field reacts in a similar way to different factors*. They may be multiple anomalies that affect an area of anatomically related structures, being monotopic field defects; or they may be anomalies in different areas of the body, being polytopic field defects. Holoprosencephaly in its different degrees is a monotopic field, such as semilobar holoprosencephaly in Morgan horses (Kock et al., 2005), and may be associated with otocephaly, as reported by Martínez et al., (2006) in a Rottweiler dog. Lumbosacral agenesis in its different degrees is a polytopic field defect and has been described in a number of domestic species, such as sheep (Denis, 1975), cattle (Jones, 1999; Son et al., 2008), pigs (Avedillo & Camón, 2007) and dogs (Araújo et al., 2008).

6.2.3 Association

Association is a *combination of two or more defects* in the same individual and occurs in the population more frequently than could be expected merely at random, but it does *not have a specific cause*. Like syndromes, associations must be defects involving more than one developmental field (or only one polytopic field), but are etiologically heterogeneous.

Example: VACTERL (or VATER) is an acronym for the non-random co-occurrence of vertebral anomalies (V), anal atresia (A), cardiac malformations (C), tracheoesophageal fistula (TE), renal anomalies (R) and limb defects (L). The presence of two of these anomalies in the same patient is considered sufficient for diagnosis (Källén et al., 2001), although other researchers are of the opinion that at least three are required (Martínez-Frías, 1994; Faivre et al., 2005). The defects that compose VACTERL association originate during blastogenesis and the existence of a characteristic pattern of abnormalities caused by different factors suggests a dysmorphogenetic response from a primary developmental field (Hersch et al., 2002). For this reason, Martínez-Frías & Frías (1999) consider it a primary, polytopic developmental field defects. In animals, the first record of a spontaneous occurrence of VACTERL association was made by Moura et al. (2010) in a female cat with costovertebral defects, anal atresia, heart and kidney defects, bilateral radial agenesis and persistent cloaca, but no tracheoesophageal fistula.

6.2.4 Sequence

This is a set of defects in an individual and results from an *initial defect* (malformation, disruption, dysplasia or deformation) that interferes in the development process, *leading to additional defects*. For example, as the result of a persistent right aortic arch, a ring is formed around the thoracic esophagus, causing an increased diameter of the esophagus in the cervical segment (a pouch is formed cranially to the point of constriction). A bilateral elbow dysplasia can cause a luxation of the elbows, which leads to medial rotation of the forearms, deforming the carpus. Micrognatia causes retroglossoptosis, which in turn can cause a cleft palate and respiratory distress (Pierre Robin sequence).

6.3 Further considerations

The same dysmorphism can appear in isolation or be part of syndromes or associations. Single defects or multiple defects of the same area (monotopic defects) without anomalies in other areas of the body are often called *nonsyndromic defects* to distinguish them from the same defects in an individual affected by a syndrome. A given defect can be a manifestation of the same anomaly expressed in different degrees, as is common in the developmental field defects. Any degree of expression of these cases is part of the total spectrum of a multiple anomaly. For instance, a single upper central incisor or an iris coloboma may be a minimum clinical sign of the total spectrum of holopresencephaly (Fig. 11-A), which at the most serious degree includes anomalies such as cyclopia, proboscis, absence of optic nerves and cleft lip and palate (Spranger, 1982; Jones, 2006). Dysmorphisms that affect the right and left side of the body (*symmetrical dysmorphisms*) are more likely to have a genetic cause than those that affect only one side (*asymmetric dysmorphisms*). However, this is not a rule (Turnpenny & Ellard, 2007). When a dysmorphism is extenal it is easily observed, especially if it is a major dysmorphism. Internal dysmorphisms, in turn, can only be confirmed by imaging tests, endoscopic viewing or a postmortem examination. Nevertheless, affected individuals will show clinical signs (Fig.11-B and C) at some time during their development, enabling a diagnosis using the aforementioned examinations. Internal congenital defects must be on the list of possible diagnoses in stillborn and critically ill newborn animals, although they may look normal externally. Internal congenital defects too must be considered a possible cause of clinical conditions identified in the first months of life. Although most of these defects are identified in the first six months, there are cases that manifest clinically later on and are diagnosed in adult life. For example, many cases of dogs with pulmonic stenosis show no clinical signs for years (Ware, 2011).

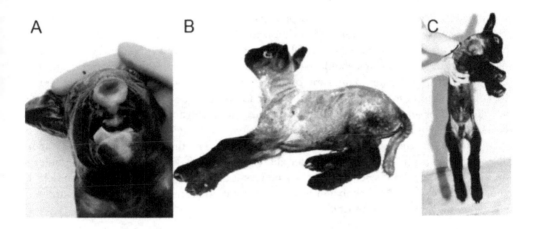

Fig. 11. A) Holoprosencephaly in a pig; B and C) Clinical signs of cerebellar disorder in a lamb (backward contraction of the neck, thoracic limbs in hyperextension and flexed pelvic limbs) as a result of cerebellar hypoplasia.

7. Medical history, physical examination and management of dysmorphic patients

In dysmorphology, the clinical activities that lead to the diagnosis (medical history, physical examination, complementary examinations, etc.) and the therapeutic procedures are that same as those of clinical medicine and/or surgery, with the inherent aspects of each specialty and any adaptations that each dysmorphic condition may require. In any situations, a correct diagnosis is very important for making the best decision. It has implications in terms of prognosis and possible treatment. All procedures should be noted according to well defined criteria in order to obtain a complete and consistent record, whose importance in terms of diagnosis and therapy transcends each case, enabling comparisons with new cases and generating innovations. The following topics introduce some general observations concerning these aspects.

7.1 Medical history

A detailed and solid medical history is one of the pillars of the diagnosis. It should include information about the environment in which the mother lives or lived, maternal diseases (metabolic disorders, infectious diseases, etc.), the mother's food, any medication given to the mother during pregnancy, and particularities of pregnancy and labor. Whenever possible, the veterinarian should seek not only similar cases but also different defects between sibs of the affected animal and other relatives. A pedigree should be drawn that is as complete as possible to facilitate the genetic analysis and enable the identification of an inheritance pattern when there is one.

7.2 Physical examination

The physical examination of a dysmorphic patient follows clinical principles, as in any specialty, and should be detailed. In addition to obvious defects, other abnormalities that the animal may have should be sought, even if they are only minimal. All anatomical regions and organic systems should be examined. All inspection and palpation should be done carefully in order not to miss any minor anomalies. One should always remember that the animal hair coat may make it difficult to see an anomaly but palpation contact facilitates detection. Minor anomalies, which may at first appear irrelevant, may help in the diagnosis. One should also remember that external defects, even if there is only one, may be a sign of an internal defect, meaning that specific examinations are required to locate them. The more minor defects at patient has, the greater the chance that it will also have major defects. Measurements of various segments of the body should be made routinely as they help to recognize patterns or define patterns of congenital malformations. An examination of normal relatives could also be useful.

7.3 Diagnostic tests

In many cases the diagnosis can be obtained with a minimum number of diagnostic tests. However, in other cases, a large number of tests is required, which significantly increases the cost, which often makes a more in-depth evaluation impossible in veterinary medicine. Some tests can only be conducted at universities, research centers or large private clinics. Imaging tests (simple X-ray, contrast X-ray, tomography, magnetic resonance imaging, ultrasound, endoscopy) are especially useful, as are karyotype analyses, biochemical examinations and, when available, DNA tests. The affected animals that do not survive should be submitted to a detailed postmortem examination. This examination provides diagnostic information and can help to develop treatment strategies for future cases.

7.4 Care and treatment

Therapy varies according to the type of defect. Very serious dysmorphisms often make life impossible, while less serious types often require no treatment. When treatment is possible, it can vary from methods that improve the quality of life of the patient to full correction of the defect. For instance, in the first case, a system of wheels for a dog that was born with no pelvic limbs (nowadays, there are "wheelchairs" for dogs and cats that are sold commercially); in the second case, a surgery to correct a cleft lip and palate or to correct a patent ductus arteriosus. There are cases where simple care is all that is required, such as giving a dog with oligodontia soft and previously cut food.

8. Prevention of dysmorphisms

Preventing dysmorphisms involves three main points: *genetic counseling, screening* and *monitoring during pregnancy*. The former two apply when the defect is hereditary or is influenced by genetic factors. The latter is useful in any situation.

8.1 Genetic counseling

The basic recommendation in the case of genetic diseases in animals is that affected individuals should not breed and that normal couples with affected descendents should not breed again. However, owners of normal animals that have had affected descendents are not usually willing to follow this advice. With this in mind, when there is a correct diagnosis and the genetic nature of the defect is known, other decisions are possible, but the risk of recurrence should be taken into consideration. To avoid autosomal recessive phenotypes, an important strategy is never to mate individuals who are known to be heterozygotes one with another, such as those who have already had an affected descendent. For recessive X-linked phenotypes, daughters of affected individuals are all carriers (heterozygotes) and should not be mated, even when the males are normal. When there is a family history of a recessive defect and the zygosity of an individual is unknown, consanguineous unions should be avoided.

8.2 Screening

When breeding small or large animals, identifying heterozygotes (recessive phenotypes and dominant phenotypes with reduced penetrance) can be an economically advantageous procedure and allows people to make appropriate preventive decisions concerning the mating of such individuals. For several recessive heredopathies commercial DNA tests are now available, significantly reducing costs. For instance, there is a test for arthrogryposis multiplex in cattle; for pulmonary hypoplasia with anasarca (PHA) in Dexter cattle; for polycystic kidney disease in cats, for Sly disease (mucopolysaccharidosis VII) in dogs; for hereditary microphthalmia in sheep. In abnormalities in which there is incomplete dominance between the mutant and normal allele, the heterozygotes can be identified visually because they have an abnormal phenotype, although it is less serious than that of homozygotes for the mutant allele. For example, there is a type of chondrodysplasia in cattle, common in the Dexter breed, in which the heterozygotes have shorter than normal limbs. If two chondrodysplasic individuals breed, there is a 50% risk of recurrence of the parents' phenotype (heterozygotes) and a 25% risk of a very serious and lethal chondrodysplasia, popularly known as a "bulldog calf", when the affected animals have very short limbs and spine, and their heads somewhat resemble that of a bulldog.

8.3 Monitoring during pregnancy

Several aspects deserve attention during pregnancy: 1) Care should be taken not to expose the pregnant animal to teratogens in the environment (mercury, herbicides, toxic plants, organochlorides, etc.); 2) The animals should not be given medicine with teratogenic potential; 3) They should not be submitted to radiographic examinations. If this cannot be avoided, the abdomen of the pregnant animal should be protected with a lead apron or the examinations should be conducted in the later stages of the pregnancy; 4) Examinations that use radioactive contrast (scintigraphy) should not be conducted; 5) Care should be taken concerning the quality and conservations of animal food. Feed that is exposed to dampness could lead to contamination by mycotoxins; 6) Food should be supplemented with folic acid[13]; 7) Pregnant animals that suffer from diabetes should be monitored. In humans, diabetes mellitus is a significant risk factor when it comes to congenital defects. This may also be the case in animals.

9. Ethical aspects in veterinary dysmorphology

When a dysmorphic animal is born, its owners can have many different reactions: pity, fear or repulsion, to name a few. They also make different decisions: some will care for the animal, while others may abandon it or kill it. Those who seek a veterinarian wish to give the animal to a new owner, treat it or sacrifice it. What will be done depends on the moral and ethical principles of each owner and each veterinarian. The most common argument is that, to avoid a life of suffering, the affected animal should be euthanatized. In this case, some points have to be considered: 1) In the case of serious malformations that are incompatible with life or when there are no technical resources to treat the animal properly, the ethical choice is undoubtedly to shorten the suffering; 2) Many cases that initially seem to be incompatible with life can be fully resolved with adequate treatment, while in other cases the animal may not even require surgery to live well, as long as it received proper care and affection. This includes some cases of conjoined twins. Unlike humans, animals have no awareness of their appearance and do not suffer because of it and can live happy lives if their owner gives them care and affection; 3) If the defects are not extensive, there are owners who decide not to submit their animal to surgery when they realize that it is living well and is not suffering and they develop an emotional tie and grow used to its different appearance; 4) There are cases when medical treatment is enough to make the animal comfortable, even though it may not completely cure the deficiency; 5) There are people who cannot bear the idea of looking after dysmorphic animals, while others do not mind and feel gratified when they see that they are keeping the animal alive. These latter are often willing to adopt animals with deficiencies; 6) The treatment and monitoring of dysmorphic animals generates technical and scientific knowledge that results in improved efficiency and quality of medical and nursing care for new cases in both animals and humans. However that may be, the decisions reflect the socioeconomic and cultural status of each society.

10. Acknowledgements

The authors would like to thank all their veterinarian colleagues who kindly provided photographs to illustrate this chapter and also those who over the years have referred patients with dysmorphisms. Dr. Moura would especially like to thank Dr. Ana Maria Della Torre (Clínica Veterinária Vida Animal), Dr. Antonia Maria do Rocio Binder do Prado (Pontifícia Universidade Católica do Paraná), Dr. Enio Celso Heller (Clínica Veterinária

---

[13] Supplementing food with folic acid has been recommended to prevent neural tube defects and cleft lip and palate in humans. This food supplement for pregnant Boston terriers, a breed of dog that is particularly susceptible to cleft lip and palate, significantly reduced the occurrence of these abnormalities in controlled studies (Elwood & Colquhoum, 1997; Guilloteau et al., 2006).

Guaíra), Dr. Jaime Trevisan Ribeiro (Clínica Veterinária Pedigree), Dr. José Leônidas Wagner (Clínica Veterinária Pet House), Dr. Joséli Maria Büchele (Pontifícia Universidade Católica do Paraná), Dr. Luiz Carlos Leite (Universidade Estadual do Centro-Oeste, PR), Dr. Marconi Rodrigues de Farias (Pontífícia Universidade Católica do Paraná), Dr. Pedro Vicente Michelloto Junior (Pontifícia Universidade Católica do Paraná), Dr. Robson Gomes da Costa Gouveia (Clínica Veterinária Guaíra), Dr. Silvana Maris Cirio (FEPAR) and Dr. Valter da Silva Queiroz (Pontifícia Universidade Católica do Paraná).

11. References

Aase, J. M. (1990). *Diagnostic dysmorphology*, Plenum Medical Book Company, ISBN 0-306-43444-X, New York, USA

Andersson, L.S.; Juras, R.; Ramsey, D.T.; Eason-Butler, J.; Ewart, S.; Cothran, G. & Lindgren, G. (2008). Equine Multiple Congenital Ocular Anomalies maps to a 4.9 megabase interval on horse chromosome 6. *BMC Genetics*, Vol.9, No.88, pp. 1-10, ISSN 1471-2156

Araújo, B. M.; Kemper, B.; Figueiredo, M. L.; Chioratto, R. & Tudury, E. A. (2008). Perosomus elumbus em cão beagle. *Ciência Veterinária nos Trópicos*, Vol.11, No.1, pp. 36-39, ISSN 1415-6326

Avedillo, L. J. & Camón, J. (2007). Perosomus elumbis in a pig. *Veterinary Record*, Vol.160, No.4, pp. 127-129, ISSN 0042-4900

Besser, T. E.; Potter, K. A.; Bryan, G.M. & Knowlen, G. G. (1990). An animal model of the Marfan syndrome. *American Journal of Medical Genetics*, Vol. 7, No.1, pp. 159-165, ISSN 0148-7299

Bingel, S.A. & Sande, R. D. (1994). Chondrodysplasia in five Great Pyrenees. *Journal of the American Veterinary Medical Association*, Vol.205, No.6, pp. 845-848, ISSN 0003-1488

Bowling, A.T. & Millon, L.V. (1990). Two autosomal trisomies in the horse: 64,XX,-26,+t(26q26q) and 65,XX,+30. *Genome / National Research Council Canada*, vol.33, No.5, pp.679-682.

Buchanan, J. W. & Patterson, D. F. (2003) Etiology of patent ductus arteriosus in dogs. *Journal of Veterinary Internal Medicine*, Vol.17, No.2, pp. 167-171, ISSN 0891-6640

Casal, M. L.; Scheidt, J. L.; Rhodes, J. L.; Henthorn, P. S., & Werner, P. (2005) Mutation identification in a canine model of X-linked ectodermal dysplasia. *Mammalian Genome*, Vol.16, No.7, pp. 524-531, ISSN 0938-8990

Cohen Jr, M. M. (2004). An introduction to sonic hedgehog signaling, In: Epstein, C. J.; Erickson, R.P. & Wynshaw-Boris, A. *Inborn errors of development*, pp. 210-228, Oxford, ISBN 0-19-514502-X, New York, USA

Davidson, E.H. (1993) Later embryogenesis: regulatory circuitry in morphogenetic fields. *Development*, Vol.118, No.3, pp. 665-90, ISSN 0950-1991

De Marco, P.; Merello, E.; Cama, A.; Kibar, Z. & Capra V. (2011) Human neural tube defects: Genetic causes and prevention. *Biofactors*, article first published online: 14 jun 2011, doi: 10.1002/biof.170, ISSN 1872-8081

Dennis, S. M. (1975) Perosomus elumbis in sheep. *Australian Veterinary Journal*, 1975 Vol.51, No.3, pp. 135-136, ISSN 0005-0423

Elwood, J.M. & Colquhoun, T.A. (1997). Observations on the prevention of cleft palate in dogs by folic acid and potential relevance to humans. *New Zealand Veterinary Journal*, Vol.45, No.6, pp. 254-6, ISSN 0048-0169

Epstein, C. J. (2004). Human Malformations and their genetic basis, In: Epstein, C. J., Erickson, R.P., Wynshaw-Boris, A. *Inborn errors of development*, pp. 3-9, Oxford, ISBN 0-19-514502-X, New York, USA

Ewart, S.L.; Ramsey, D.T.; Xu, J. & Meyers, D. (2000). The horse homolog of congenital aniridia conforms to codominant inheritance. *Journal of Heredity*, Vol.91, No.2, pp.93-98, ISSN 0022-1503

Faivre, L.; Portnoï, M.F.; Pals, G.; Stoppa-Lyonnet, D.; Le Merrer, M; Thauvin-Robinet, C.; Huet, F.; Mathew, C.G.; Joenje, H.; Verloes, A. & Baumann, C. (2005). Should chromosome breakage studies be performed in patients with VACTERL association? *American Journal of Medical Genetics A*, Vol.137, No.1, pp. 55-58, ISSN 1552-4825

Griesenbeck, J.S.; Brender, J.D.; Sharkey, J.R.; Steck, M.D.; Huber Jr, J.C.; Rene, A.A.; McDonald, T.J.; Romitti, P.A.; Canfield, M.A.; Langlois, P.H.; Suarez, L. & National Birth Defects Prevention Study. (2010). Maternal characteristics associated with the dietary intake of nitrates, nitrites, and nitrosamines in women of child-bearing age: a cross-sectional study. *Environmental Health*, Vol.9, No.10, pp.1-17, ISSN 1476-069X

Guilloteau, A.; Servet, E.; Biourge, V. & Ecochard, C. (2006). Folic acid and cleft palate in brachycephalic dogs. *WALTHAM Focus*, Vol.16, No.2, pp. 30-33

Hámori, D. (1983). *Constitutional disorders and hereditary diseases in domestic animals*, Elsevier, ISBN 0-444-99683-4, Amsterdam, Netherlands

Harada, M. (1995) Minamata disease: methylmercury poisoning in Japan caused by environmental pollution. *Critical Reviews in Toxicology*,Vol.25, No.1, pp. 1-24.

Hersh, J.H.; Angle, B.; Fox, T.L.; Barth, R.F.; Bendon, R.W. & Gowans, G. (2002) Developmental field defects: coming together of associations and sequences during blastogenesis. *American Journal of Medical Genetics*, Vol.110, No.4, pp. 320-323, ISSN 0148-7299

Herzog, A. (1974). Autosomal trisomy in lethal brachygnathia of cattle (bovine trisomia-brachygnathia-syndrome). [Abstract in English]. *Deutsche Tierärztliche Wochenschrift*, Vol.81, No.4, pp.78-80, ISSN 0012-0847

Holaday, J. W. & Berkowitz, B. A. (2009) Antiangiogenic drugs: insights into drug development from endostatin, avastin and thalidomide. *Molecular Interventions*, Vol.9, No.4, pp. 157-166, ISSN:1534-0384

Holmes, L.B. (2011) Human teratogens: update 2010. *Birth Defects Research. Part A, Clinical and Molecular Teratology*, Vol.91, No.1, pp. 1-7, ISSN 1542-0752

Jentink, J.; Loane, M.A.; Dolk, H.; Barisic, I.; Garne, E.; Morris, J.K. & de Jong-van den Berg, L.T. (2010). Valproic acid monotherapy in pregnancy and major congenital malformations. EUROCAT Antiepileptic Study Working Group. *The New England Journal of Medicine*, Vol.362, No.23, pp. 2185-2193, ISSN 0028-4793

Jones, C.J. (1999). Perosomus elumbis (vertebral agenesis and arthrogryposis) in a stillborn Holstein calf. *Veterinary Pathology*, Vol.36, No.1, pp. 64-70, ISSN 0300-9858

Jones, K. L. (2006) *Smith's Recognizable Patterns of Human Malformation*, Elsevier Saunders, ISBN 0-7216-0615-6, Philadelphia, USA

Källén, K.; Mastroiacovo, P.; Castilla, E.E.; Robert, E. & Källén, B. (2001). VATER non-random association of congenital malformations: study based on data from four malformation registers. *American Journal of Medical Genetics*, Vol.101, No.1, pp. 26-32, ISSN 0148-7299

Kemp, C.; Thiele, H.; Dankof, A.; Schmidt, G.; Lauster, C.; Fernahl, G. & Lauster R. (2009). Cleft lip and/or palate with monogenic autosomal recessive transmission in Pyrenees shepherd dogs. *Cleft Palate-Craniofacial Journal,* Vol.46, No.1, pp. 81-88, ISSN 1055-6656

Koch, T.G.; Loretti, A.P.; de Lahunta, A.; Kendall, A.; Russell, D. & Bienzle, D. (2005). Semilobar holoprosencephaly in a Morgan horse. *Journal of Veterinary Internal Medicine*, Vol.19, No.3, pp. 367-372, ISSN 0891-6640

Koren, G. & Nickel, S. (2010). Sources of bias in signals of pharmaceutical safety in pregnancy. *Clinical and investigative medicine*, Vol.33, No.6, pp. e349-355, ISSN 1488-2353

Koren, G.; & Nickel, C. (2011). Perpetuating fears: bias against the null hypothesis in fetal safety of drugs as expressed in scientific citations. *Journal of Population Therapeutics and Clinical Pharmacology*, Vol.18, No.1, pp. e28-32, ISSN 1710-6222

Kumar, P. & Burton, B. K. (2008). *Congenital malformations – Evidence-based evaluation and management*, McGraw Hill, ISBN 978-0-07-147189-3, New York, USA.

Lancaster, P. A. (2011). Causes of birth defects: lessons from history. *Congenital Anomalies*, Vol.51, No.1, pp. 2-5, ISSN 0914-3505

Lee, S.T.; Panter, K.E.; Pfister, J.A.; Gardner, D.R. & Welch, K. D. (2008). The effect of body condition on serum concentrations of two teratogenic alkaloids (anagyrine and ammodendrine) from lupines (Lupinus species) that cause crooked calf disease. *Journal of Animal Science*, Vol.86, No.10, pp. 2771-2778, ISSN 0021-8812

Mackay, D.R. (2011). Controversies in the diagnosis and management of the Robin sequence. *Journal of Craniofacial Surgery*, Vol.22, No.2, pp. 415-420, ISSN 1049-2275

Marasas, W.F.; Riley, R.T.; Hendricks, K.A.; Stevens, V.L.; Sadler, T.W.; Gelineau-van Waes, J.; Missmer, S.A.; Cabrera, J.; Torres, O.; Gelderblom, W.C.; Allegood, J.; Martínez, C.; Maddox, J.; Miller, J.D.; Starr, L.; Sullards, M.C.; Roman, A.V.; Voss, K.A.; Wang, E. & Merrill Jr, A.H. (2004). Fumonisins disrupt sphingolipid metabolism, folate transport, and neural tube development in embryo culture and in vivo: a potential risk factor for human neural tube defects among populations consuming fumonisin-contaminated maize. *Journal of Nutrition*, Vol.134, No.4, pp. 711-716, ISSN 0022-3166

Marden, P.M.; Smith, D.W. & McDonald, M. J. (1964). Congenital anomalies in the newborn infant, including minor variations. A study of 4,412 babies by surface examination for anomalies and buccal smear for sex chromatin. *Jornal de Pediatria*, Vol.64, pp. 357-371.

Martínez-Frías, M.L. (1994). Developmental field defects and associations: epidemiological evidence of their relationship. *American Journal of Medical Genetics*, Vol.49, No.1, pp. 45-51, ISSN 0148-7299

Martínez-Frías, M.L.; Frías, J.L. & Opitz, J.M. (1998). Errors of morphogenesis and developmental field theory. *American Journal of Medical Genetics*, Vol.76, No.4, pp. 291-296, ISSN 0148-7299

Martínez-Frías, M.L. & Frías, J.L. (1999). VACTERL as primary, polytopic developmental field defects. *American Journal of Medical Genetics*, Vol.83, No.1, pp. 13-16, ISSN 0148-7299

Martínez, J.S.; Velázquez, I.R.; Reyes, H. & Fajardo, R. (2006). Congenital holoprosencephaly with severe otocephaly in a rottweiler puppy. *Veterinary Record*, Vol.158, No. 15, pp. 518-519.

Moura, E. (1993). *Biologia educacional*, Editora Moderna, ISBN 85-16-00924-6, São Paulo, Brazil

Moura, E. & Cirio, S.M. (2004). Clinical and genetic aspects of X-linked ectodermal dysplasia in the dog -- a review including three new spontaneous cases. *Veterinary Dermatology*, Vol.15, No.5, pp. 269-277, ISSN 0959-4493

Moura, E.; Cirio, S. M. & Villanova Jr, J. A. (2010). VACTERL association in a cat. *American Journal of Medical Genetics A*, Vol.152, No.3, pp. 777-780, ISSN 1552-4825

Moura, E., Cirio, S. M. & Pimpão, C. T. (2011). Nonsyndromic cleft lip and palate in boxer dogs: evidence of monogenic autosomal recessive inheritance. *Cleft Palate-Craniofacial Journal*, Epub ahead of print: 2011-08-01, *ISSN* 1545-1569

Ngo, A.D.; Taylor, R. & Roberts, C.L. (2010). Paternal exposure to agent orange and spina bifida: a meta-analysis. *European Journal of Epidemiology*, Vol.25, No.1, pp. 37-44, ISSN 0393-2990

Opitz J. M. (1982). The developmental field concept in clinical genetics. *Journal of Pediatrics*, Vol.101, No.5, pp. 805-809, ISSN 0022-3476

Opitz J. M. (1984). *Tópicos recentes de genética clínica*, Sociedade Brasileira de Genética, Ribeirão Preto, Brazil.

Opitz, J. M.; Zanni, G.; Reynolds Jr, J. F. & Gilbert-Barness, E. (2002). Defects of Blastogenesis. *American Journal of Medical Genetics* (*Seminars in Medical Genetics*), Vol.115, No.4, pp. 269–286, ISSN 0148-7299

Priester, W.A.; Glass, A.G. & Waggoner, N.S. (1970). Congenital defects in domesticated animals: general considerations. *American Journal of Veterinary Research*, Vol.31, No.10, pp. 1871-1879, ISSN 0002-9645

Raudsepp, T.; Durkin, K.; Lear, T.L.; Das, P.J.; Avila, F.; Kachroo, P. & Chowdhary, B.P. (2010). Molecular heterogeneity of XY sex reversal in horses. *Animal Genetics*, Vol.41, No.2 (Suppl.), pp. 41-52, ISSN 0268-9146

Résibois, A.; Coppens, A. & Poncelet, L. (2007). Naturally occurring parvovirus-associated feline hypogranular cerebellar hypoplasia—a comparison to experimentally-induced lesions using immunohistology. *Veterinary Pathology*, Vol.44, No.6, pp. 831–841, ISSN 0300-9858

Richtsmeier, J.T.; Sack Jr, G.H.; Grausz, H.M. & Cork, L.C. (1994). Cleft palate with autosomal recessive transmission in Brittany spaniels. *Cleft Palate-Craniofacial Journal*, Vol.31, No.5, pp. 364-371, ISSN 1055-6656

Schelling, C.; Pieńkowska, A.; Arnold, S.; Hauser, B. & Switoński, M. (2001). A male to female sex-reversed dog with a reciprocal translocation. *Journal of Reproduction and Fertility. Supplement,* Vol.57, pp. 435-438, ISSN 0449-3087

Scott, F.W.; Lahunta, A.; Schultz, R.D.; Bistner, S.I. & Riis, R.C. (1975). Teratogenesis in cats associated with griseofulvin therapy. *Teratology,* Vol.11, No.1, pp. 79-86, ISSN 0040-3709

Singleton, A.C.; Mitchell, A.L.; Byers, P.H.; Potter, K.A. & Pace, J. M. (2005). Bovine model of Marfan syndrome results from an amino acid change (c.3598G > A, p.E1200K) in a calcium-binding epidermal growth factor-like domain of fibrillin-1. *Human Mutation,* Vol.25, No.4, pp. 348-352, ISSN 1059-7794

Smit, J.J.; Temwitchitr, J.; Brocks, B.A.; Nikkels, P.G.; Hazewinkel, H.A. & Leegwater, P.A. (2011). Evaluation of candidate genes as a cause of chondrodysplasia in Labrador retrievers. *Veterinary Journal,* Vol.187, No.2, pp. 269-271, ISSN 1090-0233

Son, J.M.; Yong, H.Y.; Lee, D.S.; Choi, H.J.; Jeong, S.M.; Lee, Y.W.; Cho, S.W.; Shin, S.T. & Cho, J.K. (2008). A case of perosomus elumbis in a Holstein calf. *Journal of Veterinary Medical Science,* Vol.70, No.5, pp. 521-523, ISSN 0916-7250

Spranger, J.; Benirschke, K.; Hall, J. G.; Lenz, W.; Lowry, R. B.; Opitz, J. M.; Pinsky, L.; Schwarzacher, H. G. & Smith, D. W. (1982). Errors of morphogenesis: Concepts and terms. Recommendations of an International Work Group. *Journal of Pediatrics,* Vol. 100, No.1, pp. 160-165, ISSN 0022-3476

Tarantal, A.F. & Hendrickx, A.G. (1987). Amniotic band syndrome in a rhesus monkey: a case report. *Journal of Medical Primatology,* Vol.16, No.5, pp. 291-9, ISSN 0047-2565

Traas, A.M.; Wang, P.; Ma, X.; Tittiger, M.; Schaller, L.; O'donnell, P.; Sleeper, M.M.; Vite, C.; Herati, R.; Aguirre, G.D.; Haskins, M. & Ponder K. P. (2007). Correction of clinical manifestations of canine mucopolysaccharidosis I with neonatal retroviral vector gene therapy. *Molecular Therapy: The Journal of the American Society of Gene Therapy,* Vol.15, No.8, pp. 1423-1431, ISSN 1525-0016

Turnpenny, P. & Ellard, S. (2007). *Emery's Elements of medical genetics.* Churchill Livingstone, ISBN 978-0-7020-2917-2, Edinburgh, England

Ueta, E.; Kodama, M.; Sumino, Y.; Kurome, M.; Ohta, K.; Katagiri, R. & Naruse, I. (2010). Gender-dependent differences in the incidence of ochratoxin A-induced neural tube defects in the Pdn/Pdn mouse. *Congenital Anomalies,* Vol.50, No.1, pp. 29-39, ISSN 0914-3505

Villagómez, D.A. & Alonso, R.A. (1998). A distinct Mendelian autosomal recessive syndrome involving the association of anotia, palate agenesis, bifid tongue, and polydactyly in the dog. *Canadian Veterinary Journal,* Vol.39, No.10, pp. 642-643, ISSN 0008-5286

von Moos, R.; Stolz, R.; Cerny, T. & Gillessen, S. (2003). Thalidomide: from tragedy to promise. *Swiss Medical Weekly,* Vol.133, No.5-6, pp. 77-87, ISSN 1424-7860

Ware, W. A. (2011). *Cardiovascular disease in small animal medicine,* pp. 234-238, Manson Publishing, ISBN 978-1-84076-153-5, London, England

Wiedemann, H. R. (1991). The pioneer of pediatric medicine. *European Journal of Pediatrics,* Vol.150, No.8, pp. 533, ISSN 0340-6199

Wilkerson, M.J.; Lewis, D.C.; Marks, S.L. & Prieur, D.J. (1998). Clinical and morphologic features of mucopolysaccharidosis type II in a dog: naturally occurring model of Hunter syndrome. *Veterinary Pathology*, Vol.35, No.3, pp. 230-233, ISSN 0300-9858

Wouda, W.; Peperkamp, N.H.; Roumen, M.P.; Muskens, J.; van Rijn, A. & Vellema, P. (2009). Epizootic congenital hydranencephaly and abortion in cattle due to bluetongue virus serotype 8 in the Netherlands. *Tijdschrift voor Diergeneeskunde*, Vol.134, No.10, pp. 422-427, ISSN 0040-7453

Yablokov, A.V. (2009). Chernobyl's radioactive impact on fauna. *Annals of the New York Academy of Sciences*, Vol.1181, pp. 255-280, ISSN 0077-8923

5

Steroid Hormones in Food Producing Animals: Regulatory Situation in Europe

Annamaria Passantino
Department of Veterinary Public Health,
Faculty of Veterinary Medicine,
University of Messina,
Italy

1. Introduction

Hormones are chemicals produced by animals to co-ordinate their physiological activities. They act as messengers, produced in and released from one kind of tissue to gradually stimulate or inhibit some process in a different tissue over a long period.

Steroid hormones fulfill an important role at different stages of mammalian development comprising prenatal development, growth, reproduction and sexual and social behavior.

The importance of individual hormones varies between sexes and age and a disruption of the endocrine equilibrium may result in multiple biological effects.

One hormone can have multiple actions, e.g. the male hormone testosterone controls many processes from the development of the foetus, to libido in the adult. Alternatively, one function may be controlled by multiple hormones, e.g. the menstrual cycle involves oestradiol, progesterone, follicle-stimulating hormone and luteinising hormone.

Hormones produced by the bodies of humans and animals are called endogenous or natural hormones. Compounds chemically synthesised to mimic the effect of natural hormones are called synthetic or xenobiotic hormones.

Hormones are vital in normal development, maturation and physiological functioning of many vital organs and processes in the body. However, like any other chemicals of natural or synthetic origin, hormones may be toxic to living organisms under certain circumstances. The toxicity may be due to an excess of its normal ('physiological') action. This may be the result of excessive exposure to the substance, for example following absorption of a large dose, or because the physicochemical nature of the substance gives it greater or more prolonged activity of the same type, or because the hormonal action occurs at an abnormal time during development or adult life, or is an action on an organism of the inappropriate sex. Hormones, like other chemicals, may also exert direct toxic actions not related to their endocrine ('physiological') effects.

Due to the obvious ability to improve weight gain and feed efficiency in meat producing animals, natural hormones and/or the synthetic surrogates have been used in agricultural practice for several decades (table 1).

Substances	Form	Main use - Animals
Oestrogens alone:		
DES	Feed additive	Steers, heifers
DES	Implant	Steers
DES	Oil solution	Veal calves
Hexoestrol	Implant	Steers, sheep, calves, poultry
Zeranol	Implant	Steers, sheep
Gestagens alone:		
Melengestrol acetate		Heifers
Androgens alone:		
TBA	Implant	Heifers, culled cows
Combined preparations:		
DES and Testosterone	Implant	Calves
DES and Methyl-testosterone	Feed additive	Swine
Hexoestrol and TBA	Implant	Steers
Zeranol and TBA	Implant	Steers
Oestradiol-17β and TBA	Implant	Bulls, steers, calves, sheep
Oestradiol-17β benzoate and testosterone propionate	Implant	Heifers, calves
Oestradiol-17β benzoate and progesterone	Implant	Steers

Table 1. Hormonally-active substance used in animal production (by http://www.fao.org/DOCREP/004/X6533E/X6533E01.htm, modified)

Implanting hormonal growth promoters is currently widespread in the beef cattle industry of many non-EU countries for the better performance in growth and improvement of feed efficiency. These hormonal implants may enhance growth during suckling, growing and finishing stages of production (Mader, 1997; Platter et al., 2003).

Growth hormones are implanted under the skin (usually behind the ear) of the animal in the form of depot capsules, where they release a specific dose of hormones over a fixed period of time.

The five hormone types most widely used in meat production include three natural hormones, oestradiol 17-β, testosterone, and progesterone, and two synthetic substances, trenbolone and zeranol.

Oestradiol 17-β has oestrogenic action (i.e. responsible for female characteristics); testosterone has androgenic action (i.e. responsible for male characteristics); and progesterone has gestagenic action (i.e. responsible for maintaining pregnancy). The other two hormones, as aforesaid, mimic the biological activity of the natural hormones: trenbolone mimics the action of testosterone, and zeranol mimics oestradiol 17-β.

1.1 Hormonally active substances

1.1.1 Oestradiol 17-β

Oestradiol 17-β is the most active of the female sex hormones synthesized and secreted mainly by the ovary, the adrenals and the testis.

Oestradiol is synthesized and secreted in early stages of embryogenesis and has an active role in the normal development of the female sex accessories during the lifetime of females.

It has been used to induce parturition (birth) especially in sheep, a species in which an associated oestradiol-induced increase in mothering ability has also been recorded (Poindron, 2005).

In non-pregnant animals, oestradiol has been used clinically to increase uterine contractions and cervical softening for the expulsion of unwanted uterine contents in the absence of a corpus luteum (i.e. to remove a dead fetus or infected material especially in cattle) (Elmore, 1992; Pepper &, Dobson, 1987; Sheldon & Noakes, 1998).

Oestradiol has been used in the past in turkeys and other poultry to castrate young birds. Implants would be placed subcutaneously at 5-6 weeks of age, or in slightly older birds, but certainly 4 weeks before killing. Alternatively, preparations were available as feed-additives. This approach is not now used in Europe although it was used in slower growing Spanish breeds. There are very few reproductive problems in rabbits.

Fetal mummifications and macerations occur, as do endometritis and pyometra but treatment with oestradiol has not been reported (Flecknell, 2000).

In fish, administration of oestradiol at first-fry feeding (approximately 40-70 days of age depending on species) will induce ovarian development and female characteristics in salmonids, flat-fish and eels (Shepherd & Bromage, 1988). Sex-control in this way depresses or inhibits maturation to ensure that metabolism is channelled into body growth (i.e., more saleable flesh). However, this approach is no longer commercially adopted.

Another use of very low doses of oestradiol is as a growth promoter via appetite stimulating and increased food-conversion properties. Occasionally in the past, this approach has been taken to advance the onset of puberty and thus alleviate potential gynaecological problems in slower maturing species. However, as use of hormonal growth promoters is prohibited within the European Union[1].

1.1.2 Testosterone

Testosterone and its more active metabolite, 5α-dihydrotestosterone (DHT), are the main sex hormones secreted by males. Testosterone is responsible for the early development, and the appearance and maintenance of male secondary sex accessory organs (prostate, secretory glands, penis size, etc.) during adulthood. Testosterone secretion is also affected by the complex interaction among all endocrine glands, especially with those in the brain.

Testosterone is metabolized and as a result, metabolites of different activity are generated. Some of these metabolites play a more active role in certain organs than in others.

The actions of both testosterone and DHT are mediated through their high affinity and high specificity binding and activation of an intracellular protein, the androgen receptor (AR). This AR protein is a member of the steroid hormone superfamily. The ligand-activated androgen receptor mediates its effects on cell growth and differentiation through the

[1] See the following paragraph: Background of the European Union legislation

activation and/or suppression of specific gene transcription in target organs. Androgen receptors are detected in tissues of females, as well as males. The presence of this receptor in organs such as the ovary indicates significant activity of androgens in both sexes. Furthermore, the androgen receptor is thought to be involved in ovarian tumorigenesis, as it has been detected in 67 percent of ovarian tumors. Although current information indicates the presence of only a single androgen receptor, it is known that different subsets of genes may be activated by either testosterone or DHT (Chang *et al.*, 1995).

In animals, testosterone or testosterone propionate, alone or in combination with other hormonally active substances, is used primarily to improve the rate of weight gain and feed efficiency. This effect is most likely a consequence of the anabolic action of androgens.

1.1.3 Progesterone

Progesterone is synthesized and secreted mainly by the corpus luteum in the ovary of cycling females, and, during pregnancy, by the placenta.

As all hormones, progesterone synthesis and secretion is regulated by a series of positive and negative feedback mechanisms in which polypeptidic hormones secreted by the brain (hypothalamus, pituitary) affect circulating progesterone levels.

Progesterone and synthetic progestins are used pharmacologically in women in conjunction with ovulation stimulation drugs as well as during early pregnancy in cases of luteal phase dysfunction. Although results have been conflicting, some studies find an association between pregnancy-related intake of progestins and increased risk of hypospadias (congenital malformation of the urethral opening on the penis) in the male offspring (Carmichael *et al.*, 2005). It should however be noted that this was observed in relation to pharmacological doses of progestins, and as progesterone levels are normally high during pregnancy, minor additional exogenous progestagenic activity would presumably be without significant effects in the presence of a high endogenous activity, unless the synthetic progestins act at different sites and by different mechanisms. In contrast, serum levels of progestins in children and postmenopausal women are very low. Data on effects of progesterone in the prepubertal child are scarce and no new data have been identified. Likewise, no animal studies on the effects of progesterone during the postnatal development have been published recently.

It is well established that progesterone not only serves as the precursor of all the major steroid hormones (androgens, oestrogens, corticosteroids) in the gonads and adrenals, but also is converted into one or more metabolites by most tissues in the body (Wiebe, 2006).

1.1.4 Trenbolone acetate

Trenbolone acetate (TBA) is a synthetic steroid with an anabolic potency that may exceed that of testosterone. It is a prodrug that converts into its active form 17β-trenbolone, which isomerises into 17α-trenbolone.

17β-trenbolone is the major form occurring in muscle tissue, whereas the 17α-epimer is the major metabolite occurring in liver and in the excreta including bile. It is assumed to exert its anabolic action via interaction with androgen and glucocorticoid receptors (Danhaive and Rousseau, 1986, 1988). Experiments with cattle tissues have shown that 17β-trenbolone binds to the androgen receptor with similar affinity as dihydrotestosterone. It also binds to the progesterone receptor with an affinity that exceeds that of progesterone. The other metabolites of TBA, including 17α-trenbolone (17α-hydroxy-estra-4,9,11-trien-3-one) and TBO (estra-4,9,11-triene-3,17-dione) show a significantly lower binding affinity to both types of receptors (Bauer et al., 2000).

Reports regarding the (mis)use of TBA as an anabolic agent in sports people describe several adverse effects, including liver cell injury with an increase in liver-specific enzymes in serum, cholestatic jaundice, peliosis hepatitis and various neoplastic lesions. Moreover, decreased endogenous testosterone production and spermatogenesis, oligospermia and testicular atrophy may be associated with the repeated use of TBA as anabolic (Bahrke and Yesalis, 2004; Maravelias et al., 2005).

1.1.5 Zeranol

Zeranol is derived from the naturally occurring mycoestrogen zearalenone, and is a potent oestrogen receptor agonist *in vivo* and *in vitro* (Leffers et al., 2001; Le Guevel and Pakdel, 2001; Takemura et al., 2007; Yuri et al., 2006). Its actions resemble those of oestradiol. (Leffers et al., 2001).

Zeranol stimulates the proliferation of ER-dependent cell proliferation in MCF-7 human breast cancer cells (which are widely used in the assessment of estrogenic activity) and in transfected cells (Leffers et al., 2001; Le Guevel and Pakdel, 2001; Liu and Ling, 2004).

It is used alone or in combination with TBA as a hormonal growth promoter in various products.

2. Background of the European Union legislation

The use of hormonal growth promoters in food-producing animals has been a sensitive issue of debate in the EU and elsewhere for several decades.

Prior to 1981, the EC had no universal policy on the use of growth promoting hormones in meat animals.

The use of hormones had been banned in Italy since 1961, in Denmark since 1963, and in Germany since 1977. Belgium and Greece had never permitted the use of hormones for fattening purposes. However, Spain, the United Kingdom, France and Netherlands permitted the use of most hormones for speeding growth in beef cattle[2].

The move to impose a Europe wide ban was spurred by the worrying discovery in 1977 of breast enlargement in girls and boys attending a school in Milan (Italy) (Scaglioni et al., 1978). Although oestrogen contamination was not detected when samples of school meals were tested, an uncontrolled supply of poultry and beef was hypothesized as being the cause of this outbreak (Fara et al., 1979).

---

[2] See http://www.fao.org/DOCREP/004/X6533E/X6533E03.htm#refeecstr Accessed August 19, 2011.

In 1980 the discovery of 30,000 jars of baby food containing dethylstilboestrol, commonly known as DES, contaminated French veal was reported. European consumer organizations called for a boycott of veal, and the market for veal was severely affected. On September 20, 1980, the EC Council of Agriculture Ministers adopted a declaration in favor of a ban on the use of oestrogen and endorsed the principle of greater harmonization of legislation on veterinary medicines and of greater control on animal rearing, both at the production and slaughtering stages.

On October 31, 1980, the EC Commission proposed even more rigorous legislation that would ban the use of all hormone products in meat production, except for therapeutic purposes[3]. This proposal was expanded later by documents COM(80)920 and COM(80)922, presented on 6 January 1981. These allowed for the controlled use for therapeutic and zootechnical purposes of three natural hormone products, and introduced a number of control measures on the production and handling of such products, together with proposals on the testing of animals. Discussions in the European Parliament revealed that three EC member States (Belgium, Ireland and the United Kingdom) favored the use of some hormones to promote growth in meat animals, and Ireland and the United Kingdom also argued for the retention of the synthetic hormones, trenbolone and zeranol. Third countries, including The United States, Argentina, Australia, Canada, New Zealand and South Africa raised concerns concerning the potential impact of a ban on their exports to European Communities[4].

Subsequently, the European Council adopted its first directive on the hormones issues in July 1981 (Directive 81/602/EEC)[5].

Directive 81/602/EEC prohibits the administering to farm animals of substances having a *thyrostatic action* or substances having an *oestrogenic, androgenic or gestagenic* action; the placing on the market or slaughtering of farm animals to which these substances have been administered; the placing on the market of meat from such animals; the processing of meat from such animals and the placing on the market of meat products prepared from or with such meat. The Directive provides two exceptions to the prohibition: one exception is provided for substances with an oestrogenic, androgenic or gestagenic action when they are used for therapeutic or zootechnical purposes and administered by a veterinarian or under a veterinarian's responsibility. The other exception was for oestradiol-17β, progesterone, testosterone, TBA and zeranol - when they were used for growth promotion purposes and their use was governed according to the individual regulatory schemes maintained by EC member States. This exception was made pending an examination of the effects of these hormones on the health of consumers and the adoption of an EC rule. EC member States are obliged to apply their regulatory schemes to imports from third countries in a manner not more favorable than that applied to intra-EC trade.

---

[3] Commission of the European Communities 1980. Proposal for a Council Regulation (EEC) Concerning the Uses of Substances with a Hormonal Action and those having a Thyrostatic Action in Domestic Animals. COM (80) 614, 31 October, Brussels: Commission of the European Communities.

[4] WTO, 1997. EC measures concerning meat and meat products (hormones), complaint by the United States. Report of the WTO Panel, WT/DS26/R/USA, August 18, 1997, 2: 26-28. Available at http://www.sice.oas.org/dispute/wto/horm-us.asp, Accessed August 20, 2011.

[5] Council Directive 81/602/EEC of 31 July 1981 concerning the prohibition of certain substances having a hormonal action and of any substances having a thyrostatic action. Official Journal of the European Communities, L Series, No. 222, pp. 32-33.

The relevant international organizations - FAO, WHO, OIE and Codex - started to seriously examine the safety of these hormones in meat production only during the 1980s.

The first substantive scientific report had been published by OIE in 1983. The Joint FAO/WHO Expert Committee on Food Additives (JECFA)[6] had discussed and issued a scientific report on these hormones only in 1988[7].

There were two other international reports comprising collective scientific work: the 1984 Scientific Report published by the European Commission (based on the Lamming Report[8]) and the Proceedings of the 1995 EC Scientific Conference[9].

---

[6] It is an independent expert group which deals with specific commodity issues or general health and safety matters related to food. The JECFA focuses on the scientific evaluation of a veterinary drug and does not consider government policies and politics.

[7] The JECFA Report, on which the Codex standard for zeranol is based, noted that zeranol was a weak oestrogen which mimicked the action of oestradiol-17β. The report concluded that the toxic (in casu tumorigenic) effect of zeranol is associated with its hormonal (i.e. oestrogenic) properties and that an ADI could thus be established on the basis of a no-hormonal-effect level. Adopting what it considered to be a conservative approach by using as a basis studies on ovariectomized female cynomolgus monkeys (highly sensitive to oestrogenic substances) and using a safety factor of 100, JECFA set an ADI for human beings of 0-0.5 μg/kg of body weight. For a 70 kg person consuming 500 g of meat daily over an entire lifetime, the maximum permissible or safe level of zeranol residues in meat would then, according to JECFA, be 70 μg/kg of edible tissue. However, the report noted that when zeranol is administered to cattle according to good animal husbandry practice, the maximum mean residue levels did not exceed 0.2 μg/kg in muscle, 10 μg/kg in liver, 2 μg/kg in kindney, and 0.3 μg/kg in fat at any time after implantation. These residue levels obtained on the basis of good animal husbandry practice are thus below the maximum permissible level of 70 μg/kg. However, in order to set a level which is detectable by routine residue analysis methods, the Codex MRL was increased to 2 μg/kg in muscle and set at 10 μg/kg in liver.
With respect to trenbolone acetate (TBA), the Report concluded that its potential toxic effects only arise as a consequence of its hormonal activity. The report further concluded that, therefore, an ADI could be established on the basis of a no-hormonal-effect level. Adopting what it considered to be a conservative approach by using as a basis studies on castrated male rhesus macaque monkeys (which are highly sensitive to compounds with antigonadotropic activity) and pigs (which are a sensitive model for assessing hormonal effects of TBA) and using a safety factor of 100, JECFA later set an ADI for human beings of 0-0.02 μg/kg of body weight (34th JECFA Report of 1989). The maximum ADI for a 60 kg person would thus be 1.2 μg of TBA residues. JECFA then set MRL's for -trenbolone in muscle and -trenbolone in liver of 2 μg/kg and 10 μg/kg, respectively, based on average residue levels in heifers at 15-30 days after implantation of 300 mg TBA, noting that concentrations would be even lower at proposed GPVD. According to JECFA, the MRL's thus obtained on the basis of conservative estimates should not exceed the Codex ADI or safe level at any time after implantation of the drug, that is, irrespective of the withdrawal period used.

[8] The Lamming Group's interim report, issued in September 1982, found that the three natural hormones (oestradiol-17β, testosterone and progesterone) "would not present any harmful effects to the health of the consumer when used under the appropriate conditions as growth promoters in farm animals".
For the findings of the scientific working group, see Lamming, G.E., Ballarini, G., Baulieu, E.E. et al., (1987). Scientific Report on Anabolic Agents in Animal Production. The Veterinary Record, 121, at 389-392.

[9] The 1995 EC Scientific Conference on Growth Promotion in Meat Production concluded that: "At present, there is no evidence for possible health risks to the consumer due to the use of natural sex hormones for growth promotion, since: Residue levels of these substances measured in meat of treated animals fall within the physiological range observed in meat of comparable untreated animals. The daily production of sex hormones by humans is much higher than the amounts possibly consumed from meat, even in the most sensitive humans (prepubertal children and menopausal women).

The European Communities stressed, however, that these reports did not constitute the entire body of scientific knowledge on the issue of safe use of these hormones for growth promotion. There were also important studies made by individual scientists, and other specialized institutions like the International Agency for Research on Cancer (IARC).

The EC Scientific Veterinary Committee gave its reaction to the Lamming Report on November 9, 1982, followed by the EC Scientific Committee for Animal Nutrition on November 17, 1982 and by the EC Scientific Committee for Food on February 4, 1983. These Committees supported the conclusions and recommendations of the Lamming Report, but stressed the need to lay down provisions regarding the establishment of proper programmes to control and monitor the use of anabolic agents with regard, in particular, to instructions for use, surveillance programmes and analysis methods. In January 1984, the Commission asked a group of experts within the EC Scientific Committee on Anabolic Agents to review the information on trenbolone and zeranol. On June 12, 1984, the Commission published a proposal (COM(84)295 final) for a Council Directive amending Directive 81/602/EEC, which envisaged the controlled use of the three natural hormones for growth promotion purposes and proposed re-examining the ban on the two synthetic hormones after their scientific evaluation had been completed. However, the European Parliament, the EC Economic and Social Committee and the EC Council of Ministers rejected the Commission's proposal.

The EC Commission amended its proposal accordingly and on December 31, 1985 the EC Council adopted Directive 85/649/EEC[10]. This Directive banned the use of all the substances concerned for growth promotion purposes and established more detailed provisions concerning authorized therapeutic uses. Its preamble began by emphasizing that differing rules on hormone use in different member countries had distorted trade in the European market and that "[...] these distortions of competition and barriers to trade must therefore be removed [...]".

The Directive was challenged in the European Court of Justice, which annulled it on procedural grounds. The proposals were re-introduced by the EC Commission and re-adopted by the EC Council as Council Directive 88/146/EEC on March 7, 1988[11]. This Directive extends the prohibition imposed by Directive 81/602/EEC to the administration to farm animals of trenbolone acetate and zeranol for any purpose, and oestradiol-17β,

---

Due to an extensive first-pass metabolism, the bioavailability of ingested hormones is low, thus providing a further safety margin".

With regard to the synthetic hormones, zeranol and trenbolone, the 1995 EC Scientific Conference concluded that: "At the doses needed for growth promotion, residue levels [of trenbolone and zeranol] are well below the levels regarded as safe (the MRLs). There are, at present, no indications of a possible human health risk from the low levels of covalently-bound residues of trenbolone".

See Assessment of Health Risk - Working Group II", in 1995 EC Scientific Conference Proceedings, pp. 20-21.

[10] Council Directive 85/649/EEC of 31 December 1985 prohibiting the use in livestock faring of certain substances having hormonal action. *Official Journal of the European Communities*, L Series, No. 382, pp. 228-231.

[11] Council Directive 88/146/EEC of 7 March 1988 prohibiting the use in livestock farming of certain substances having a hormonal action. *Official Journal of the European Union*, L Series, No. 70, pp. 16-18.

testosterone and progesterone for fattening purposes. However, the Directive maintains the permission to administer these three natural hormones to animals for therapeutic and zootechnical purposes under prescribed conditions; in particular, therapeutic treatment is defined to mean the administering to an individual animal of any of the substances which are authorized to treat a fertility problem diagnosed on examination by a veterinarian. The products which are used for therapeutic treatment may be administered only by a veterinarian, in the form of an injection (to the exclusion of implantation) to farm animals which have been clearly identified. Such treatment must be registered by the veterinarian and these animals may not be slaughtered before expiry of the period fixed. In the case of animals at the end of their reproductive career, the treatments are prohibited from being administered during the fattening period following the end of their breeding life. Article 4 of Directive 88/146/EEC explicitly requires that undertakings in the EC member States producing the prohibited hormones, those companies authorized to market these hormones for whatever purposes and undertakings producing pharmaceutical and veterinary products based on those substances, must keep a detailed register recording (in chronological order) the quantities produced or acquired and those sold or used for the production of pharmaceutical and veterinary products. The importation from third countries of animals and meat from animals to which have been administered substances with thyrostatic, oestrogenic, androgenic or gestagenic action is prohibited. However, under certain conditions, Article 7 of Directive 88/146/EEC allows trade in those animals and meat from those animals treated for therapeutic or zootechnical purposes, including imports from third countries.

Directive 88/299/EEC[12] lays down the conditions for applying the derogations, provided for in Article 7 of Directive 88/146/EEC, from the prohibition on trade in certain categories of animals and their meat. The first derogation of the Directive requires EC member States to authorize trade in animals intended for reproduction and reproductive animals at the end of their career (and of meat of such animals) which, during their reproductive career, have undergone one of two categories of treatments. The first category is therapeutic treatment with one of the following substances: oestradiol-17β, testosterone and progesterone; and those derivatives which readily yield the parent compound on hydrolysis after absorption at the site of application which appear in a list of approved products. The second category is the administration of substances having an oestrogenic, androgenic or gestagenic action for synchronization of oestrus, termination of unwanted gestation, the improvement of fertility and the preparation of donors and recipients for the implantation of embryos, provided that the products in which they are contained appear on a list of approved products and with the respect of strict conditions of use concerning, in particular, the respect of the withdrawal period, the monitoring of those conditions of use and of the means of identification of the animals. In addition, Articles 3 and 4 of this Directive provide that trade between the EC member States of the European Communities in animals intended for reproduction and reproductive animals and meat from such animals is allowed only if all the conditions laid down in the Directive are respected, in particular as regards the waiting period and the requirement that animals have not received any of the above treatments with any of the

---

[12] Council Directive 88/299/EEC of 17 May 1988 on trade in animals treated with certain substances having a hormonal action and their meat, as referred to in Article 7 of Directive 88/146/EEC. *Official Journal of the European Union*, Series L, No. 87, pp. 36-38.

above substances during the fattening period following the end of their breeding life. The EC stamp may be affixed to the meat only if the waiting time ended before the animals are slaughtered. The second derogation in Directive 88/299/EEC allows imports from third countries of treated animals and meat of such animals under guarantees equivalent to those for domestic animals and meat.

Following reports of significant use of illegal growth-promoting hormonal substances in a number of EC member States, on September 26, 1988 the European Parliament established a Committee of Enquiry into the Problem of Quality in the Meat Sector. The conclusions of this Committee were published in a document known as the "Pimenta Report", which recognized the ban on the use of hormones[13]. On March 29, 1989, the European Parliament adopted its recommendations to maintain and expand the ban.

The European Parliament adopted another report on the issue of use of hormones for animal growth promotion, the "Collins Report" of February 7, 1989[14]. This report argued that: "Current licensing systems for the regulation of veterinary medicines (including at present, growth promoting products) require that a new product satisfy three criteria: safety, quality and efficacy. These criteria may well be satisfactory for therapeutic drugs. They are by no means sufficient for growth promoting products. For the latter it is proposed here that the Community's veterinary medicine licensing system be adapted to include a "fourth hurdle", entailing an objective socio-economic and environmental impact assessment". In the Commission's July 1988 draft proposals for the reform of veterinary medicine licensing in the Community this idea was accepted in principle. The final version of the proposals (December 1988) does not include this concept. It is clear, however, that the social, agricultural and environmental implications of the use of growth and yield promoting pharmaceuticals require a licensing system somewhat different from that which exists for these products when used for therapeutic purposes.

Directive 96/22/EC[15] replaces Directives 81/602/EEC, 88/146/EEC and 88/299/EEC. It maintains the prohibition on the use of these hormones for growth promotion purposes; extends the prohibition on the use of beta-agonists; restricts the use of the hormones at issue for therapeutic or zootechnical purposes, reinforcing in particular the role of the

---

[13] The scientific conclusions regarding the use of natural hormones rested upon strict conditions of use which it believed could not in reality be attained. The Committee was of the opinion that use of the natural/nature-identical hormones carries the risk of inexperienced application, incorrect dosage and unsupervised injection which could pose a risk to the animal and the consumer, and also noted doubts with regard to long-term cumulative and interactive potential carcinogenicity. In addition, the Committee believed that proven necessity and socio-economic desirability should be criteria of acceptability for the use of (bio)chemical growth promoters in animal-rearing. In brief, the essential findings of the Pimenta Report were that the prohibition of hormonal substances for non-therapeutic (i.e. growth-promoting) purposes must be maintained and expanded.

[14] European Parliament, Committee on the Environment, Public Health and Consumer Protection, Report on "The USA's Refusal to comply with Community legislation on slaughterhouses and hormones and the consequences of this refusal", EP 128 381/B, 7 February 1989, named after its reporter Mr. Collins, MEP.

[15] Council Directive 96/22/EC of 29 April 1996 concerning the prohibition on the use in stockfarming of certain substances having a hormonal or thyrostatic action and of beta-agonists, and repealing Directives 81/609/EEC, 88/146/ECC and 88/299/EEC. Official Journal of the European Union, L Series, No. 125, pp. 5-9.

veterinarian; and reinforces the provisions on control and testing. Penalties and sanctions in case of violations are to be increased where checks detect the presence of prohibited substances or products or residues of substances administered illegally.

In Directive 96/23/EC measures are specified to control the ban[16] (Passantino *et al.*, 2001). The control should be performed by special, dedicated institutes. Analysis of the samples taken is performed by routine or field laboratories (RFLs). In each member state the RFLs are coordinated and controlled by at least one national reference laboratory (NRL) designated by the national government.

Finally, the NRLs are supported, advised and controlled by four community reference laboratories (CRLs), which were designated in 1991 by the EU and implemented in 1993 (Stephany *et al.*, 1994). Annually a residue monitoring programme must be made in which the results of the controls of the previous year and the targets for control in the new year are given. People working on the farms and veterinarians are made co-responsible for the control of the ban. Samples can be taken at production plants for banned substances and animal feeds, and at farms, slaughterhouses and butchers. There should be at least one national reference laboratory for every banned substance. Indications should be available for sampling and analysis. The main sanction on the use of banned substances is the destruction of the positive animals. The farmer has to pay for the additional controls that are performed. When meat is imported from third countries, it must also be controlled. When the products give a positive result the European Commission should be informed and additional controls are indicated. Eventually this could lead to a ban on the import from a certain country.

It is important underlines that the Opinion of the Scientific Committee on Veterinary Measures relating to Public Health (SCVPH)[17] of 30 April 1999 on potential adverse effects to human

---

[16] A principal objective of Council Directive 96/23/EC is to detect illegal use of substances in animal production as well as detecting the misuse of authorized veterinary medicinal products. The Directive lays down measures requiring European Member States to monitor the substances and their residues in both live animals and animal products, listed in Annex I to the Directive.
In particular, this directive describes guidelines for residue control and divides all pharmacologically active substances into two groups:
· Group A compounds, which comprise prohibited substances (listed in the Directive 96/22/EC and in Annex IV of the Regulation 2377/90/EC);
· Group B compounds, which comprise substances with final and provisional MRLs (listed in Annexes I and III of the Regulation 2377/90/EC). See, Council Directive 96/23/EC of 29 April 1996 on measures to monitor certain substances and residues thereof in live animals and animal products and repealing Directives 85/358/EEC and 86/469/EEC and Decisions 89/187/EEC and 91/664/EEC. Official Journal of the European Union, L Series, No. 125, pp. 10-32.

[17] The United States and Canada contested the prohibition imposed by the European Communities on the import from third countries of treated animals with the hormones and, in 1997, a panel of the World Trade Organisation (WTO) ruled that the measure was not in line with the Agreement on the Application of Sanitary and Phytosanitary Measures (SPS). The EU appealed against this ruling and, in 1998, the WTO Appellate Body reversed most of the findings of the panel. The WTO Appellate Body only upheld the finding that prohibition of imports of meat from hormone-treated animals to the EU did not comply with the requirement that such a measure should be based on a relevant assessment of the risks to human health. In reaction to these findings, the EU carried out a complementary risk assessment and mandated the Scientific Committee on Veterinary measures relating to Public Health (SCVPH) to evaluate the risks to human health from hormone residues in bovine meat and meat products treated with six hormones for growth promotion.

health from hormone residues in bovine meat and meat products (which was reviewed on 3 May 2000 and confirmed on 10 April 2002[18]) established that there is a substantial body of recent evidence suggesting that oestradiol 17ß has to be considered as a complete carcinogen, as it exerts both tumour-initiating and tumour-promoting effects, and that the data currently available do not make it possible to give a quantitative estimate of the risk to human health[19].

In the light of the conclusions of the 1999, 2000, and 2002 Opinions, the European Communities adopted Directive 2003/74/EC[20], which amends Directive 96/22/EC in relation to the prohibition permanently of the use of hormones in stockfarming.

Directive 2003/74/EC maintains the permanent prohibition of the placing on the market of meat and meat products from animals treated with oestradiol-17β for growth-promotion purposes originally contained in Directive 96/22/EC[21].

---

[18] The EU Scientific Committee confirmed that the use of hormones as growth promoters for cattle poses a potential health risk to consumers, following a review of 17 studies and other recent scientific data.

Subsequent to the adoption of the 1999 Opinion, additional scientific information was made available to the European Commission in the form of scientific studies conducted by: (i) the United Kingdom's Veterinary Products Committee sub-group on the 1999 Opinion (October 1999); (ii) the Committee for Veterinary Medicinal Products ("CVMP") of the European Union (a subcommittee of the European Medicines Agency (EMEA)) (December 1999); and (iii) the Joint FAO/WHO Expert Committee on Food Additives ("JECFA") (February 2000). At the request of the European Commission, the SCVPH examined this scientific information and, on 3 May 2000, issued a review of its 1999 Opinion in which it declined to alter the conclusions contained therein (the "2000 Opinion").

On 10 April 2002, a second review of the 1999 Opinion was issued by the SCVPH (the "2002 Opinion") on the basis of more recent scientific data collected since the previous review. The scientific data reviewed by the SCVPH included the final results of all 17 studies that had been commissioned by the European Commission. Publishing its third opinion on the risks to human health from hormone residues in beef products, the SCVPH found no reason to change its previous opinions of 1999 and 2000.

See, Opinion of the Scientific Committee on Veterinary Measures relating to Public Health on "Assessment of potential risks to human health from hormone residues in bovine meat and meat products, adopted on 30 April 1999. Available at

http://ec.europa.eu/food/fs/sc/scv/out21_en.pdf Accessed August 19, 2011.

See also Opinion of the Scientific Committee on Veterinary Measures relating to Public Health on "Review of specific documents relating to the SCVPH opinion of 30 April 1999 on the potential risks to human health from hormone residues in bovine meat and meat products", adopted on 3 May 2000, and on "Review of specific documents relating to the SCVPH opinion of 30 April 1999 and 3 May 2000 on the potential risks to human health from hormone residues in bovine meat and meat products", adopted on 10 April 2002. Available at http://ec.europa.eu/food/fs/sc/scv/out50_en.pdf Accessed August 19, 2011.

[19] In this context, it is important underlines that Article 168 of the Treaty establishing the European Union (EU) states that a high level of human health protection shall be ensured in the definition and implementation of all EU policies and activities. A comprehensive body of EU legislation has been put in place to achieve this objective. All of this legislation is publicly available at http://eur-lex.europa.eu/en/index.htm Accessed August 23, 2011.

[20] Directive 2003/74/EC of the European Parliament and of the Council of 22 September 2003 amending Council Directive 96/22/EC concerning the prohibition on the use in stockfarming of certain substances having a hormonal or thyrostatic action and of beta-agonists. Official Journal of the European Union, L Series, No. 262, pp. 17-21.

In relation to the five other hormones (testosterone, progesterone, TBA, zeranol, and MGA) Directive 2003/74/EC continues to apply the prohibition contained in Directive 96/22/EC, but on a provisional basis[22].

This Directive specifies that, even though the scientific information available showed the existence of risks associated with these substances, "the current state of knowledge does not make it possible to give a quantitative estimate of the risk to consumers"[23]. Accordingly, the prohibition of these five hormones should apply "while the Community seeks more complete scientific information from any source, which could shed light and clarify the gaps in the present state of knowledge of these substances"[24].

On 27 October 2003, the European Communities notified the Dispute Settlement Body (DSB) of the adoption, publication, and entry into force of Directive 2003/74/EC, as well as the 1999, 2000, and 2002 Opinions, which it considered to be risk assessments that sufficiently justified the permanent and provisional import prohibitions under the *SPS Agreement* (Agreement on the Application of Sanitary and Phytosanitary Measures)[25].

The latter use has to be phased out by until 14 October 2006 and for the rest of the uses the Commission was to present a report in October 2005.

The report was presented on 11 October 2005 to Council and Parliament. It comes to the conclusion that the use of the alternative substances such as prostaglandins is already common.

Veterinarians predict an insignificant impact of future unavailability of oestradiol 17β and its ester like derivates on farmers and on animal welfare. It was moreover observed that the unavailability of oestradiol and its ester like derivates would have minimal economic effect. This is because the incidence of fetal mummification and fetal maceration is low, and although the incidence of pyometra is higher, methods of prevention not involving use of oestradiol do exist and would be preferable.

Article 11a of Council Directive 96/22/EC as amended by Council Directive 2003/74/EC requires the presentation of a report on the necessity of the use of the hormone oestradiol 17β in food animal production. A report concerning the availability of alternative veterinary medicinal products to those containing oestradiol 17β or its ester-like derivatives for the treatment of fetal maceration or mummification in cattle, and for the treatment of pyometra prepared (later addressed as the Report) by an independent scientist has been presented by the Commission in October 2006[26]. The Report concludes that oestradiol 17β is not essential in food animal production.

---

[21] Directive 2003/74/EC, supra, footnote 20, Recital 10 and Article 1 (amending Articles 2 and 3 of Directive 96/22/EC).
[22] Ibid.
[23] Directive 2003/74/EC, supra, footnote 20, Recital 7.
[24] Ibid., Recital 10.
[25] European Communities – Measures concerning meat and meat products (hormones), Communication from the European Communities, WT/DS26/22, WT/DS48/20, 28 October 2003. Available at http://trade.ec.europa.eu/doclib/docs/2003/november/tradoc_114641.pdf Accessed August 23, 2011.
[26] See, Report concerning the availability of alternative veterinary medicinal products to those containing oestradiol 17β or its ester-like derivatives for the treatment of fetal maceration or

3. Situation in other countries

Whereas the EU has banned the use of all hormones, other countries do allow the use of steroid hormones and hormone-like substances in various combinations with the aim to improve weight gain and feed efficiency in livestock farming. Recommended application occurs in the form of small implants or devices, containing the active hormones, into the subcutaneous tissue of the ears. Both ears are completely discharged at slaughter[27] (Galbraith, 2002). Pharmaceutically, these implants represent slow-release devices, containing relatively large quantities of hormones, which are fractionally released over a period of several months.

In the United States[28], Canada, Australia, New Zealand and in some countries in South America, Asia and Africa the natural hormones - testosterone, 17ß-oestradiol and progesterone - and the (semi-) synthetic hormones trenbolone, zeranol and melengestrol acetate can be used to promote growth.

In particular, in the USA[29] five hormones are authorized as the active component of solid ear implants (17β-estradiol - as such or as benzoate, testosterone - as such or as propionate,

---

[27] mummification in cattle, and for the treatment of pyometra. Commission of the European Communities – SEC(2005) 1303 of 11.10.2005.

[27] See European Commission, 1999. Scientific Committee on Veterinary Measures relating to Public Health (SCVPH). Assessment of potential risks to human health from hormone residues in bovine meat and meat products. Available at http://europa.eu/comm/food/fs/sc/scv/out21_en.html Accessed August 23, 2011.

[28] The U.S. Food and Drug Administration (FDA) and the U.S. Department of Agriculture (USDA) cooperate in regulating growth promotants for livestock. Both of these agencies maintain that hormones in beef from an implanted animal have no physiological significance for humans. All animal drug products are approved for safety and effectiveness under the Federal Food, Drug, and Cosmetic Act (21 U.S.C. 301 et seq.). Information on approved hormone products are at 21 CFR Parts 522, 556, and 558. FDA requirements for the review and approval of new animal drug applications is at http://www.fda.gov/AnimalVeterinary/GuidanceCompliance Enforcement/GuidanceforIndustry/ucm123821.htm Accessed August 26, 2011.

[29] The United States continues to maintain that U.S. beef from cattle treated with certain approved growth hormones pose no public health risk. Overall, the official U.S. position is that "there is a clear world-wide scientific consensus supporting the safety of these approved and licensed hormones when used according to good veterinary practice".
The United States claims that this position is supported by "scientific reviews of the six hormones, international standards pertaining to their use, and a longstanding history of administering the six hormones to cattle for growth promotion purposes". Accordingly, the United States claims that the use of these hormones as growth promoters in beef production is safe, when applied in accordance with good veterinary practices.
The United States has criticized the EU's scientific opinions for focusing on only one growth promotant, estradiol-17β, and on its potential genotoxicity, while directing relatively little attention toward the other natural and synthetic hormones. The United States also claims that the "EU failed to use solid evaluative methods in their studies and completely disregarded the large body of evidence from epidemiological studies that indicate that estradiol does not contribute to any increased cancer risk and that meat from animals tested with estradiol is safe for consumers".
Regarding the EU's more recent reviews, the United States claims they fail to provide any new evidence that would call into question the findings and conclusions of other authoritative reviews.
More broadly, the United States also disputes whether the EU's scientific reviews serve as a risk assessment. The United States claims: "There has been no new risk assessment based on scientific information and reasoning presented by the EU," further claiming that the "17 studies" funded by the Commission beginning in 1998 were "not intended as a to serve as a risk assessment, but instead were

progesterone, trenbolone acetate and zeranol) and two hormones as feed additives: melengestrol acetate (MGA) for feedlot heifers[30] (Berende & Ruitenberg, 1983; Meissonnier & Mitchell-Vigneron, 1983) and ractopamine for swine (Marchant Forde *et al.*, 2003).

As aforementioned, the hormone ban of the EU is currently the cause of a dispute between the EU and these third countries, led by the United States and Canada. The reason for this dispute is that those countries want to export meat to EU nations from animals treated with in their view acceptable hormones. In their opinion the EU blocks international trade on improper grounds and against international law.

The National Cattlemen's Beef Association (NCBA), the largest national group of cattle producers, has long opposed the EU's ban on imports of U.S. hormone-treated beef, claiming that the ban is scientifically unjustified and fails to satisfy the EU's WTO requirements under the SPS. Similar concerns have been expressed by other U.S. farm groups, including American Farm Bureau Federation (AFBF), the Animal Health Institute (AHI), and the American Meat Institute (AMI)[31]. Many trade analysts believe that the United States has a strong case against the hormone ban under WTO rules that require SPS restrictions to be based on risk assessment and to have a scientific justification. These various interest groups have continued to exert pressure on U.S. trade policy officials to hold to their position regarding the EU's meat hormone ban.

Recently, On May 13, 2009, following a series of negotiations, the United States and the EU signed a memorandum of understanding (MOU) implementing an agreement that could resolve this long standing dispute[32]. On July 13, 2009, the EC adopted regulations opening a tariff quota for imports of High Quality Beef, effective August 1, 2009[33]

4. Existing community legislation

Currently Council Directive 2008/97/EC[34] has been published amending Council Directive 96/22/EC concerning the prohibition on the use in stock farming of certain substances

---

to fill in the gaps". Accordingly, the United States claims, the EU's 2003 update to its hormone ban is not in compliance with its WTO obligations and should be discontinued.

For more detailed discussion see USDA, Foreign Agriculture Service, Historic Overview and Chronology of EU's Hormone Ban, GAIN Report E23206, Nov. 7, 2003, available at http://www.fas.usda.gov/gainfiles/200311/145986773.pdf Accessed August 26, 2011; USDA, FAS, EU Presentation on Hormone Ban Directive (2003/74/EC), GAIN Report E23217, Nov. 13, 2003, available at http://www.fas.usda.gov/gainfiles/200311/145986807.pdf Accessed August 26, 2011.

[30] http://www.fda.gov/AnimalVeterinary/SafetyHealth/ProductSafetyInformation/ucm055436.htm Accessed August 23, 2011.

[31] See, "Coalition Statement on EU's Latest Pronouncement on Hormones," May 14, 2002 by AFBF, AHI, AMI, and NCBA, Available at http://www.meatami.com/ht/d/sp/i/1482/pid/1482 Accessed August 23, 2011.

[32] For other information, see WTO, European Communities – Measures Concerning Meat And Meat Products (Hormones), Joint Communication from the European Communities and the United States, WT/DS26/28, September 30, 2009; 74 Federal Register 40864, August 13, 2009; 74 Federal Register 48808, September 24, 2009; and USTR press releases.

[33] Council Regulations (EC) No 617/2009 of 13 July 2009 opening an autonomous tariff quota for imports of high-quality beef. Official Journal of the European Union, L series, No. 182, 1..

[34] Directive 2008/97/EC of the European Parliament and of the Council of 19 November 2008 amending Council Directive 96/22/EC concerning the prohibition on the use in stockfarming of certain substances

having a hormonal or thyreostatic action and of β-agonists, to exclude companion animals from the prohibition.

In fact, experience gained in particular with national residue plans submitted under Directive 96/23/EC has shown that the misuse of product presentations intended for pet animals does not play a role as a source of abuse or misuse. That is partly because it is economically unattractive to use presentations intended for pet animals for growth promotion in food-producing animals.

It was considered therefore appropriate to limit the scope of Directive 96/22/EC only to food-producing animals and withdraw the prohibition for pet animals, as well as to adjust the definition of therapeutic treatment.

5. Conclusions

The EU continues to maintain that "there is a lack of data on the type and amount of [growthpromoting hormone] residues in meat on which to make a quantitative exposure assessment" that would change the EU's understanding of the "possible risks to human health" associated with hormone-treated meat and meat products. It claims that this position is supported by a series of commissioned research studies and scientific reviews conducted by the EU, although there has been no conclusive testing on the issue.

The most recent review, conducted in 2007 by the European Food Safety Authority (EFSA), cites evidence supporting that estradiol-17β be considered as a carcinogen, and states that all six hormones may pose endocrine, developmental, immunological, neurobiological, immunotoxic, genotoxic, and carcinogenic effects, particularly for susceptible risk groups (such as prepubertal children). The toxicological and epidemiological data reviewed by the Commission panels do not allow a quantitative estimate of the risk, leading to the panel's conclusions that no threshold levels can be defined for any of the six hormones

Based on this series of reviews, the Commission maintains that these reviews "reaffirmed public health concerns about the large scale use of hormones administered to cattle for growth promoting purposes," and therefore "provided the scientific basis for community legislation not allowing the use of hormones for growth promoting purposes in the EU".[35]

6. References

Bahrke, M.S., & Yesalis C.E. (2004). Abuse of anabolic androgenic steroids and related substances in sport and exercise. *Current Opinion in Pharmacology*, 4, 614-620, ISSN: 1471-4892.

Bauer, E.R., Daxenberger, A., Petri, T., Sauerwein, H., &Meyer, H.H. (2000). Characterization of the affinity of different anabolic and synthetic hormones to the human androgen receptor, human sex hormone binding globulin and to the bovine progestin

---

having a hormonal or thyrostatic action and of beta-agonists. Official Journal of the European Union, L series, No. 318, 9-11.

[35] EFSA, "EFSA Concludes Review of New Scientific Data on Potential Risks to Human Health from Certain Hormone Residues in Beef," Press Release dated July 18, 2007, Available at http://www.efsa.europa.eu/EFSA/efsa_locale-1178620753812_1178622723847.htm. Accessed August 26, 2011.

receptor. *Acta Pathologica Microbiologica et Immunologica Scandinavica*, 108, 838-846, ISSN: 0903-4641.

Berende, P.L.M., & Ruitenberg, E.J. (1983). Domestication, conservation and use of animal resources. Elsevier, Amsterdam, pp 191-233, ISBN: 0-444.42068-1.

Carmichael, S.L., Shaw, G.M., Laurent, C., Croughan, M.S., Olney, R.S., & Lammer, E.J. (2005). Maternal progestin intake and risk of hypospadias. *Archives of Pediatrics & Adolescent Medicine*, 159(10), 957-62, ISSN: 1072-4710.

Chang, C., Saltzman, A., Yeh, S., Young, W., Keller, E., Lee, H-J, Wang, C., & Mizokami, A. (1995). Androgen Receptor: an overview. *Critical Reviews in Eukaryotic Gene Expression*, 5, 97-125, ISSN: 1045-4403.

Danhaive, P.A., & Rousseau, G.G. (1986). Binding of glucocorticoid antagonists to androgen and glucocorticoid hormone receptors in rat skeletal muscle. *The Journal of Steroid Biochemistry and Molecular Biology*, 24, 481-487, ISSN: 0960-0760.

Danhaive, P.A., & Rousseau, G.G. (1988). Evidence for sex-dependent anabolic response to androgenic steroids mediated by muscle glucocorticoid receptors in the rat. *The Journal of Steroid Biochemistry and Molecular Biology*, 29, 575-581, ISSN: 0960-0760.

Elmore, R.G. (1992). Focus on bovine reproductive disorders: managing cases of fetal mummification. *Veterinary Medicine*, 87, 155-159, ISSN: 8750-7943.

Fara, G.M., Del Corvo, G., Bernuzzi, S., Bigatello, A., Di Pietro, C., Scaglioni, S., & Chiumello, G. (1979). Epidemic of breast enlargement in an Italian school. *Lancet*, 314, 295-297, ISSN: 0140-6736.

Flecknell, P. (2000). Manual of rabbit medicine and surgery. Publishers: British Small Animal Veterinary Association, ISBN-10: 0905214463, Quedgeley, Gloucs (UK).

Galbraith, H. (2002). Hormones in international meat production: biological, sociological and consumer issues. *Nutrition Research Reviews*, 15, 243-314, ISSN: 0954-4224.

Le Guevel, R., & Pakdel, F. (2001). Assessment of oestrogenic potency of chemicals used as growth promoter by in-vitro methods. *Human Reproduction*, 16, 1030-6, ISSN: 0268-1161.

Leffers, H., Naesby, M., Vendelbo, B., Skakkebaek, N.E., & Jorgensen, M. (2001).Oestrogenic potencies of zeranol, oestradiol, diethylstilboestrol, bisphenol-A and genistein: implications for exposure assessment of potential endocrine disrupters. *Human Reproduction*, 16, 1037-45, ISSN: 0268-1161.

Liu, S., & Lin, Y.C. (2004). Transformation of MCF-10A human breast epithelial cells by zeranol and estradiol-17beta. *The Breast Journal*, 10(6), 514-21, ISSN: 1075-122X.

Mader, T.L. (1997). Carryover and lifetime effects of growth promoting implants. Proc. OSU Symposium: Impact of implants on performance and carcass value of beef cattle, pp 88-94, Oklahoma Agric. Exp. Stn., Stillwater, OK, 21-23 November 1996.

Maravelias, C., Dona, A., Stefanidou, M., & Spiliopoulou, C. (2005). Adverse effects of anabolic steroids in athletes. A constant threat. *Toxicology Letters*, 158, 167-175, ISSN: 0378-4274.

Marchant Forde, J.N., Lay, D.C. Jr, Pajor, E.A., Richert, B.T., & Schinckel, A.P. (2003). The effects of ractopamine on behavior and physiology of finishing pigs. *Journal of Animal Science*, 81, 416-422, ISSN:0021-8812.

Meissonnier, E., & Mitchell-Vigneron, J. (1983) Anabolics in animal production. Office International des Epizooties, ISBN 92-9044-118-6, Paris.

Passantino, A., Fenga, C., Venza, M., Maressa, P., & Passantino M. (2001). The future of hormonal substances in zootechnical breeding: legislative aspects. Preprints of III

Congress of the European Society for Agricultural and Food Ethics, Florence (Italy), 3-5 October 2001, 483-484.

Pepper, R., & Dobson, H. (1987). Preliminary results of treatment and endocrinology of chronic endometritis in the dairy cow. *The Veterinary Record*, 120, 53-56, ISSN: 0042-4900.

Platter, W.J., Tatum, J.D., Belk, K.E., Scanga, J.A., & Smith, G.C. (2003). Effects of repetitive use of hormonal implants on beef carcass quality, tenderness, and consumer ratings of beef palatability. *Journal of Animal Science*, 81, 984-996, ISSN:0021-8812.

Poindron, P. (2005). Mechanisms of activation of maternal behaviour in mammals. *Reproduction Nutrition Development*, 45, 341-51, ISSN: 0926-5287.

Scaglioni, S., Di Pietro, C., Bigatello, A., & Chiumello, G. (1978). Breast enlargement in an Italian school. *Lancet*, 311, 551-552, ISSN: 0140-6736.

Sheldon, I.M., & Noakes, D.E. (1998). Comparison of three treatments for bovine endometritis. *The Veterinary Record*, 142, 575-579, ISSN: 0042-4900.

Shepherd, C.J., & Bromage, N.R. (1988). Intensive fish farming. Pub: BSP Professional Books, pp 103-105, ISBN: 0632019042, Oxford, Boston.

Stephany, R.W., van Ginkel, L.A., & Schothorst, R.C. (1994). Perspective. European Union reference laboratories for residue analysis: a quality challenge. *Analyst*, 119, 2707-2711, ISSN: 0003-2654.

Takemura, H., Shim, J.Y., Sayama, K., Tsubura, A., Zhu, B.T., & Shimoi, K. (2007). Characterization of the estrogenic activities of zearalenone and zeranol in vivo and in vitro. *The Journal of Steroid Biochemistry and Molecular Biology*, 103(2), 170-7, ISSN: 0960-0760.

Wiebe, J.P. (2006). Progesterone metabolites in breast cancer. *Endocrine-Related Cancer*, 13, 717-738, ISSN: 1351-0088.

Yuri, T., Tsukamoto, R., Miki, K., Uehara, N., Matsuoka, Y., & Tsubura, A. (2006). Biphasic effects of zeranol on the growth of estrogen receptor-positive human breast carcinoma cells. *Oncology Reports*, 16(6), 1307-12, ISSN: 1021335X-.

6

Use of Dual-Energy X-Ray Absorptiometry (DXA) with Non-Human Vertebrates: Application, Challenges, and Practical Considerations for Research and Clinical Practice

Matthew D. Stone and Alec J. Turner
Kutztown University,
USA

1. Introduction

The applications of Dual-energy X-ray Absorptiometry (DXA) to vertebrate research and veterinary practice are many. DXA has been used successfully to rapidly and non-invasively quantify bone density and body composition in a variety of animals. The use of DXA has been limited, primarily, to basic and applied research, but DXA technology has great promise for clinical practice involving animals. Despite this potential, a number of limitations hinder its use in veterinary practice. These issues must be resolved before DXA can be widely used in traditional veterinary practice and a goal of this chapter is to discuss these limitations. This chapter reviews the past and current uses of DXA in basic and applied research involving non-human vertebrates.

2. DXA theory

DXA is a non-invasive technique for the determination of body composition. Users of DXA are able to rapidly quantify lean tissue mass, fat mass, total body mass, bone mineral mass, and bone mineral density. A comprehensive review of how DXA quantifies body composition can be found in (Adams, 1997; Jebb, 1997; Peppler & Mazess, 1981; Pietrobelli et al., 1996). The method by which DXA estimates body composition is based on the principle that the intensity of X-rays as they pass through tissues is attenuated in proportion to tissue mass (Figure 1).

The attenuation of a single intensity X-ray beam, as it passes through a single-tissue model (e.g. bone) of unknown mass, can be calculated based on the equation below (modified from Jebb, 1997):

$$R = M_B(R_B) \tag{1}$$

where R is the degree of attenuation, M_B is the mass of the tissue (e.g. bone), and R_B is the tissue-specific attenuation coefficient. In this scenario, bone mass is the unknown of interest

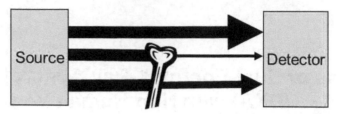

Fig. 1. Depiction of X-ray intensity attenuation as it passes through a tissue. X-ray attenuation is proportional to tissue mass.

while the degree of attenuation is determined by measuring the difference in intensity of X-rays between the source and detector. The attenuation coefficient is a known constant for a particular tissue that has been derived theoretically and empirically (Jebb, 1997). If more than one tissue type is present, the attenuation of the X-ray is a function of each of the individual tissue components contribution to the total beam attenuation (Figure 2).

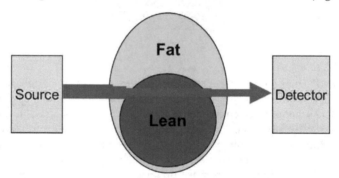

Fig. 2. Depiction of X-ray intensity as it passes through two tissue types. The total beam attenuation is a combination of the individual contributions of the two tissues, each at a different rate.

The relationship between the individual tissue contributions to total beam attenuation in a two tissue model (e.g. fat and lean tissue) can be summarized in the following equation, which is an extension of equation 1 (modified from Jebb, 1997).

$$R = M_F(R_F) + M_L(R_L) \tag{2}$$

Subscripts F and L denote fat and lean tissue contributions to total beam attenuation. In this equation there are two tissues of unknown mass contributing to beam attenuation. Directly solving for both of these unknowns is impossible, so the use of single energy X-ray absorptiometry is limited by its ability to distinguish various tissue components. DXA technology was developed to overcome this limitation. DXA utilizes X-rays of two different peak energies (high and low) and the attenuation of these beams can be used to calculate both unknowns. Each of these beams is attenuated differently when they pass through specific tissues, as indicated in equation 3.

$$R_{High} = M_F(R_F) + M_L(R_L) \tag{3}$$

$$R_{Low} = M_F(R_F) + M_L(R_L)$$

When more than two tissue components exist (e.g. bone, fat, and lean tissue) DXA cannot directly estimate the relative proportion of all three components. DXA indirectly estimates these three components by first distinguishing areas of the scan that contain soft tissue (lean & fat mass combined) from areas containing bone and soft tissue (Figure 3).

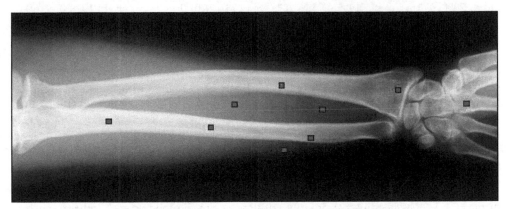

Fig. 3. X-ray image depicting the method by which DXA estimates body composition from a scan. DXA distinguishes regions (pixels) containing bone (red squares) from regions without bone (blue pixels).

In areas lacking bone, DXA can directly estimate the proportion of fat and lean tissue. For areas that contain bone, DXA determines the proportion of bone and soft tissue. Since DXA cannot distinguish between lean and fat tissue in these areas, DXA applies the proportion of fat and lean tissue, determined at neighboring non-bone areas, to the soft-tissue component of bone containing regions (Pietrobelli et al., 1996).

3. Basic applications of DXA

DXA is a non-invasive technique that was originally designed for the purpose of predicting current and future risk of bone fracture in humans by measuring bone mineral density (Grier et al., 1996). DXA can rapidly quantify total body mass, fat mass, lean tissue mass, and bone content and density, so it has potential applications in a variety of research and clinical fields. DXA has been used in and/or has practical applications to the fields of nutrition, sports and exercise science, physical therapy, animal science and nutrition, food science, pharmacology, pathology, metabolism, endocrinology, dentistry, and veterinary medicine. Because DXA is a non-invasive technique it is well suited for longitudinal studies. This advantage allows for reduced sampling error and potentially reduces required sample sizes and reduces those associated costs.

4. DXA use with animals

To date DXA has been applied to a diversity of small and large animal species, representing most major taxonomic groups. Of the major taxonomic groups, mammals have received the most attention, in part, due to their role as human models of osteoporosis or their role in the food industry. Even though mammals have received the most attention, other taxa are becoming increasingly well represented.

In mammals, DXA has been used most extensively with rodents. Due to the extent of published studies covering the use of DXA with rodents we elected to avoid their inclusion in this chapter except in a few instances for comparison. DXA has been used with species of agricultural concern including sheep (Mercier et al., 2006; Ponnampalam et al., 2007; Pouilles et al., 2000; Turner et al., 1995a), pigs (Clarys et al., 2010; Elowsson et al., 1998; Lee et al., 2011; Losel et al., 2010; Lukaski et al., 1999; Mitchell et al., 1998; Nielson et al., 2004), horses (McClure et al., 2001; Secombe et al., 2002), goats (Corten et al., 1997), and cattle (Zotti et al., 2010). Additionally, DXA has been applied to wildlife such as the grizzly bear (Felicetti, 2003 as cited in Stevenson & van Tets, 2008). DXA has been used to analyze excised bones of several species of marine mammals including Blainville's beaked whale (Zotti et al., 2009), Mediterranean monk seals (Mo et al., 2009), and bottlenose dolphins (Lucic et al., 2010). Finally, DXA has been applied to domestic pets including cats (Buelund et al., 2011; Turner et al., 1995b), rabbits (Castaneda et al., 2006; Hanafusa et al., 1995), guinea pigs (Fink et al., 2002), and dogs (Lorinson, 2009; Markel & Bogdanske, 1994a, 1994b; Mawby et al., 2004; Schneider et al., 2004; Toll et al., 1994; Zotti et al., 2004a). The use of DXA with ferrets has been noted (Grier et al., 1996); however few published studies have been cited.

In birds, DXA has been used primarily with species in the food science industry such as domestic poultry, including the red junglefowl (Jensen et al., 2005), white leghorns (Kim et al., 2006; Jensen et al., 2005), and turkey (Zotti et al., 2003). It has also been applied to wildlife including wild turkey, ruffed grouse, bobwhite quail (Dirrigl et al., 2004) and small passerines (Korine et al., 2004).

In reptiles, fewer species have been used with DXA, but most major taxonomic groups are represented, including snakes (Secor & Nagy, 2003); turtles (Fledelius et al., 2005; Stone et al., 2010), and lizards (Zotti et al., 2004b). The focus of these studies was validating the use of DXA with these species; however, Zotti et al., (2004b) used DXA to study metabolic bone disease in the green iguana (*Iguana iguana*) and Fledelius et al, (2005) used DXA to investigate how supplementing calcium in the diet of tortoises impacts bone density.

DXA has been used successfully and/or validated in a diverse number of animal species; however, there are a number of common household pets and research model species to which DXA has never been applied. This is especially true for exotic animals. Further research is needed to validate the use of DXA with these species before DXA can be put into practical use in animal research or medicine. To our knowledge, DXA has not been used or validated with amphibians or fish, despite the importance of these groups to animal research. In addition to filling in these "species gaps," further research is needed with species to which DXA has already been applied. Establishing a series of reference intervals for body composition in these species will provide important baseline data for future studies and will provide a frame of reference from which clinicians can use to diagnose pathology (Jebb, 1997).

5. Applications to veterinary medicine

5.1 Patient monitoring of bone density and body composition

As a non-invasive methodology, DXA is effective for longitudinal quantification of bone health and nutritional status of patients. Thus, DXA has potential to be a powerful tool for preventative and post-operative health care because it allows veterinary practitioners to quantify and systematically monitor patients' body condition and bone health over time.

DXA has been previously used to monitor bone density changes during fracture healing in rodents (Millett et al., 1998). Significant increases in femur bone density were measured during fracture healing of Sprague-Dawley rats. The region of the bone closest to the callus showed the largest difference in bone mineral density between the experimental and control groups (non-fractured). A similar study was conducted in dogs, where DXA was used to quantify changes in bone mineral density at the site of fracture following ostectomies of various widths (Markel & Bogdanske, 1994b). The results of these and other studies suggest that DXA can be used to effectively monitor changes in bone density after fracture. The ability to conduct analyses at particular regions of interest (ROIs), in addition to whole body analyses, makes this an extremely effective tool for post-operative monitoring.

In addition to post-operative monitoring of bone healing, DXA shows great promise in preventative medicine, such as early identification/diagnosis of metabolic bone diseases. This would serve an important service to exotic animal practice, because metabolic bone disease is the most common disease of some captive reptiles (Raiti & Haramati, 1997). Furthermore, DXA has the potential for diagnosing increases in bone density found in third carpal bone disease of horses; however, its utility was not deemed practical due to the logistical issues of scanning time with large animals (Secombe et al., 2002).

Monitoring of changes in fat mass in patients is another effective use of DXA. In the domestic dog and cat, obesity is the most common nutritional disorder (Mawby et al., 2004; German, 2006). Therefore, DXA is potentially a useful tool to monitor the efficacy of therapies, nutrition, and weight reduction regimes for obese or overweight pets. Effective monitoring programs have been shown to be critical for successful weight loss (Yaissle et al., 2004 as cited in German, 2006) and long-term maintenance of a healthy body mass (Laflamme & Kuhlman, 1995 as cited in German, 2006).

5.2 Visual diagnosis of gravidity & foreign objects

Because DXA scanners provide a digital image of the patient, DXA can be used for basic radiographic applications. The resolution of images produced by DXA is relatively poor compared to traditional X-ray radiography; therefore, DXA scanning is unlikely to replace traditional radiography for most applications requiring high resolution imaging (e.g. diagnosing of minor stress fractures). The poor resolution of images produced by DXA is a software issue, rather than a technological limitation of the technique per se. For instance, certain DXA imaging procedures provide sufficient resolution for visual diagnosis for minute quantities of calcification such as with aortic atherosclerosis (Wilson, 2006). Despite the limitations in resolution of routinely produced DXA images, image quality is sufficient to diagnose a variety of conditions. For example, in our research we have used DXA to determine if female turtles are gravid (Figure 4).

Additionally, we have used DXA to visually detect the presence of foreign objects in wildlife. Specifically, we have identified the ingestion of fish hooks in turtles (Figure 5). Fishhook injuries are common in aquatic wildlife such as turtles. Swallowing of fishhooks in household pets is also relatively common (Michels et al., 1995).

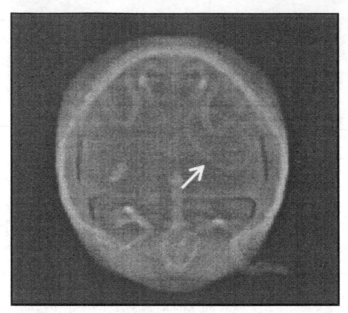

Fig. 4. X-ray image of a gravid female Eastern Box Turtle (*Terrapene carolina*). Arrow identifies a single egg.

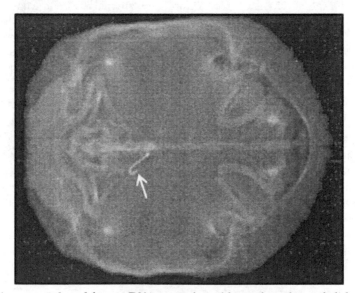

Fig. 5. X-ray image produced from a DXA scan of a wild-caught red-eared slider turtle (*Trachemys scripta*). Arrow indicates the presence of a fish hook lodged in the gastrointestinal tract.

Finally, we have used DXA to diagnose a gunshot wound in an adult wild-caught red-eared slider turtle (*Trachemys scripta;* Figure 6). In this case the subject showed no obvious signs of trauma and the external wound had completely healed. Upon our initial external inspection of the subject we failed to recognize the injury. It wasn't until we performed a DXA scan that we discovered a bullet located in the forelimb. After the diagnosis from the X-ray image, we visually identified the object as a hard palpable mass. The 0.22 caliber bullet was encysted in connective tissue surrounding the humerus, which was fractured and had not healed from the gunshot wound.

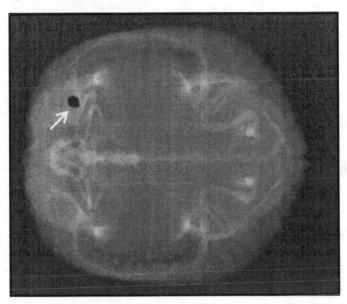

Fig. 6. X-ray image of a red-eared slider turtle (*Trachemys scripta*) that had been shot by a 0.22 caliber bullet (yellow arrow).

Even though DXA scans typically result in lower image quality, there are benefits to using it over traditional X-ray radiography. For instance, DXA offers important health benefits over traditional radiography for both the radiographer and the patient. X-ray exposure using DXA is a fraction of that produced by other means. Patient X-ray exposure during a typical whole-body DXA scan is a fraction of that during a typical chest X-ray. Furthermore, the technician's exposure to X-rays is generally negligible if the unit is operated several meters away from the source, where scatter radiation is minimal.

6. DXA precision in non-human vertebrates

Critical to the successful use of DXA in clinical and research settings is its ability to make accurate and, more importantly, precise estimates of body composition. Accuracy is of lesser importance because estimates can be corrected when systematic biases exist with a particular technique (Stone et al, 2010). On the other hand, precise estimates of body composition are critical to be able to detect longitudinal changes. We reviewed the precision of DXA in estimating body composition among a variety of taxa (Table 1). The precision among taxa was relatively low in most cases. Fat mass tended to be the least precisely estimated parameter of body composition; however, in most cases was within ranges seen in humans. A notable exception is with turtles. DXA's poor ability to estimate fat content is a result of the relatively high proportion of bone in turtles (Stone et al., 2010, discussed below).

Source	Study Animal	Location	Subject Treatment	Subject moved between scans? (#scans)	CV%			
					Lean Tissue Mass	Fat Mass	Bone Mineral Content	Bone Mineral Density
Secor & Nagy, 2003	Snake	Whole body	Euthanasia	No (2)	0.6	9.2	1.0	NR
Zotti et al., 2004b	Iguana	Femur[1]	Anesthesia	Yes (5)	NR	NR	NR	1.7
Zotti et al., 2004b	Iguana	Lumbar Spine	Anesthesia	Yes (5)	NR	NR	NR	1.6
Zotti et al., 2004b	Iguana	Head	Anesthesia	Yes (5)	NR	NR	NR	1.3
Stone et al., 2010	Turtle	Whole body	Anesthesia	No (2)	1.05	28.54	1.00	0.97
Nagy & Clair, 2000	Mouse	Whole body excluding head	Anesthesia	Yes (3)	0.86	2.20	1.60	0.84
Rose et al., 1998	Zucker Rat	Whole body	Anesthesia	Yes (3)	2.88	12.16	6.34	NR
Kastl et al., 2002	Lewis Rat	Humerus	Excised bone	No (6)	NR	NR	0.90	0.76
Kastl et al., 2002	Lewis Rat	Humerus	Excised bone	Yes (6)	NR	NR	1.32	0.86
Stevenson & van Tets, 2008	Vole	Whole body	Euthanized	Yes (>5)	1.6	6.8	2.3	3.6
Elowsson et al., 1998	Pig	Processed carcass	Euthanized	No (3)	0.94	13.51	1.91	NR
Lukaski et al.,1999	Pig	Whole body	Anesthesia	(3)	0.72	2.37	1.12	NR
Korine et al., 2004	Bird	Whole body	Physical restraint	? (2-3)	1.28	4.92	NR	NR
Korine et al., 2004	Bird	Whole body	Euthanized	? (2-3)	0.47	1.71	NR	NR
Korine et al., 2004	Bird	Whole body (feathers removed)	Euthanized	? (2-3)	0.16	2.06	NR	NR
Castaneda et al., 2006	Rabbit	Lumbar spine	Anesthesia	Yes (3)	NR	NR	NR	7.8
Black et al., 2001	Rhesus Monkey	Whole body	Anesthesia	Yes (5)	2.3	10.3	1.2	NR
Toll et al., 1994	Dog	Whole body	Anesthesia	No (6)	0.51	1.55	1.40	0.79

Table 1. Literature review of the precision, as determined by mean intraindividual coefficients of variation, of DXA estimates of lean tissue mass, fat mass, bone mineral content, and bone mineral density in various non-human vertebrates. NR = not reported. Table adapted from Stone (2009).

7. Limitations/impediments for use of DXA in clinical practice

Even though there are a variety of important applications of DXA to veterinary research and clinical practice, there are a number of logistical issues that preclude its widespread use. These limitations include the expense to purchase, operate, and maintain DXA equipment, the space required to house a unit, the time to scan a subject, the need to restrain the test subjects during scanning, and the potential for certain confounding variables to influence accurate/precise estimates of body composition as a result of technological limitations of DXA. In this section we discuss these limitations and offer some potential solutions.

7.1 Expense

In most veterinary practices the purchase of DXA equipment is likely to be cost prohibitive. The cost of a new unit averages $35,000 USD (Walpert, 2000). Additionally, there are a number of hidden costs such as software upgrades, equipment repair and maintenance, technician training, and remodeling costs associated with installation (e.g. electrical, space, etc.) Also, considering that the majority of diagnosis in a veterinary clinic would utilize traditional X-ray units, it is unlikely that clinics will purchase both traditional X-ray equipment and a dual-energy X-ray absorptiometer. Even though the costs of purchasing a DXA unit might be prohibitive, alternatives might exist. Potential users might be able to contract DXA services from local clinical or academic institutions.

7.2 Size

Space limitations are potentially major impediments for use of DXA in small animal practice. Since most DXA scanners are designed to be large enough to perform a whole body scan of an adult human, the housing of DXA equipment necessitates a dedicated room, which will likely deter or preclude its use in most small animal veterinary businesses. Some manufacturers, after recognizing this limitation, have designed DXA models that double as an exam table when not in use. Smaller models exist (e.g. PIXImus, GE Medical Systems), but are limited to small rodent-sized species, and not likely useful for most veterinary applications. Despite the space demands that a full-size DXA scanner necessitates, the size offers potential for its use with large-animal practices and has already proven useful for food-industry research. Even though there are benefits of the large scanner size for these applications, there are upper limits in body size that DXA can handle. Although DXA has been used previously with horses and cattle, its uses have been limited to analyses of bone density on excised bones (Secombe et al., 2002; Zotti et al., 2010). Currently, scanners are not large enough to allow for full-body scanning of larger animals, with the exception of carcass analysis.

7.3 Time

The use of DXA incurs a variable, and in some cases a significant, time component; however, the total time involved might not vary much more than it takes to produce a traditional X-ray radiograph. The total time it takes to scan an individual will vary depending on the type of equipment, its application, and the species under investigation. The time involved in producing a completed DXA scan of a patient involves four separate phases, with the vast majority of time allocated to machine and subject preparation. Phase 1 includes unit powering, calibration, and quality control. Phase 2 includes subject preparation, handling, orientation, and restraint. Phase 3 includes subject scanning time. Phase 4 is computational analyses. Subject scanning time can vary depending on a variety of factors including scanner brand, beam type (pencil vs. fan-beam), scanner resolution, and subject size/region of interest. Phase 1 is typically performed once each day that scanning takes place. The total time to power the unit and perform calibrations and quality control will likely vary depending on the unit manufacturer. In our experience this takes approximately 20-30 minutes. Phase 2 is likely to vary drastically with the patient under investigation due to the nuances on each organism's physiology and their body size. For instance, larger organisms pose more of a challenge to manipulate and orient on the scanner bed and may require more advanced planning. Phase 3 will vary primarily with patient size. For small patients such as rodents, where high-resolution small-animal software is necessary, scan time will take up to a few minutes. Scan time will increase with body size of the subject. The completion of DXA computational analyses (Phase 4) exemplifies the power of this tool. DXA nearly instantaneously calculates body composition at the completion of scanning. The relatively rapid scanning time combined with quick analyses makes DXA a potentially powerful tool in a clinical setting.

7.4 Need for chemical/physical restraint

Despite the relatively rapid scanning time of DXA, the accuracy and precision of DXA estimates of body composition are sensitive to the movements of subjects on the scanner bed (Cawkwell, 1998; Engelke et al., 1995). Due to this caveat, chemical or physical restraint of subjects is typically required with the use of DXA. The choice and efficacy of a particular method of restraint will vary among taxonomic groups. Use of restraint for full - body scanning of mammals and birds will invariably require general anesthesia to prevent movement artifacts. In birds, other methods of restraint have been used. Korine et al. (2004) covered the heads of small birds to immobilize them during scanning, but they found this method decreased precision in estimating lean tissue and fat mass compared to estimates determined after euthanasia (Table 1). In other exotic animals, reptiles in particular, additional methods are available. Cooling of body temperature is an effective method to immobilize subjects during scanning (Stone et al., 2010). This method requires planning on the part of the practitioner because safe cooling of core body temperature can take several hours for large reptiles. Despite its potential as a viable source of restraint, cooling of body temperature in reptiles tended to result in less precise estimates of body composition compared to anesthesia and euthanasia. (Stone et al., 2010)

7.5 Intestinal artifacts: A case study on the ingestion of foreign particles and their associated impacts on DXA estimates of body composition

DXA estimates of body composition from whole body scans are likely to be influenced by superimposing the contents of the gastrointestinal tract with the composition of the subject's tissues. Even though the effects of intestinal contents are thought to have a negligible impact on DXA estimates of body composition in humans, the consumption of certain items in animals might impact DXA estimates. For instance, the consumption of calcified particles such as sand, stones, or bone might influence estimates of bone mineral content because they will result in similar beam attenuation as bone. In reptiles and birds the consumption of calcified particles is common as these items might aid in digestion or provide particular nutrients (Walde et al., 2007). In this study we investigated whether ingestion of intestinal artifacts (sand in this case) impacts DXA estimates of body composition in turtles.

To determine the effects of intestinal artifacts on DXA estimates of body composition, we performed DXA analysis on 55 captive box turtles, *Terrapene carolina*. This captive population of turtles was housed outdoors in a pen with a sand substrate. Prior to scanning, straight carapace length (SCL) and mass were recorded for each individual. All specimens, who were not fasted prior to analysis, were then cooled for a minimum of eight hours at 4°C to prevent movement artifacts while scanning. Following the same procedure for turtles as Stone et al. (2010), scanning was performed using a Hologic QDR-4500A fan-beam scanner equipped with a small-animal software program on three occasions: 13 May 2004, 15 October 2005, and 10 May 2005. During each scanning day, duplicate scans, without movement between scans, were performed on each individual. If the same individual was scanned on multiple dates, only scans from the first day were used in analyses. Prior to statistical analyses, duplicate DXA estimates of body composition (bone mineral content (BMC), fat mass (FM), lean tissue mass (LTM), and body mass (BM)) were averaged for each individual. All turtles were qualitatively scored based on the amount of sand in the gastrointestinal tract. Turtles were scored as having zero (n=27), moderate (n=20), or heavy levels (n=8) of intestinal artifacts (Figure 7). Following DXA analyses, fecal samples were collected to confirm the presence of sand in the intestine.

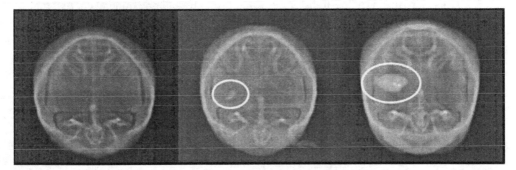

Fig. 7. DXA scans of box turtles (*Terrapene carolina*) showing, from left to right, (a.) zero, (b.) moderate, and (c.) heavy levels of intestinal artifacts (yellow circles).

To examine the effects of intestinal artifacts on DXA estimates of bone mineral content and lean tissue mass, we performed analysis of covariance (ANCOVA). Prior to analyses, we $\log_{10}$ transformed bone mineral content and lean tissue mass (dependent variables) to linearize the relationship between covariate (straight carapace length) and the response variable. Prior to analysis, all assumptions of ANCOVA were tested and not violated, including the assumption of parallelism (BMC, $F_{2,48}=0.24$, p>0.05; LTM, $F_{2,48}=0.11$, p=0.89). To compare fat mass among turtles with different artifact scores we used ANOVA, because body size did not significantly influence fat mass in this study. Data were left untransformed. For all analyses, when significant differences among intestinal artifact levels were found, Tukey multiple-comparisons were used to determine where differences occurred. Statistical analyses were performed using the general linear model procedure on Minitab version 13.2.

DXA estimates for bone mineral content were significantly different among turtles with intestinal artifact scores (ANCOVA; $F_{2,50}$=3.12, p=0.05). Bone mineral content was not different between turtles with zero and moderate levels of intestinal sand (T=1.12, p=0.52), as well as between turtles with moderate and heavy levels (T=1.62, p=0.25). A significant difference was found in mean BMC between turtles with zero and heavy levels of intestinal artifacts (T=2.48, p=0.04; Figure 8).

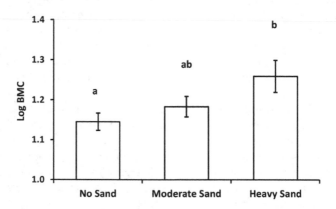

Fig. 8. Least square means of log-transformed DXA estimates of bone mineral content for turtles with no sand, moderate sand, and heavy sand in the gastrointestinal tract. Significant differences (P<0.05) are indicated by different letters. Data are presented as mean ± 1SE.

DXA estimates for lean tissue mass were not significantly different among turtles with different intestinal artifact scores ($F_{2,50}$=1.73, p=0.19; Figure 9).

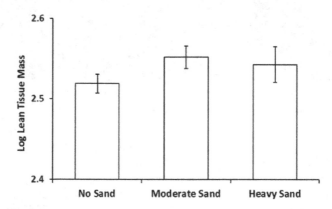

Fig. 9. Least square means of log-transformed DXA estimates of lean tissue mass for turtles with no sand, moderate sand, and heavy sand in the gastrointestinal tract. Data are presented as mean ± 1SE.

The effects of intestinal artifacts on estimates of fat mass followed similar trends to lean tissue mass. We observed a no significant effect of intestinal contents on DXA estimates of fat mass (F = 1.76, P=0.18; Figure 10).

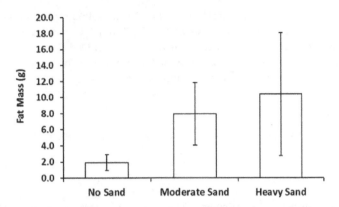

Fig. 10. Mean fat mass estimates for turtles with no sand, moderate sand, and heavy sand in the gastrointestinal tract. Data are presented as mean ± 1SE.

The results of this study suggest that DXA estimates of bone mineral content are influenced by ingestion of mineralized foreign particles. DXA tended to overestimate bone mineral content in individuals that ingested sand. Therefore, it is important to consider whether individuals have access to foreign particles when utilizing DXA to quantify bone mineral content in exotic animal practice or wildlife research involving birds or reptiles. In cases where ingestion of foreign particles is possible, fasting may be required to ensure evacuation of the gastrointestinal tract prior to DXA scanning.

7.6 Taxon-specific considerations

Technological limitations exist with the use of DXA with certain taxa. As we discussed previously, DXA is unable to directly estimate the proportion of lean, fat, and bone when they occur concurrently at a single pixel on the scan. This is a limitation with the use of two peak energies. To distinguish all three tissue components a third peak energy would be required (Swanpalmer et al., 1998). DXA overcomes this limitation by using neighboring pixels without bone to estimate the proportion of fat and lean tissue and then applies them to pixels containing bone. This limitation presents a serious impediment for the use of this technique with species that contain a high proportion of bone. Stone et al. (2010) found that DXA was unable to accurately or precisely predict fat mass in turtles as a result of the high proportion of pixels containing bone. Despite the limitation, DXA was able to effectively estimate bone and lean tissue mass, and so this methodology could be useful in a clinical setting for predicting and monitoring metabolic bone diseases in turtles (Stone et al, 2010).

8. Conclusions

Dual-energy X-ray absorptiometry can effectively quantify lean tissue, fat, and bone mineral mass in humans and most animals. As a result of its high degree of precision and accuracy, it has proven useful for research in fracture risk and healing, obesity, metabolism, pathology, and nutrition. Despite the plethora of potential and realized uses for DXA in veterinary research, the use of DXA remains restricted, primarily, to the human health industry or animal research. Currently, a number of limitations exist that prevent the widespread use of DXA in veterinary medicine. Most notably, the high purchase and maintenance costs and relatively short life-span of DXA units, combined with their size, are major limitations for DXA and hinder its widespread use in traditional veterinary practice. Until these limitations are resolved, DXA will continue to be restricted to human-based clinical settings or with animal research institutions.

9. Acknowledgment

We thank the Oklahoma State University Department of Nutritional Sciences for providing logistical support and access to their DXA equipment.

10. References

Adams, J.E. (1997). Single and dual energy X-ray absorptiometry. *European Radiology*, Vol. 7, Suppl. 2, pp. (S20-S31), ISSN: 0938-7994

Buelund, L., Nielsen, D., Mcevoy, F., Svalastoga, E., & Bjornvad, C. (2011). Measurement of body composition in cats using computed tomography and dual energy X-ray absorptiometry. *Veterinary Radiology and Ultrasound*, Vol. 52, No. 2, (March-April 2011), pp. (179-184), ISSN: 1058-8183

Black, A., Tilmont, E.M., Baer, D.J., Rumpler, W.V., Ingram, D.K. Roth, G.S., & Lane, M.A. (2001). Accuracy and precision of dual-energy X-ray absorptiometry for body composition measurements in Rhesus monkeys. *Journal of Medical Primatology*, Vol. 30, pp. (94-99), ISSN:0047-2565

Castaneda, S., Largo, R., Calvo, E., Rodriguez-Salvanes, F., Marcos, M.E., az-Curiel, M., & Herrero-Beaumont, G. (2006). Bone mineral measurements of subchondral and trabecular bone in healthy and osteoporotic rabbits. *Skeletal Radiology*, Vol. 35, No. 1, (January 2006), pp. (34-41), ISSN: 0364-2348

Cawkwell, G.D. (1998). Movement artifact and dual X-ray absorptiometry. *Journal of Clinical Densitometry*, Vol. 1, No. 2, pp. 141-147, ISSN 1094-6950

Clarys, J.P., Scafoglieri, A., Provyn, S., Louis, O., Wallace, J.A., & De Mey, J. (2010). A macro-quality evaluation of DXA variables using whole dissection, ashing, and computer tomography in pigs. *Obesity*, Vol. 18, No. 8, (August 2010), pp. (1477-1485), ISSN: 1930-7381

Corten, F.G.A., Caulier, H., van der Waerden, J.P.C.M., Kalk, W., Corstens, F.H.M., & Jansen, J.A. (1997). Assessment of bone surrounding implants in goats: Ex vivo measurements by dual X-ray absorptiometry. *Biomaterials*, Vol. 18, No. 6, (March 1997), pp. (495-501), ISSN: 0142-9612

Dirrigl, F.J., Dalsky, G.P., & Warner, S.E. (2004). Dual-energy X-ray absorptiometry of birds: An examination of excised skeletal specimens. *Journal of Veterinary Medicine: Series A*, Vol. 51, No. 6, (August 2004), pp. (313-319), ISSN: 0931-184X

Elowsson, P., Forslund, A.H., Mallmin, H., Feuk, U., Hansson, I., & Carlsten, J. (1998). An evaluation of dual-energy X-ray absorptiometry and underwater weighing to estimate body composition by means of carcass analysis in piglets. *The Journal of Nutrition*, Vol. 128, No. 9, (September 1998), pp. (1543-1549), ISSN: 0022-3166

Engelke, K., Gluer, C.C., & Genant, H.K. (1995). Factors influencing short-term precision of dual X-ray bone absorptiometry (DXA) of spine and femur. *Calcified Tissue International*, Vol. 56, No. 1, (January 1995), pp. (19-25), ISSN: 0171-967X

Use of Dual-Energy X-Ray Absorptiometry (DXA) with Non-Human Vertebrates: Application, Challenges, and Practical
Considerations for Research and Clinical Practice
113

Felicetti, L.A., Robbins, C.T., & Shipley, L.A. (2003). Dietary protein content alters energy expenditure and composition of the mass gain in grizzly bears (*Ursus arctos horribilis*). *Physiological and Biochemical Zoology*, Vol. 76, No. 2, (March-April 2003), pp. (256-261), ISSN: 1522-2152

Fink, C., Cooper, H.J., Huebner, J.L., Guilak, F., & Kraus, V.B. (2002). Precision and accuracy of a transportable dual-energy X-ray absorptiometry unit for bone mineral measurements in guinea pigs. *Calcified Tissue International*, Vol. 70, No. 3, (March 2002), pp. (164-169), ISSN: 0171-967X

Fledelius, B., Jorgensen, G.W., Jensen, H.E., & Brimer, L. (2005). Influence of the calcium content of the diet offered to leopard tortoises (*Geochelone pardalis*). *Veterinary Record*, Vol. 56, No. 26, (June 2005), pp. (831-835), ISSN 0042-4900

German, A.J. (2006). The growing problem of obesity in dogs and cats. *The Journal of Nutrition*, Vol. 136, No. 7, (July 2006), pp. (1940S-1946S), ISSN: 0022-3166

Grier, S.J., Turner, A.S., & Alvis, M.R. (1996). The use of dual-energy x-ray absorptiometry in animals. *Investigative Radiology*, Vol. 31, No. 1, (January 1996), pp. (50-62), ISSN: 0020-9996

Hanafusa, S., Matsusue, Y., Yasunaga, T., Yamamuro, T., Oka, M., Shikinami, Y., & Ikada, Y. (1995). Biodegradable plate fixation of rabbit femoral-shaft osteotomies: A comparative study. *Clinical Orthopaedics and Related Research*, Vol. 315, (June 1995), pp. (262-271), ISSN: 0009-921X

Jebb, S.A. (1997). Measurement of soft tissue composition by dual energy X-ray absorptiometry. *British Journal of Nutrition*, Vol. 77, No. 2, (February 1997), pp. (151-163), ISSN: 0007-1145

Jensen, P., Keeling, L., Schutz, K., Andersson, L., Mormede, P., Brandstrom, H., Forkman, B., Kerje, S., Fredriksson, R., Ohlsson, C., Larsson, S., Mallmin, H., & Kindmark, A. (2005). Feather pecking in chickens is genetically related to behavioural and developmental traits. *Physiology and Behavior*, Vol. 86, (September 2005), pp. (52-60), ISSN: 0031-9384

Kastl, S., Sommer, T., Klein, P., Hohenberger, W., & Engelke, K. (2002). Accuracy and precision of bone mineral density and bone mineral content in excised rat humeri using fan beam dual-energy X-ray absorptiometry. *Bone*, Vol. 30, No. 1, (January 2002), p. (243-246), ISSN 8756-3282

Kim, W.K., Donalson, L.M., Mitchell, A.D., Kubena, L.F., Nisbet, D.J., & Ricke, S.C. (2006). Effects of alfalfa and fructooligosaccharide on molting parameters and bone qualities using dual energy X-ray absorptiometry and conventional bone assays. *Poultry Science*, Vol. 85, No. 1, (January 2006), pp. (15-20), ISSN: 0032-5791

Korine, C., Daniel, S., van Tets, I.G., Yosef, R., & Pinshow, B. (2004). Measuring fat mass in small birds by dual-energy X-ray absorptiometry. *Physiological and Biochemical Zoology*, Vol. 77, No. 3, (May-June 2004), pp. (522-529), ISSN: 1522-2152

Laflamme, D.P., & Kuhlman, G. (1995). The effect of weight loss regimen on subsequent weight maintenance in dogs. *Nutrition Research*, Vol. 15, No. 7, (July 1995), pp. (1019-1028), ISSN: 0271-5317

Lee, C.Y., Chan, S.H., Lai, H.Y., & Lee, S.T. (2011). A method to develop an in vitro osteoporosis model of porcine vertebrae: Histological and biomechanical study Laboratory investigation. *Journal of Neurosurgery: Spine*, Vol. 14, No. 6, (June 2011), pp. (789-798), ISSN: 1547-5654

Lorinson, K., Lobcke, S., Skalicky, M., & Lorinson, D. (2009). Densitometric properties of canine appendicular bones based on dual-energy X-ray absorptiometry measurements. *Wiener Tierarztliche Monatsschrift*, Vol. 96, pp. (72-77), ISSN 0043-535X

Losel, D., Kremer, P., Albrecht, E., & Scholz, A.M. (2010). Comparison of a GE Lunar DPX-IQ and a Norland XR-26 dual energy X-ray absorptiometry scanner for body composition measurements in pigs - in vivo. *Archiv Tierzucht*, Vol. 53, No. 2, pp. (162-175), ISSN 0003-9438

Lucic, H., Vukovic, S., Posavac, V., Gomercic, M.D., Gomercic, T., Galov, A., Skrtic, D., Curkovic, S., & Gomercic, H. (2010). Application of dual energy X-ray absorptiometry method for small animals in measuring bone mineral density of the humerus of bottlenose dolphins (*Tursiops truncatus*) from the Adriatic Sea. *Veterinarski Arhiv*, Vol. 80, No. 2, pp. (299-310), ISSN 0372-5480

Lukaski, H.C., Marchello, M.J., Hall, C.B., Schafer, D.M., & Siders, W.A. (1999). Soft tissue composition of pigs measured with dual X-ray absorptiometry. *Nutrition*, Vol. 15, No. 9, (September 1999), pp. (697-703), ISSN 0899-9007

Markel, M.D., & Bogdanske, J.J. (1994a). Dual-energy X-ray absorptiometry of canine femurs with and without fracture fixation devices. *American Journal of Veterinary Research*, Vol. 55, No. 6, (June 1994), pp. (862-866), ISSN 0002-9645

Markel, M.D., & Bogdanske, J.J. (1994b). The effect of increasing gap width on localized densitometric changes within tibial ostectomies in a canine model. *Calcified Tissue International*, Vol. 54, No. 2, (February 1994), pp. (155-159), ISSN 0171-967X

Mawby, D.I., Bartges, J.W., d'Avignon, A., Laflamme, D.P., Moyers, T.D., & Cottrell, T. (2004). Comparison of various methods for estimating body fat in dogs. *Journal of the American Animal Hospital Association*, Vol. 40, No. 2, (March-April 2004), pp. (109-114), ISSN 0587-2871

McClure, S.R., Glickman, L.T., Glickman, N.W., & Weaver, C.M. (2001). Evaluation of dual energy X-ray absorptiometry for in situ measurement of bone mineral density of equine metacarpi. *American Journal of Veterinary Research*, Vol. 62, No. 5, (May 2001), pp. (752-756), ISSN 0002-9645

Mercier, J., Pomar, C., Marcoux, M., Goulet, F., Theriault, M., & Castonguay, F.W. (2006). The use of dual-energy X-ray absorptiometry to estimate the dissected composition of lamb carcasses. *Meat Science*, Vol. 73, No. 2, (June 2006), pp. (249-257), ISSN 0309-1740

Michels, G.M., Jones, B.D., Huss, B.T., & Wagner-Mann, C. (1995). Endoscopic and surgical retrieval of fishhooks from the stomach and esophagus in dogs and cats: 75 cases (1977-1993). *Journal of the American Veterinary Medical Association*, Vol. 207, No. 9, (November 1995), pp. (1194-1197), ISSN 0003-1488

Millett, P.J., Cohen, B., Allen, M.J., & Rushton, N. (1998). Bone mineral density changes during fracture healing: a densitometric study in rats, In: *Internet Journal of Orthopedic Surgery and related Subjects*, 18.8.2011, Available from: http://www.rz.uni-duesseldorf.de/WWW/MedFak/Orthopaedie/journal/, ISSN 0949-2607

Mitchell, A.D., Scholz, A.M., & Conway, J.M. (1998). Body composition analysis of small pigs by dual-energy X-ray absorptiometry. *Journal of Animal Science*, Vol. 76, No. 9, (September 1998), pp. (2392-2398), ISSN 0021-8812

Mo, G., Zotti, A., Agnesi, S., Finola, M.G., Bernardini, D., & Cozzi, B. (2009). Age classes and sex differences in the skull of the Mediterranean monk seal, *Monachus monachus* (Hermann, 1779): A Study Based on Bone Shape and Density. *Anatomical Record: Advances in Integrative Anatomy and Evolutionary Biology*, Vol. 292, No. 4, (April 2009), pp. (544-556), ISSN 1932-8486

Nagy, T.R., & Clair, A.L. (2000). Precision and accuracy of dual-energy X-ray absorptiometry
for determining in vivo body composition of mice. *Obesity Research*, Vol. 8, No. 5,
(August 2000), p. (392-398), ISSN 1071-7323

Nielson, D.H., McEvoy, F.J., Poulsen, H.L., Madsen, M.T., Buelund, L.E., & Svalastoga, E.
(2004). Dual-energy X-ray absorptiometry of the pig: Protocol development and
evaluation. *Meat Science*, Vol. 68, No. 2, (October 2004), pp. (235-241), ISSN 0309-
1740

Peppler, W.W., & Mazess, R.B. (1981). Total body mineral and lean body mass by dual-
photon absorptiometry: theory and measurement procedure. *Calcified Tissue
International*, Vol. 33, No. 1, (December 1981), pp. (353-359), ISSN 0171-967X

Pietrobelli, A., Formica, C., Wang, Z.M., & Heymsfield, S.B. (1996). Dual-energy X-ray
absorptiometry body composition model: Review of physical concepts. *American
Journal of Physiology: Endocrinology and Metabolism*, Vol. 271, No. 6, (December 1996),
pp. (E941-E951), ISSN 0193-1849

Ponnampalam, E.N., Hopkins, D.L., Dunshea, F.R., Pethick, D.W., Butler, K.L., & Warner,
R.D. (2007). Genotype and age effects on sheep meat production: Carcass
composition predicted by dual energy X-ray absorptiometry. *Australian Journal of
Experimental Agriculture*, Vol. 47, No. 10, pp. (1172-1179), ISSN 0816-1089

Pouilles, J.M., Collard, P., Tremollieres, F., Frayssinet, P., Railhac, J.J., Cahuzac, J.P.,
Autefage, A., & Ribot, C. (2000). Accuracy and precision of in vivo bone mineral
measurements in sheep using dual-energy X-ray absorptiometry. *Calcified Tissue
International*, Vol. 66, No. 1, (January 2000), pp. (70-73), ISSN 0171-967X

Raiti, P., & Haramati, N. (1997). Magnetic resonance imaging and computerized
tomography of a gravid leopard tortoise (*Geochelone pardalis pardalis*) with
metabolic bone disease. *Journal of Zoo and Wildlife Medicine*, Vol. 28, No. 2, (June
1997), p. (189-197), ISSN 1042-7260

Rose, B.S., Flatt, W.P., Martin, R.J., & Lewis, R.D. (1998). Whole body composition of rats
determined by dual energy X-ray absorptiometry is correlated with chemical
analysis. *Journal of Nutrition*, Vol. 128, No. 2, (February 1998), pp. (246-250), ISSN
0022-3166

Schneider, S., Breit, S.M., Grampp, S., Kunzel, W.W.F., Liesegang, A., Mayrhofer, E., &
Zentek, F. (2004). Comparative assessment of bone mineral measurements obtained
by use of dual-energy X-ray absorptiometry, peripheral quantitative computed
tomography, and chemical-physical analyses in femurs of juvenile and adult dogs.
American Journal of Veterinary Research, Vol. 65, No. 7, (July 2004), pp. (891-900),
ISSN 0002-9645

Secombe, C.J., Firth, E.C., Perkins, N.R., & Anderson, B.H. (2002). Pathophysiology and
diagnosis of third carpal bone disease in horses: A review. *New Zealand Veterinary
Journal*, Vol. 50, No. 1, (February 2002), pp. (2-8), ISSN 0048-0169

Secor, S.M., & Nagy, T.R. (2003). Non-invasive measure of body composition of snakes
using dual-energy X-ray absorptiometry. *Comparative Biochemistry and Physiology A:
Molecular and Integrative Physiology*, Vol. 136, No. 2, (October 2003), pp. (379-389),
ISSN 1095-6433

Stevenson, K.T., & van Tets, I.G. (2008). Dual-energy X-ray absorptiometry (DXA) can
accurately and nondestructively measure the body composition of small, free-living
rodents. *Physiological and Biochemical Zoology*, Vol. 81, No. 3, (May-June 2008), pp.
(373-382), ISSN 1522-2152

Stone, M.D. (2009). Effects of season, sex, and age on the calcium physiology and bone
dynamics of turtles. Oklahoma State University, Ph.D. dissertation, Stillwater, OK

Stone, M.D., Arjmandi, B.H., & Lovern, M.B. (2010). Dual-energy X-ray absorptiometry (DXA) as a non-invasive tool for the prediction of bone density and body composition of turtles. *Herpetological Review*, Vol. 41, No. 1, (March 2010), pp. (36-42), ISSN 0018-084X

Swanpalmer, J., Kullenberg, R., & Hansson, T. (1998). Measurement of bone mineral using multiple-energy X-ray absorptiometry. *Physics in Medicine and Biology*, Vol. 43, pp. (379-387), ISSN 0031-9155

Toll, P.W., Gross, K.L., Berryhill, S.A., & Jewell, D.E. (1994). Usefulness of dual energy X-ray absorptiometry for body composition measurement in adult dogs. *The Journal of Nutrition*, Vol. 124, Suppl. 12, (December 1994), pp. (2601S-2603S), ISSN 0022-3166

Turner, A.S., Mallinckrodt, C.H., Alvis, M.R., & Bryant, H.U. (1995a). Dual-energy X-ray absorptiometry in sheep: Experiences with in-vivo and ex-vivo studies. *Bone*, Vol. 17, No. 4, (October 1995), pp. (S381-S387), ISSN 8756-3282

Turner, A.S., Norrdin, R.W., Gaarde, S., Connally, H.E., & Thrall, M.A. (1995b). Bone mineral density in feline mucopolysaccharidosis VI measured using dual-energy X-ray absorptiometry. *Calcified Tissue International*, Vol. 57, No. 3, (September 1995), pp. (191-195), ISSN 0171-967X

Walde, A.D., Delaney, D.K., Harless, M.L., & Pater, L.L. (2007). Osteophagy by the desert tortoise (*Gopherus agassizii*). *Southwestern Naturalist*, Vol. 52, No. 1, (March 2007), pp. (147-149), ISSN 0038-4909

Walpert, B. (2000). With ancillary services, you can do well by doing good. In: *American College of Physicians Observer*, October, 8.2.2011, Available from: http://www.acpinternist.org

Wilson, K.E. (2006). Detection of abdominal aortic calcification with IVA. 8.1.2011, Available from: http://www.hologic.com/data/W_158_AAC_05-06.pdf

Yaissle, J.E., Holloway, C., & Buffington, C.A.T. (2004). Evaluation of owner education as a component of obesity treatment programs for dogs. *Journal of the American Veterinary Medical Association*, Vol. 224, No. 12, (June 2004), pp. (1932–1935), ISSN 0003-1488

Zotti, A., Gianesella, M., Ceccato, C., & Morgante, M. (2010). Physiological values and factors affecting the metacarpal bone density of healthy feedlot beef cattle as measured by dual-energy X-ray absorptiometry. *Journal of Animal Physiology and Animal Nutrition*, Vol. 94, No. 5, (October 2010), pp. (615-622), ISSN 0931-2439

Zotti, A., Isola, M., Sturaro, E., Menegazzo, L., Piccinini, P., & Bernardini, D. (2004a). Vertebral mineral density measured by dual-energy X-ray absorptiometry (DEXA) in a group of healthy Italian boxer dogs. *Journal of Veterinary Medicine: Series A*, Vol. 51, No. 5, (June 2004), pp. (254-258), ISSN 0931-184X

Zotti, A., Poggi, R., & Cozzi, B. (2009). Exceptional bone density DXA values of the rostrum of a deep-diving marine mammal: A new technical insight in the adaptation of bone to aquatic life. *Skeletal Radiology*, Vol. 38, No. 12, (December 2009), pp. (1123-1125), ISSN 0364-2348

Zotti, A., Rizzi, C., Chiericato, G., & Bernardini, D. (2003). Accuracy and precision of dual-energy X-ray absorptiometry for ex vivo determination of mineral content in turkey poult bones. *Veterinary Radiology and Ultrasound*, Vol. 44, No. 1, (January-February 2003), pp. (49-52), ISSN 1058-8183

Zotti, A., Selleri, P., Carnier, P., Morgante, M., & Bernardini, D. (2004b). Relationship between metabolic bone disease and bone mineral density measured by dual-energy X-ray absorptiometry in the green iguana (*Iguana iguana*). *Veterinary Radiology and Ultrasound*, Vol. 45, No. 1, (January 2004), pp. (10-16), ISSN 1058-8183

Part 2

Clinical Attention in Pets

7

Periodontal Disease in Dogs

Fábio Alessandro Pieri, Ana Paula Falci Daibert,
Elisa Bourguignon and Maria Aparecida Scatamburlo Moreira
Federal University of Viçosa,
Brazil

1. Introduction

Periodontics is a science that aims to study the periodontium and the diagnosis, prevention and treatment of periodontal diseases, in order to promote and restore the periodontal health (Harvey & Emily, 1993; Roman et al., 1995).

The periodontium is the set of adjacent structures to the teeth that provides them with support and protection. These structures are: gingiva, cementum, alveolar bone and periodontal ligament (Harvey & Emily, 1993; Roman et al., 1995; De Marco & Gioso, 1997; Clarke, 2001).

Periodontal disease is the most common oral disease in dogs with up of 80% of animals affected (Riggio et al., 2011). This disease is progressive and involves two stages: gingivitis (reversible) and periodontitis (irreversible, but often controllable). It is caused by plaque buildup on teeth. The plaque is a smooth membrane, adhesive, contaminated with saliva bacteria and debris. Bacteria and bacterial products cause inflammation of soft tissue. The plaque becomes mineralised to form calculus, which migrates into the gingival sulcus, causing additional inflammation, loss of periodontal ligament, bone loss and ultimately tooth loss (Ford & Mazzaferro, 2007).

Medical problems that affect the oral cavity should be identified in its early stages, so that the animals can be treated before showing serious secondary systemic disorders related to malnutrition and/or infections (Pachaly, 2006). One should also be aware of ways to prevent the disease, as animal tooth brushing and the use of antimicrobials as an adjunct in periodontal therapy (De Marco & Gioso, 1997).

2. Dental anatomy of dogs

As in most domestic mammals and in humans, dogs have diphyodont dentition, featuring two sets of teeth, a deciduous or primary and a permanent, although edentulous at birth (Harvey, 1992).

The oral anatomy of dogs has subdivisions and similar structures to those of humans (Figure 1), differing in the shape of the cavity, which also varies between breeds (Roza, 2004), anatomy and quantity of teeth and in the teeth apex (Harvey & Emily, 1993). Dogs have, like humans, incisors, canines, premolars and molars, differing among themselves in functions and numbers of roots (Roza, 2004; Mitchell, 2005).

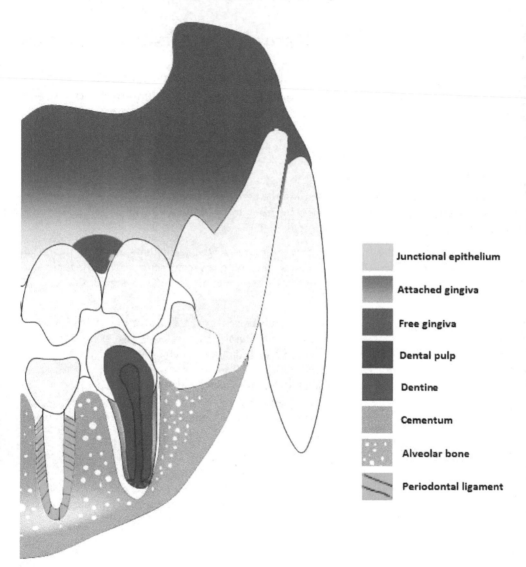

Fig. 1. Structures of dental organ in dogs

Domestic dogs have in their primary teeth, 28 teeth (12 incisors, four canines, 8 premolars and 4 molars), and in the permanent, 42 teeth (12 incisors, four canines, 16 premolars and 10 molars) (Roza, 2004). Regardless of the number of roots, function, size and shape, the teeth have subdivisions that are common to all types (Roza, 2004), and form the dental organ together with some adjacent structures (Gioso, 2007).

For a better understanding of periodontal disease it is important to have further information about a set of structures that constitute the alveolar-dental joint, the periodontium (Picosse, 1987).

The periodontium (peri, around; dental, tooth) (Lindhe & Karring, 1997) is the set of hard and soft tissues (Mitchell, 2005) that support (Harvey & Emily, 1993, Domingues et al., 1999), by fixing, adhering (Lindhe & Karring, 1997; Roza, 2004) and protecting the tooth in the alveolar bone (Roza, 2004). The structures that comprise the periodontium are the periodontal ligament, cementum, gingiva and alveolar bone (Carranza, 1983; Lindhe & Karring, 1997; Wiggs & Lobprise, 1997). There is a division of these structures according to their functions, so there is a periodontal support formed by the cementum, the periodontal ligament, alveolar bone, and gingiva that besides participating in the support also comprises the protection periodontium (Roza, 2004).

The gingiva (Figure 1) is the part of the masticatory mucosa that surrounds the cervical portion of the tooth and covers the alveolar process (Lindhe & Karring, 1997). Its main function is to protect structures adjacent to the tooth, being the first line of defence against periodontal disease (Harvey & Emily, 1993). Two parts can be distinguished: the free and attached gingiva (Harvey & Emily, 1993; Lindhe & Karring, 1997).

The free gingiva can be pink or pigmented in some breeds, with firm consistency and an opaque surface (Lindhe & Karring, 1997). The margin of the free gingiva is the edge of it. Between the free gingiva and the tooth, a groove is formed (Mitchell, 2005) known as the gingival sulcus, which, in normal conditions in the dogs, varies in depth from one to three millimeters (Harvey & Emily, 1993; Roza, 2004). The sulcus is surrounded by an adhered epithelium that secretes a fluid with inflammation mediatory cells, immunoglobulins and antibacterial substances important in the physical and immunological protection of the junctional epithelium and deeper tissues (Pope, 1993).

The junctional epithelium (Figure 1) is located at the bottom of the sulcus, with flat and elongated cells (Hennet, 1995; Wiggs & Lobprise, 1997) adhering to the enamel through hemidesmosomes, promoting the junction between the gingiva and the tooth (Harvey & Emily, 1993). The junctional epithelium ends in the cementum-enamel junction (Roza, 2004).

In processes such as inflammation, hyperplasia or in both, the junctional epithelium can recede apically or the gingiva can increase, making deeper the gingival sulcus (Harvey & Emily, 1993). In gingival hyperplasia the deepening of the sulcus occurs without loss of periodontal tissue, named false pocket, although when there is a loss of the support tissue and protection of the tooth, the sulcus is called periodontal pockets, which can be of two types: suprabone, when the bottom of the sulcus is coronal to the support alveolar bone, and intrabone, when the bottom is located apically in relation to the adjacent alveolar bone. The pocket depth can vary between regions of the mouth and even between neighbouring teeth (Newman et al., 2004).

The attached gingiva (Figure 1) is the continuation of the free gingiva, that, is firmly attached to the underlying bone, and extends to the mucogingival junction (Carranza, 1983).

Cementum (Figure 1) is a hard tissue with no vascularity (Harvey et al. 1994; Hennet, 1995) that covers the tooth root (Mitchell, 2005), is composed of collagen fibres embedded in an organic matrix, and has in its mineral portion, which is responsible for about 65% of its weight, hydroxyapatite crystals (Lindhe & Karring, 1997). It has as its main functions the insertion of periodontal ligament fibres into the root of the tooth (Harvey & Emily, 1993; Lindhe & Karring, 1997; Roza, 2004), the contribution to the process of repair of the root surface and the maintenance of the periodontal ligament fibres (Picasso, 1987; Lindhe & Karring, 1997).

There are two types of cementum: the first, called primary or acellular cementum, is formed in association with root formation and teeth eruption (Lindhe & Karring, 1997). It occupies the coronal and middle thirds of the tooth root and is constituted mostly of Sharpey's fibres, which are the periodontal ligament collagen fibres that attach at one end to the cementum and at the other to the alveolar bone (Roza, 2004). The other type of cementum is called secondary or cellular cementum, formed after the teeth (Lindhe & Karring, 1997) and usually located in the periapical region. It is secreted by cementocytes or cementoblasts, which are cells that are trapped into the organic matrix of cementum. It does not have vascularization, therefore is nourished from the periodontal ligament. The cells secrete cellular cementum in response to functional demands (Wiggs & Lobprise, 1997). Despite the description of the location of each type of cementum, in some cases they can occur alternately in some areas of the root surface (Lindhe & Karring, 1997).

The alveolar bone (Figure 1) involves the maxilla, incisor bone and jawbone that support the teeth in cavities where they are inserted. These cavities are called alveolus (Picasso, 1987; Harvey & Emily, 1993; Roza, 2004).

Composed of 65% minerals (Wiggs & Lobprise, 1997), this bone has a hard consistency and is very dense and compact, but differs from the root cementum because it has innervation, blood and lymphatic vasculature (Lindhe & Karring, 1997).

The interior of the alveolus is where the cribriform plate is located, which radiographically is known as lamina dura, characterised as a radiopaque line around the alveolus. The fibres of the periodontal ligament that attach to the tooth are connected to this plaque and it is where the vessels pass for ligament irrigation and for the nutrition of the cementum organic matrix (Harvey & Emily, 1993; Roza, 2004)

The alveolar bone can be resorbed or remodelled, according to the stimuli that it may suffer (Harvey & Emily, 1993; Roza, 2004).

The periodontal ligament (Figure 1) is a connective tissue structure that binds the tooth to its alveolus, fixing it (Lindhe & Karring, 1997; Figueiredo & Parra, 2002). It originates from mesenchymal cells of the dental sac (Picasso, 1987; Wiggs & Lobprise, 1997).

The periodontal ligament contains nerves and great vascularity, with vessels emanating from the maxillary artery in the case of the maxilla and from the inferior alveolar artery in the case of the jaw, and other cells. It is located between the root cementum and the cribriform plate. Its height, width, quality and condition are crucial to give the tooth its characteristic mobility (Harvey & Emily, 1993; Lindhe & Karring, 1997; Roza, 2004).

There are three different categories of fibres in the periodontal ligament: the fibres of the gingival grouping, composed by dental gingival fibres (connect the cementum to the gingiva), the alveologingival fibres (connects the cribriform plate to the gingiva), the circular (surrounding the tooth at the free gingiva), the transseptal fibres (connects the supra cementum alveolus of neighbour teeth), the fibres of the dental alveolar group, which are the fibres of the alveolar ridge (connecting the alveolar ridge to the cementum, obliquely), the horizontal fires (connect the cementum to the ridge, horizontally), the oblique fibres (connect the cementum to the alveolar bone, has a higher number of ligaments), apical fibres (connecting the bone to the cementum around the apex) and the inter-root fibres (that are between roots of multirooted teeth) (Wiggs & Lobprise 1997; Roza, 2004).

The periodontal ligament plays several roles in the tooth, such as:

- physical features, support, shock absorption caused by the chewing strength and transmission of occlusal forces to the bone (Figueiredo & Parra, 2002);
- formation, by osteoblasts, cementoblasts and fibroblasts (Clarke, 2001);
- reabsorption by osteoclasts, cementoclast and fibroclasts (Clarke, 2001);
- sensory, because it is abundantly innervated by sensory nerve fibres that are able to transmit tactile sensations of pressure and pain by the trigeminal pathways (Carranza, 1983; Figueiredo & Parra, 2002);
- nutritive, since it has blood vessels that provide nutrients and other substances required by the ligament tissues by the cementocytes and the more superficial osteocytes of alveolar bone (Carranza, 1983; Figueiredo & Parra, 2002);
- and homeostasis, because of its ability to absorb and synthesise the intercellular substance of the ligament connective tissue, alveolar bone and cementum (Carranza, 1983; Figueiredo & Parra, 2002).

In cases where the complete avulsion of tooth occurs, there is a possibility of reintegration of the tooth to the body (Pieri, 2004) if it returns to the alveolus quickly, since the periodontal ligament has ability to rejoin the cementum (Harvey & Orr, 1990). In these cases the endodontic treatment should be performed since the apical vascularisation of the tooth was ruptured (Pieri, 2004).

3. Periodontal disease

Periodontal disease is a condition that affects the periodontium, therefore the structures that surrounds the teeth, whose role is to protect and provide support to it (De Marco & Gioso, 1997). It is an infectious disease (Mitchell, 2005) that affects more than 80% of dogs (Riggio, 2011), and climbing to about 85% of dogs over four years old (Roman et al., 1995; De Marco & Gioso, 1997). This fact makes it the most prevalent disease in dogs (Harvey & Emily, 1993; Gioso & Carvalho, 2004; Mitchell, 2005). It has been described as a multifactorial infection with aetiological factors such as bacterial plaque, microflora, immune status, the amount of saliva, breed, age, routine of prophylactic cleaning and type of food. However, plaque is the primary aetiological agent, which consists predominantly of gram-positive, aerobic, non-motile bacteria early in the infection, and anaerobic, gram-negative and motile bacteria in the later stages of infection (Harvey & Emily, 1993; Gioso, 2007).

The disease is caused by the accumulation of bacterial plaque on teeth and gingiva (Harvey & Emily, 1993; Gioso & Carvalho, 2004), by toxic metabolism products of these microorganisms and the host immune response against infection (Mitchell, 2005) that triggers the inflammatory process. Initially this process affects only the gingiva tissue, which characterises the gingivitis that later may worsen and develop into a process of periodontitis which involves changes in other periodontium tissues and can cause bone, periodontal ligament, and in some cases, cementum or even tooth loss (Harvey & Emily, 1993).

Bacterial plaque is a sticky, yellowish material that colonises the entire mouth (Gioso, 2007), the faces of the teeth in their enamel structure (Slee & O'Connor, 1983; Katsura et al., 2001) and gingival sulcus (Domingues et al., 1999). This plaque is a biofilm (Dupont, 1997; Roza, 2004) or an undefined microbial community associated with the tooth surface (Wilderer; Charaklis, 1989, Lang et al., 1997), and is considered the leading cause of pathological process (aetiologic agent) (Tanzer et al. 1977; McPhee & Cowley, 1981). The plaque has as its main constituents: salivary glycoproteins, minerals, oral bacteria, extracellular polysaccharides that adhere to the tooth surface, desquamated epithelial cells, leukocytes, macrophages and lipids (Harvey & Emily, 1993; Roza, 2004)

Initially there is a pellicle formation upon the tooth surfaces and other areas of the mouth, called attached pellicle, which is an organic film derived from the saliva that, at first, has no micro-organisms (Sans & Newman, 1997). In the acquired pellicle begins the formation of a biofilm through the adhesion of the first microorganisms that are mostly gram-positive aerobic bacteria (Figure 2) (Lang et al. 1997; Sans & Newman, 1997; Gioso, 2007), mainly of the *Streptococcus* genus, which produce an exopolysaccharide, a substance that acts like a "glue", facilitating the attachment of these bacteria to the surfaces in question (Wiggs & Lobprise, 1997; Gioso, 2007; Roza, 2004) especially in places where there are small irregularities, cracks or roughness (Sans & Newman, 1997).

The first layer is usually single-celled and appears irregularly distributed on the tooth surface. With the microbial growth, the layer starts to come out of these areas of irregularities onto the enamel surface and increases in volume. The isolated plaques start to coalesce, forming a single plate. Over time in the process of plaque formation, a new phase is present, where new microbial strains with less ability to adhere to tooth structure, adhere to the already formed plaque, featuring new microcolonies and increasing the biodiversity of the plaque (Figure 2) (Sans & Newman, 1997). This process is called the organisation of the bacterial plaque, in which the bacteria need approximately 24 to 48 hours to get organised enough to cause the disease (Gioso, 2007). At this stage, the fight against bacterial plaque, with the simple disruption of it, is able to stall and reverse the process (Slee et al., 1983).

According to the location, the plaque can be classified as supra or sub-gingival. The supragingival plaque corresponds mainly to microbial aggregates found on tooth surfaces (mostly in the gingival third of the crown), however may extend into the gingival sulcus, where they are in immediate contact with the marginal gingiva. The subgingival plaque corresponds to bacterial aggregates found entirely within the gingival sulcus or periodontal pockets (Harvey & Emily 1993).

The bacterial constituents present in dental plaque are modified according to the disease evolution. In healthy gingiva, the cocci represent nearly two-thirds of the bacteria, followed by non-motile small rods. The bacteria present are mostly gram-positive and there is no significant representation of more virulent bacterial types. A new work from Federal University of Viçosa, Brazil, identified bacteria that are present in initial supra-gingival plaque in ten young dogs and found the genera *Streptococcus*, *Staphylococcus* and *Enterococcus* as the main components (personal data). At the stage of gingivitis, the gram-positive rods (non-motile) gradually increase, surpassing the cocci, and the number of gram-negative bacteria also grows. This change continues to go on until the periodontium involvement phase (periodontitis), when the more pathogenic gram-negative microorganisms become the majority, so that the spirochetes represent almost half of the bacteria, while gram-positives are underrepresented (Niezengard et al., 1997; Riggio et al., 2011).

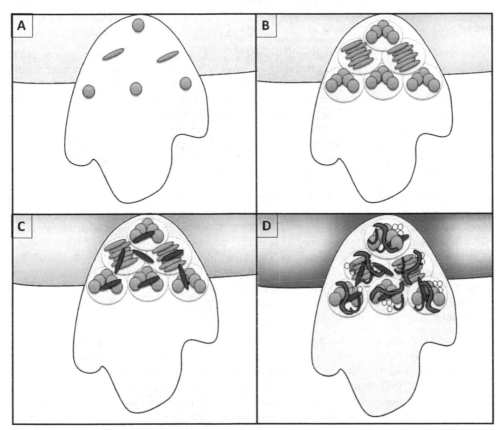

Fig. 2. Formation phases of dental plaque: A) Adhesion of Gram-positive cocci and rods; B) cellular proliferation and exopolysaccharide production; C) adhesion of Gram-negative bacteria; D) maturation of plaque with increase of bacterial biodiversity.

Without interference in the plaque formation an inflammatory process can occur, which marks the beginning of a periodontal disease and that provides a favourable environment for change in the microbial composition of the plaque, that become a biofilm with more pathogenic characteristics, continuing with later stages of the disease (Sans & Newman, 1997; Loesche & Grossman, 2001; Gioso, 2007).

The main bacteria involved in the formation of dental plaque are *Streptococcus* sp. (Gibbons, 1972; Tanzer et al. 1974; Duchin & Houte, 1978; Slee & O'Connor, 1983; Slee et al. 1983; Corner et al., 1988; Murray et al., 1992; Harvey & Emily, 1993; Lang et al., 1997; Loesche &

Grossman, 2001; Katsura et al., 2001; Drummond et al., 2004; Swerts et al., 2005), *Actinomyces* sp. (Slee & O'Connor, 1983; Katsura et al., 2001), and *Lactobacillus* sp. (Drummond et al. 2004; Roza, 2004). These colonise initially the adhered film of the enamel and then start to multiply and aggregate. Thereafter, surface receptors on the cocci and gram-positive rods allow adherence of gram-negative bacteria and, over time, they present the greatest biodiversity and pathogenic potential (Lang et al., 1997). In dogs, the most important bacteria of this group are *Veillonella, Bacterioides, Prevotella* (Domingues et al., 1999), *Fusobacterium* (Murray et al., 1992; Braga et al., 2005) and *Porphyromonas* (Domingues et al., 1999; Katsura et al., 2001; Braga et al., 2005; Senhorinho et al., 2011).

The bacteria involved in the periodontal disease process may migrate to other regions of the body by bacteraemia and colonise there, causing various diseases such as endocarditis, nephritis (Harvey & Emily, 1993; Debowes, 1996; Gioso, 2007), hepatitis (Debowes, 1996; Gioso, 2007) and myocarditis (Harvey & Emily, 1993). Another disease that can be caused by the microorganisms involved in periodontal disease, is a pathological process known as periodontic-endodontic lesion. There is an infection and inflammation of the dental pulp caused by the migration of periodontal bacteria at the apex of the tooth and root canal penetration through the foramen, which are small holes through which the vascular supply, lymphatics and nerves of the tooth passes (Pieri, 2004).

In dogs, the progression of periodontal disease can be divided into stages based on the clinical appearance of the gingiva (classified according to an index ranging from zero degree representing healthy gingiva, to four, when there is severe involvement of it (Roza, 2004; Mitchell, 2005) and loss of adherence of the periodontium, which is measured by inserting a millimeter probe into the gingival sulcus. This measure represents how much the junctional epithelium has migrated toward the apex of the tooth. The result in millimeters is the distance between the bottom of the gingival sulcus or periodontal pocket to the cementoenamel junction. The rate of adhesion loss is expressed by the ratio between the loss and the total normal adhesion (Mitchell, 2005).

In the process of disease formation, the healthy periodontium is considered stage 0 (Figure 3) (Harvey & Emily, 1993) when the gingiva presents a uniform colour, the bacterial plaque is imperceptible and there are little pathogenic characteristics, and there is no halitosis (De Marco & Gioso, 1997). With the increase in bacterial plaque and its change regarding the amount and specificity of the present microorganisms, such as its pathogenicity, begins to emerge an inflammation that marks the beginning of periodontal disease itself, which can be divided into stages of gingivitis (stage 1), initial periodontitis (stage 2), moderate periodontitis (stage 3) and severe periodontitis (stage 4) (Harvey & Emily, 1993).

The first stage of periodontal disease begins with the emergence of bacteria which, through its metabolites, cause inflammation of the gingival tissue, called gingivitis (Figure 3 and Figure 4). This is the first defence of the tooth, without much pathogenicity and without damaging the structures of the support periodontium. Such inflammation is similar to that seen in other connective tissues. Vasodilation, leukocyte marginalisation, cell migration, production of prostaglandins and destructive enzymes also occurs (Gioso, 2007), making the gingiva red, swollen and painful, and may cause halitosis (De Marco & Gioso, 1997). At this stage the possibility of regression of the disease remains through the proper management of the oral health of the animal with measures such as brushing, promoting removal of the aetiological agent (bacterial plaque) (Gorrel & Rawlings, 1996; Gioso, 2007). At this moment it is also possible to use mouthwash in conjunction with brushing to obtain increased efficiency of bacterial removal (Clarke, 2001). Periodontal disease can remain in this state or progress to the loss of insertion of the gingiva to the tooth, thus, the loss of the junctional epithelium adhesion and consequently the formation of periodontal pockets characterising the beginning of the pathologic stage called initial periodontitis (Hennet, 2002).

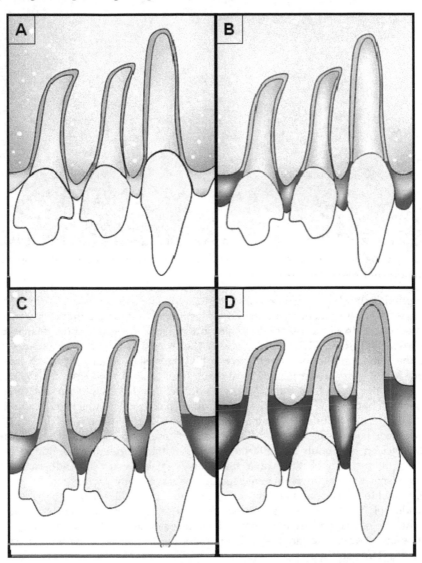

Fig. 3. Periodontal disease progression: A) healthy periodontium; B) gingivitis; C) Initial periodontitis – begins with the loss of periodontal tissue; D) moderate and severe periodontitis - The loss of periodontal tissue is more severe (25 to 50% loss) and the gum can appear cyanotic..

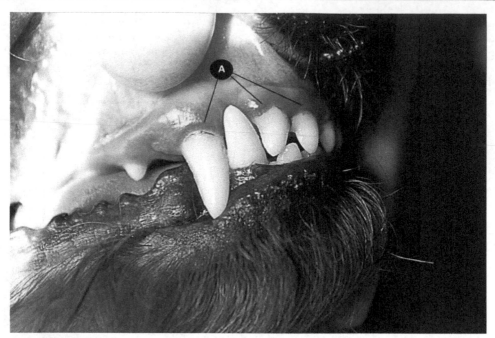

Fig. 4. Dog with gingivitis: A) red line on the cervical region of the tooth indicating gingival inflammation in a two years old poodle

Initial periodontitis (Figure 3) is a sequel of the untreated gingivitis. It is the phase that begins with loss of the junctional epithelium insertion considered the first irreversible phase of the disease, and from this point it becomes only possible to stabilise it (De Marco & Gioso, 1997; Gioso, 2007; Roza, 2004). This phase is the extension of the inflammatory process toward the supporting periodontium (periodontal ligament, cementum and alveolar bone) and leads to progressive destruction of the reported tissues (Harvey & Emily, 1993; Hennet, 2002). The gingiva is still in its normal topography and may have slight gingival recession in some breeds, but when it is very sore it may bleed when touched. There is mild inflammation in the periodontal ligament and little evidence of bone loss (Harvey & Emily, 1993). Intensive halitosis is presented (De Marco & Gioso, 1997). There is also the formation of dental calculus, commonly called tartar, which is nothing more than the mineralisation of dental plaque by salts of the saliva that makes it easier for the adherence of new microorganisms with more pathogenic features, subsequently increasing the severity of injuries caused to the periodontal tissues. The amount of calculus should not be used for the classification of the disease, since it is not the aetiologic agent, but the bacterial plaque. Large amounts of calculus are not indicative of the stage of the disease, and the diagnosis must be established in the gingival poll to assess the loss of adhesion of the epithelium (Gioso, 2007; Roza, 2004).

Moderate (Figure 5) and severe (Figure 6) periodontitis are the most advanced stages of periodontal disease and differ only in the degree of injury (Harvey & Emily, 1993). Some authors do not report the presence of moderate periodontitis, considering only the severe periodontitis after the initial process of aggression to the support tissues of the teeth (De

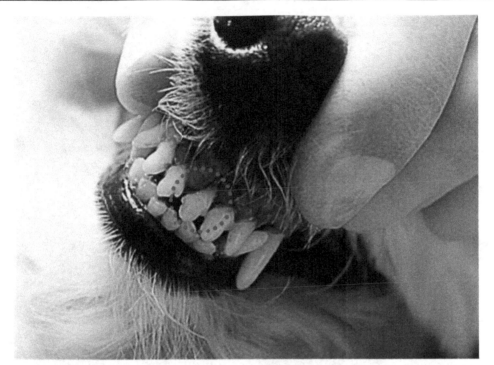

Fig. 5. Into de red circle: root exposure in the upper left central incisor, indicating moderate periodontitis in a poodle with five years.

Marco & Gioso, 1997). In these stages the microbiota of dental plaque is completely different from the initial one, having only a small amount of non-motile gram-positive cocci and large percentages of motile gram-negative spirochetes, virtually absent in healthy individuals (Niezengard et al., 1997). This phase shows severe inflammation, eventually cyanotic (Figure 3), with bleeding in response to the minimum stimulus, greater accumulation of bacterial plaque, intense halitosis (De Marco & Gioso, 1997), mild (in moderate) or large (in severe) tooth mobility (Harvey & Emily, 1993), and in most cases, there is also receding gingiva and a large accumulation of dental calculus. The bacteria enter the bloodstream and cause damage to the heart, liver, kidneys, joints and other organs (De Marco & Gioso, 1997; Gioso, 2007). In moderate periodontitis, there is between a 25 and 50% loss of supporting periodontium (which can be masked by large gingival hyperplasia in some animals), creating the need for treatment and care for the maintenance of the teeth in the socket. In severe periodontitis there is a loss of more than 50% of the supporting periodontal tissue and furcation may be exposed in multirooted teeth and in many cases leading to exfoliation of teeth (Harvey & Emily, 1993).

4. Prevention of periodontal disease

Prevention s considered essential for the maintenance of the animals' teeth throughout their lives, making it impossible for the formation of the periodontal disease process (Lyon, 1991). Brushing, chewable products, promoters of friction and the use of antimicrobial substances

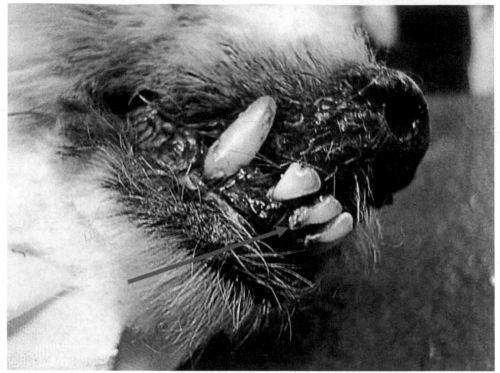

Fig. 6. At the end of the red arrow: extensive root exposure with dental calculus in the lower right medial incisor, indicating severe periodontitis in an old mongrel dog.

are considered preventive techniques that remove supra and sub-gingival plaque. The effectiveness of the preventive technique should be monitored by a veterinarian and in most cases will require their intervention, performing dental prophylaxis in order to eliminate residual plaque and calculus in places of difficult access in the teeth (Lima et al., 2004).

The tooth brushing (Figure 7), which acts by removing the biofilm through friction (Dupont, 1998), is considered a technique with greater effect to reduce the buildup of plaque on the tooth (Hennet, 2002). The frequency of tooth brushing in the animals should be daily, to constantly avoid the formation of dental plaque (Niemiec, 2008) and to establish a routine between the owner and the animal. However, because less than 10% of owners agree with these recommendations for the dental care of their dogs (Lima et al., 2004) and because of the time required for the organisation of the plaque, dog tooth brushing procedure has been recommended three times a week with satisfactory results (Dupont, 1998; Niemiec, 2008).

There are numerous veterinary toothbrushes on the market today, but a child brush with soft bristles is considered effective for removal of the biofilm in dogs. Many veterinary toothpastes are also available, with flavours to facilitate animal acceptance of the brushing, besides the fact that it increases friction promoted with brushing (Niemiec, 2008). It is clear, however, that the use of correct brushing techniques minimises the need for this additive effect of toothpaste on the attrition of the teeth (Lima et al., 2004). Antimicrobial substances

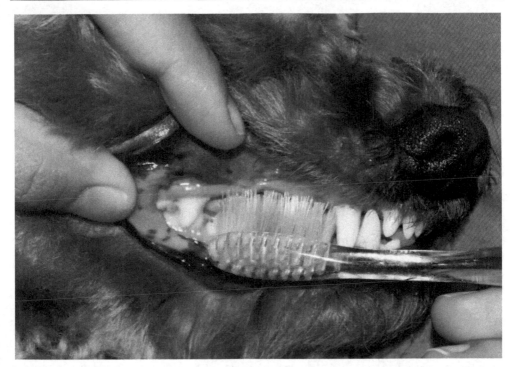

Fig. 7. Dog's Tooth brushing by an owner.

may also help in effective biofilm removal (Jensen et al., 1995; Lima et al. 2004; Niemiec, 2008), used in conjunction with a toothbrush, added to toothpaste or employed as solutions, minimising the ineffective brushing technique in some inaccessible places in the animal's mouth.

The brushing technique should be used properly because inappropriate use can increase the prevalence of periodontal disease, as occurs in humans (Jongenelis & Wiedemann, 1997). One of the indicated techniques uses circular movements on the dental surfaces, with the brush tilted at an angle of 45 ° from the gingival margin (Niemiec, 2008).

Some studies have been conducted with the intention of establishing new therapies to combat dental plaque accumulation on the face of the tooth, both for the aid in brushing as for the use as a preventive agent of choice against periodontal disease when the practice of brushing is inefficient, as in wayward animals that do not allow the mechanical handling of oral practices (Gioso & Carvalho, 2004; Pieri, 2010).

Various forms of introduction of these therapies in the animal management have been tested, including the use of cookies and chewing objects for oral hygiene (Gioso & Carvalho, 2004; Niemiec, 2008), additives to drinking water with an inhibitory effect on the growth of bacteria (Clarke, 2006) and oral rinse solutions as well as leather and biscuits with the addition of antimicrobial agents (Addy, 1997; Niemiec, 2008).

Topical application of a drug to control the disease is considered desirable, in view of the lower incidence of side effects when compared to other routes of application. For the prevention of periodontal disease, taking into account the least harmful nature of bacteria in the onset of the disease and higher prevalence of supragingival plaque, it is recommended that the use of topical oral solutions such as mouthwashes is sufficient to combat bacteria in question with great advantage because of its easy application in most patients (Ciancio & Niezengard, 1997).

Among the chemicals, that can be used this way to reduce the accumulation of plaque on dental surfaces, the bisguanids, quaternary ammonia and phenols have been widely evaluated. Chlorhexidine appears as a substance that has the greatest efficacy in the inhibition of oral plaque (Hennet, 2002) and has good antiseptic activity against all oral pathogens, more directly on the bacterial plaque organisms (Harvey & Emily, 1993). Its main concentration is the commercial use of alcoholic solution at 0.12% and it is also found in alcohol-free solutions and in gel form (Robinson, 1995).

Despite the above indications for the use of chlorhexidine in the fight against dental plaque, it presents a series of unpleasant effects when used for prolonged therapy, such as loss of taste by the patient, pigmentation of the enamel, burning and even ulceration of the buccal mucosa (Zanini et al., 1995). These effects justify the use of this material only for few days (Gioso, 2007), which makes its application not recommended in the prevention of periodontal disease, which requires a prolonged use of the antimicrobial agent chosen for this purpose (Lascala & Moussalli, 1995).

The natural sweetener xylitol has been used in human patients in chewing gum, mouthwashes and toothpastes in order to reduce plaque. There is also one xylitol based product in the veterinary market today, which when added to the animal drinking water has a lowering effect on oral bacterial plaque formation (Dunayer & Gwaltney-Brant, 2006).

Recently, the ozonised sunflower oil was tested, with positive results on microbial reduction in human patients with periodontal disease (Fiorini et al., 2006) and copaiba oil was applied topically on dogs and the results were equal to those obtained with chlorhexidine on the oral microbial population (Pieri, 2010). Additionally, some in vitro tests were performed to analyse the antimicrobial activity of Copaiba oil on plaque-forming bacteria (Simões, 2004; Pieri, 2010; Valdevite et al., 2007) and the evaluation of the inhibition of *Streptococcus* sp. adherence in glass capillaries caused by the same phytotherapic (Pieri, 2010), obtaining in both cases positive results. A actual work has been conduced to evaluate the copaiba oil as antimicrobial against bacterial isolates from initial dental plaque of dogs, aiming identify a potential drug to prevent the plaque formation and consequently the periodontal disease (personal data).

Many researchers continue their analysis looking for natural drugs as propolis (Swerts et al., 2005), *Camellia sinensis* (Chang et al., 2009), *Mimosa tenuiflora* (Macedo-Costa, 2009), *Vitis amurensis* (Yim et al., 2010), *Rhinacanthus nasutus* (Puttarak et al., 2010), *Murraya koenigii*, *Allium sativum* and *Melaleuca alternifolia* (Prabhakar et al., 2009) to its use in the prevention of periodontal disease by inhibiting plaque formation.It important that this drug combine properties such as antimicrobial activity that does not induce bacterial resistance, and inhibition of microbial adherence on tooth surfaces that suggest a great potential for use in therapies in the oral cavity and as an aid in oral hygiene (Sudo et al., 1986; Corner et al., 1988; Pieri, 2010). For the use in the treatment of domestic animals it is suggested the inclusion of this antimicrobial and non-adherent agent in formulations containing the base flavours of chicken, beef, fish, etc. (De Marco & Gioso, 1997).

5. Diagnosis

The diagnosis of periodontal disease is based on history, clinical examination and radiological evaluation. Any changes in apprehension and chewing of food, as well as in general conditions and in the behaviour of animals, can be associated with oral disorders. Certain physical and behavioral changes are highly suggestive of dental disorders, including abnormal ways of eating and drinking, acute reactions to the ingestion of cold water, selective appetite (preference for soft foods), anorexia and weight loss, salivation, bleeding, epitaxy, digging of the ground, behavior of rubbing their feet on the face, shaking of the head, oronasal fistulas, abnormal aggressive behavior (because of pain) and distress and anguish (Emily & Penman, 1994; Pachaly, 2006; Gorrel, 2004). When it comes to periodontal disease, the main complaint of the owner will always be halitosis (Emily & Penman, 1994; Gorrel, 2004; Gioso, 2007) due to tissue decay and bacterial fermentation in the sulcus or periodontal pocket (Gioso, 2007).

Like any other clinical examination, the examination in dentistry should be preceded by thorough history and general physical examination. At the end, the oral cavity should be examined. It is necessary to do a complete oral examination to assess the presence of periodontal disease and other diseases, such as fractures or dental malocclusions. The intra- and extraoral structures should be assessed, including bone surfaces, the jaw muscles, salivary glands and regional cervical lymph nodes (Gorrel., 2004). Ideally, the complete periodontal examination should be performed in anaesthetised dogs (Harvey, 1992; Gorrel, 2004; Gioso, 2007). The evaluation of the tooth must be made with an explorer and periodontal probe (Gioso, 2007). The examination must be careful; incorrect handling of the probe may damage the soft tissues and lead to misdiagnosis of periodontal lesions (Gorrel, 2004). The changes observed should be recorded in an appropriate medical record and serve as the basis for the therapeutic treatment (Pachaly, 2006).

The periodontal examination includes the evaluation of teeth mobility, of injuries or furcation exposure, gingival retracting or hyperplasia, the evaluation of the depth, the presence of dental plaque, of gingivitis and dental calculus The furcation is the area between the roots of teeth that have more than one root. This area is usually filled with alveolar bone. During exploration, a depression can be felt while passing the extremity of a probe perpendicular to the tooth crown and below the gingival margin. In the presence of periodontitis, the furcation bone can be resorbed and probe inserted between the roots. Changes in the furcation are classified on a scale ranging from 0 to 3, where in grade 3 lesions the probe passes freely through the furcation, from the vestibular part to the lingual/palatal tooth (Gorrel, 2004).

The gingival sulcus is the space between the free gingiva and the tooth crown. In dogs, the depth of the gingival sulcus should be less than 3mm, and in giant breed dogs less than 4 mm (Gioso, 2007). When periodontitis is established, the junctional epithelium, the region of the gingival tissue inserted to the tooth surface, migrates apically along the root. If the apical migration is not accompanied by a receding gingiva then the periodontal pocket is formed, which has a depth greater than 3mm (Gorrel, 2004). Values above 3 mm mean loss of clinical attachment of the junctional epithelium with bone destruction (periodontitis) and periodontal pocket formation (Gioso, 2007)

The periodontal probe is essential in the examination and diagnosis of periodontal disease. This thin probe has a tip calibrated in millimetres, measuring the depth of the gingival sulcus when it is inserted between the gingiva and the tooth (Grove, 1998). The probe depth is defined as the distance between the coronal margin of the free gingiva and apical junctional epithelium (Gorrel, 2004). It is measured by positioning the tip of the periodontal probe parallel to the long axis of the tooth (or following the contour of the crown), and gently inserting between the teeth and free gingiva until the bottom of the sulcus is felt. In cases of gingival recession, periodontal destruction usually does not cause the formation of periodontal pockets. Gingival recession is measured in millimetres from the cementoenamel junction, where the gingival attachment should be normally at the gingival margin. The most profound measure for each tooth must be registered in the dental chart. Normally the junctional epithelium is located near the cementoenamel junction. In cases of gingival hyperplasia, in other words, in the presence of excessive amounts of soft tissues, the pseudopocket formed is measured with the probe, defined as the distance between the junctional epithelium and gingival margin. Since the areas deeper than 5 mm are difficult to clean mechanically, surgery might be needed to remove the deep pockets and pseudopockets, depending on the care undertaken by the owner (Gorrel, 2004).

The accumulation of dental deposits (plaque and calculus) and the severity of gingivitis can be quantified by standardised indices that correspond to the numerical expression of the presence or absence of disease severity. These indexes are extremely useful when there is a need for assessment of periodontal disease. The accumulation of plaque and calculus can be quantified in terms of coverage or thickness for all teeth (Gorrel, 2004).

The plaque is not always visible to the dental inspection, therefore solutions that highlight the plaque may be used (Gorrel, 2004; Gioso, 2007). The calculus is evident, presenting as a hard mass on the tooth surface, intra-or extra-sulcular, yellowish, brownish, sometimes greenish, which is not removed by scraping or brushing with gauze. The calculus most frequently occurs in fourth premolar and first superior molar teeth, as close to them are the openings of the parotid ducts and zygomatic glands, however, over time, almost all teeth can be affected (Gioso, 2007).

Bleeding during the survey, which indicates an inflammatory process in the connective tissues within the junctional epithelium, is a particularly useful method for evaluating an active gingivitis (Grove, 1998). Dogs rarely show signs of pain due to periodontal disease, even when there is loss of many teeth or exposed root dentine, which can cause sensitivity. There may be ulcers on the buccal mucosa (cheek) or on the tongue, because of the direct contact with areas of severe periodontal disease (Gioso, 2007). However, to form a definitive diagnosis, loss of tooth support must be present (Grove, 1998). The full-mouth radiographic examination is mandatory for patients with periodontal disease to get information from bone and periodontal structures (Gorrel, 2004). The results obtained by clinical and radiographic examinations are complementary and the diagnosis requires the completion of both (Harvey & Emily, 1993). Although radiographs provide essential data for determining the state of periodontal disease, this diagnostic test has low sensitivity to assess the progression of periodontitis. This is due to the inability to accurately repeat the positions, exposure and development time. Thus, any comparison between two different radiographs of the same animal becomes limited (Gorrel, 2004).

Radiographs are evaluated for changes in alveolar bone, interdental bone height, presence of lamina dura, trabecular pattern, periodontal ligament and severity of bone loss. X-rays show two-dimensional representation of three-dimensional structures. Sometimes, the radiographs do not show adequately the severity of the disease. Early lesions of bone destruction are sometimes not observed radiographically. Buccal and lingual alveolar bones are particularly difficult to assess because of the overlap. In addition to the radiological findings, the clinician must rely on clinical examination, including sulcular depths, tooth mobility, and gingival appearance, in order to decide on the diagnosis and treatment plan (Bellows, 2001).

The earliest radiographic sign of periodontitis is loss of definition of the bone ridge. In healthy animals, the bony ridge appears as a radiopaque line, which follows one or two millimetres in the apical direction, in parallel to an imaginary line drawn between the cementoenamel junction of two adjacent teeth (Harvey, 1992). This loss of definition of the bone ridge is always accompanied by progressive demineralisation of the lamina dura (Harvey & Emily, 1993). Other radiographic signs of periodontal disease include rounding of the alveolar margin, the discontinuity of the lamina dura, widening of the periodontal space and the gradual disappearance of the alveolar bone (Gorrel, 2004).

In some cases, pathological fractures of the jaw are seen as a consequence of severe bone loss. This situation occurs especially in small breed dogs, typically in the inferior first molar, whose roots reach the ventral cortex of the lower jaw (Gorrel, 2004).

Once the diagnosis is established, treatment plan should be developed that will range from just dental curettage and polishing to extraction. In some situations the extraction of the involved tooth is the best treatment option, especially if the loss of adhesion and mobility is very pronounced. However, for moderate disease cases there are a variety of other treatment strategies (Wiggs & Lobprise, 1997).

6. Treatment

Harvey and Emily (1993) described that the goal of periodontal treatment is to control microorganisms, restore normal anatomy and physiology and avoid new adhesion of bacterial plaque on tooth surfaces. Furthermore, periodontal pockets should be eliminated and re-adhesion of tissue to the tooth should be promoted, aiming, wherever possible, to do this by destroying the minimum of healthy tissue and keeping the gingiva.

The periodontal soft tissues quickly re-adhere to the cementum after the debridement, which removes the dead space of the pocket. However, this union could be weaker than the original depending on the type of tissue that repopulates the root surface; gingival epithelium, gingival connective tissue, alveolar bone and periodontal ligament; the latter being more desirable. When replacement by the alveolar bone occurs, the result is root resorption or ankylosis. Epithelium and gingival connective tissue are not desirable because they are extremely weak. Grafts or barrier materials can be used to delay or exclude the gingival tissue growth, favouring the growth of periodontal ligament growth (Wiggs & Lobprise, 1997).

According to Gioso (2007), treatment is based on the elimination of plaque or calculus, normal gingival depth restoration and monitoring through a preventive program. General anaesthesia is essential to perform the scraping and it is a procedure that can last around 2 to 3 hours in more advanced cases. The main treatment options for periodontal curettage are supragingival curettage, subgingival curettage, root planing, gingivectomy, gingivoplasty and gingival grafts.

Manfra-Marretta et al. (1992) highlighted the importance of subgingival curettage, where the plaques accumulated in the marginal gingiva that cause inflammation and affect the supporting structures of the tooth are removed. A curette to subgingival scrapping may be used. In some cases it is necessary to do a gingivectomy of periodontal pockets.

After removing all of the dental calculus, teeth must undergo a polishing with a rubber cup. It is not necessary to put a lot of pressure on the tooth and polishing should not exceed 15 seconds per tooth (Manfra-Marretta et al., 1992).

If there is severe bone loss, with roots exposure, an elevation of a gingival flap, complete curettage and displacement of the gingival margin closer to the apex of the tooth may be necessary, followed by fixating it with sutures. In the case of failure of this treatment, the extraction is the next step (Gioso, 2007).

Some surgical techniques are also indicated in the treatment of periodontal disease. According to Gioso (2007), when the periodontal pocket has more than 2 mm depth, partial gingivectomy is indicated, eliminating the pocket and re-forming the normal depth of the gingival sulcus (gingivoplasty). Another indication of the gingivectomy is gingival hyperplasia. In this surgery, excess gingiva is excised with a scalpel blade or electrocautery, which controls bleeding and is therefore preferred.

Another surgical technique described is the simple gingiva flap (or retail), which is indicated to obtain access to deeper periodontal structures through the creation of mucogingival flap. For its realisation an incision along the longitudinal axis of the root should be made, preserving the interdental papillae. Subsequently, the gingival flap should be completely translocated with the aid of a periosteum elevator and then root planing and repair of bone defects should be proceeded with. At the end of the procedure the flap should be sutured to its source with separate sutures (Wiggs & Lobprise, 1997).

The sliding flap can also be done in order to cover the root in cases of secondary exposure to gingival defect or periodontal disease. In order to do this an adjacent donor site must be identified and a flap at least 2.5 times wider than the defect to be covered must be created. The flap should contain full thickness of the epithelium and connective tissues. The periosteum should be maintained at the donor site, which will be left exposed. The proceeding finishes with the lateral slip of the flap and its suturing with simple interrupted technique, with stitches 1.5 mm apart, in its receptor place (Wiggs & Lobprise, 1997). This surgical technique is also indicated for closure of oronasal fistulas, which are abnormal communications between the oral and nasal cavities. In these cases it is very important to provide hermetic sealing of the suture without tension (Bolson & Pachaly, 2004).

7. Acknowledgments

The authors would like to thank Pró-Reitoria de Extensão e Cultura from Federal University of Viçosa (UFV), FAPEMIG (Fundação de Amparo à Pesquisa do Estado de Minas Gerais), CAPES (Coordenação de Aperfeiçoamento de Pessoal de Nível Superior) and CNPq (Conselho Nacional de Desenvolvimento Científico e Tecnológico) for financial support8.
References

Addy, M. (1997). Anti-sépticos na terapia periodontal. In: Lindhe J. *Tratado de periodontia clínica e implantologia oral*. 3ed. p.332-349, Guanabara Koogan, Rio de Janeiro..

Bellows, J. (2001) *All pets dental - The why, when, and how of small animal dental radiology*. Avaiable from:
http://www.dentalvet.com/vets/basicdentistry/whywhenhow_radiology.htm

Bolson, J.; Pachaly, J.R. (2004) Fístula oronasal em cães (*Canis familiaris* Linnaeus, 1758) – Revisão de literatura. *Arquivos de Ciências Veterinárias e Zoologia*, Vol.7 No.1 pp. 53-56.

Braga, C.; Rezende, C.; Pestana, A.; Carmo, L.; Costa, J.; Silva, L.; Assis, L.; Lima, L.; Farias, L.; Carvalho, M. (2005) Isolamento e Identificação da microbiota periodontal de cães da raça pastor alemão. *Ciência Rural*, Vol.35, pp.385-390.

Carranza, F.A. (1983) *Periodontia Clínica de Glickman*. Editora interamericana, Rio de Janeiro, Brazil.

Chang, H.; Hwang, H.; Kang, E.; Lee, J.; Chung, D.; Yang, W.; Chung, W.; Kim, H. (2009) The effect of Green tea bag in dogs with periodontal disease. *Journal of Veterinary Clinics*, Vol.26, pp.41-47.

Ciancio, S.; Niezengard, R. (1997) Controle e prevenção da doença periodontal In: Niezengard, R.; Newman, M. *Microbiologia oral e imunologia*. 2ed. Guanabara Koogan, pp.309-330, Rio de Janeiro.

Clarke, D.E. (2006) Drinking water additive decreases plaque and calculus accumulation in cats. *Journal of Veterinary Dentistry*, Vol.23, pp.79-82.

Clarke, D.E. (2001) Clinical and microbiological effects of oral zinc ascorbate gel in dogs. *Journal of Veterinary Dentistry*, Vol.18, pp.177-183.

Corner, A.; Dolan, M.M.; Yankell, S.L.; Malamud, D. (1988) C31G, a new agent for oral use with potent antimicrobial and antiadherence properties. *Antimicrobial Agents and Chemotherapy*, Vol.32, pp.350-353.

Debowes, L.; Mosier, D.; Logan, E.; Harvey, C.E.; Lowry, S.; Richardson, D.C. (1996) Association of periodontal disease and histologic lesions in multiple organs from 45 dogs. *Journal of Veterinary Dentistry*, Vol.13, pp.57-60.

De Marco, V.; Gioso, M.A. (1997) Doença periodontal em cães e gatos: profilaxia e manejo dietético. *Clinica Veterinária* (São Paulo), Vol.2, pp.24-28.

Domingues, L.M.; Alessi, A.C.; Schoken-Iturrino, R.P.; Dutra LS (1999) Microbiota saprófita associada à doença periodontal em cães. *Arquivo Brasileiro de Medicina Veterinária e Zootecnia*, Vol.51, pp.329-332.

Drumond, M.R.; Castro, R.D.; Almeida, R.V.; Pereira, M.S.; Padilha, W.W. (2004) Comparative study in vitro of the antibacterial activity from phytotherapeutic products against cariogenical bacteria. *Pesquisa Brasileira em Odontopediatria e Clínica Integrada*, Vol.4, pp.33-38.

Duchin S; Houte V (1978) Colonization of teeth in humans by Streptococcus mutans as related to its concentration in saliva and host age. *Infection and Immunity*,Vol.20, pp.120-125.

Dunayer, E.K.; Gwaltney-Brant, S.M. (2006) Acute hepatic failure and coagulopathy associated with xylitol ingestion in eight dogs. *Journal of the American Veterinary Medical Association*, Vol.229, pp.1113-1117.

Dupont, G.A. (1997) Understanding dental plaque: biofilm dynamics. *Journal of Veterinary Dentistry*, Vol.14, pp.91-94.

Dupont, G.A. (1998) Prevention of periodontal disease. *Veterinary Clinics of North American: small animal practice*, Vol.28, pp.1129-1145.

Emily PP; Penman S (1994) *Handbook of small animal dentistry*. Pergamon, p.35-53, Oxford.

Figueiredo, M.C.; Parra, S.L. (2002) *Aspectos normais da membrana periodontal e osso alveolar*. Avaiable from: http://www.odontologia.com.br.

Fiorini, J.M.; Cardoso, C.; Macedo, S.; Schneedorf, J.M.; Fiorini, J.E. (2006) Ação do óleo ozonizado como coadjuvante na terapia da doença periodontal. *Revista Internacional de Periodontia Clínica*, Vol.3, pp.55-99.

Ford, R.B.; Mazzaferro, E.M. (2007) *Manual de procedimentos veterinários e tratamento emergencial segundo Kirk e Bistner*. Editora Roca, pp.279-365, São Paulo.

Gibbons, R.J. (1972) Ecology and cariogenic potential of oral streptococci. In: Wannamaker, L.W.; Matsen, J. *Streptococci and streptococcal diseases*. Academic press Inc, pp.371-385, New York.

Gioso, M.A. (2007) *Odontologia para o clínico de pequenos animais*. Ed.Manole, São Paulo.

Gioso, M.A.; Carvalho, V.G. (2004) Métodos Preventivos para a manutenção da boa saúde bucal em cães e gatos. *Clínica Veterinária (São Paulo)*, Vol.9, pp.68-76.

Gorrel, C.; Rawlings, J.M. (1996) The role of dental hygiene chew in maintaining periodontal health in dogs. *Journal of Veterinary Dentistry*, Vol.13, pp.31-34.

Gorrel, C. (2004) *Veterinary dentistry for the general practitioner*. W.B. Saunders, pp.87- 110, Philadelphia.

Grove, T.K. (1998) Treatment of periodontal disease. *Veterinary Clinics North American*: small anim pract, Vol.28, No.5, pp.1147-1164,

Harvey, C.E. (1992) Distúrbios orais, faringianos e das glândulas salivares. In: Ettinger, S.J. *Tratado de medicina interna veterinária*. Ed. Manole, pp.1265-1290, São Paulo.

Harvey, C.; Emily, P. (1993) *Small Animal Dentistry*. Mosby – year book inc, St. Louis.

Harvey, C.E.; Orr, S. (1990) *Manual of small animal dentistry*. British small animal veterinary association, Cheltenham;

Harvey, C.; Shofer, F.S.; Laster, L. (1994) Association of age and body weight with periodontal disease in north American dogs. *Journal of Veterinary Dentistry*, Vol.11, pp.94-105.

Hennet, P. (1995) Dental anatomy and physiology of small carnivores. In: Crossley, D.A.; Penmann, S. *Manual of Small Animal Dentistry*. British small animal veterinary association pp. 93-104, Cheltenham.

Hennet, P. (2002) Effectiveness of a dental gel to reduce plaque in beagle dogs. *Journal of Veterinary Dentistry*, Vol.19, pp.11-14.

Jensen, L.; Logan, E.; Finney, O.; Lowry, S.; Smith, M.; Hefferren, J.; Simone, A.; Richardson, D. (1995) Resuction in accumulation of plaque, stain, and calculus in dogs by dietary means. *Journal of Veterinary Dentistry*, Vol.12, pp.161-163.

Jongenelis, A.P.; Wiedemann, W (1997) A comparison of plaque removal effectiveness of electric versus a manual toothbrush in children. *Journal of Dentistry for Children*, Vol.64, pp.176-182.

Katsura, H.; Tsukiyama, R.; Suzuky, A.; Kobayashi, M.; (2001) In vitro antimicrobial activities of bakuchiol against oral microorganisms. *Antimicrobial agents and chemotherapy*, Vol.45, pp.3009-3013.

Lang, N.; Mombelli, A.; Attström, R. (1997) Placa e cálculo dentais. In: Lindhe, Jan. *Tratado de periodontia clínica e implantologia oral*. 3.ed. Guanabara Koogan. pp.66-91, Rio de Janeiro.

Lascala, N. T.; Moussalli, N.H. (1995) *Compêndio terapêutico periodontal*. 2.ed. Editora Artes Médicas, São Paulo.

Lima, T.B.; Eurides, D.; Rezende, R. Milken, V; Silva, L.; Fioravanti, M. (2004) Escova dental e dedeira na remoção da placa bacteriana dental em cães. *Ciência Rural*, Vol.34, pp.155-158.

Lindhe, J; Karring, T. (1997) *Tratado de periodontia clínica e implantologia oral*. 3ed. Guanabara Koogan, Rio de Janeiro.

Loesche, W.; Grossman, N. (2001) Periodontal disease as a specific, albeit chronic, infection: diagnosis and treatment. *Clinical Microbiologicals Reviews*, Vol.14, pp.727-752.

Lyon, K.F. (1991) Dental home care. *Journal of Veterinary Dentistry*,Vol.8, pp.26-30.

Macêdo-Costa, M.; Pereira, M.; Pereira, L.; Pereira, A.; Rodriques, O. (2009) Atividade Antimicrobiana do Extrato da mimosa tenuiflora. *Pesquisa Brasileira de Odontopediatria Clínica Integrada*, Vol.9, pp.161-165.

Manfra-Marretta, S.; Cchloss, A.J.; Klippert, L.S. (1992) Classification and prognostic factors of endodontic-periodontic lesions in the dog. *Journal of Veterinary Dentistry*, Vol.9, No.2, pp.27-30.

McPhee, T.; Cowley, G. (1981) *Essentials of periodontology and periodontics*. 3ed. Blackwell scientific, Oxford.

Mitchell, P. (2005) *Odontologia de Pequenos Animais*. Editora Roca, São Paulo.

Murray, P.; Prakobphol, A.; Lee, T.; Hoover, C.; Fisher, S. (1992) Adherence of oral streptococci to salivary glycoproteins. *Infection and Immunity*, Vol.60, pp.31-38.

Newman, M.G.; Carranza, F.A.; Takei, F.A.; Henry, H. (2004) *Periodontia Clínica*. 9.ed. Guanabara Koogan, Rio de Janeiro..

Niemiec, B.A. (2008) Periodontal Therapy. *Topics in Companion Animal Medicine*, Vol.23, pp.81-90.

Niezengard, R.; Newman, M.G.; Zambom, J.J. (1997) Doença Periodontal In: Niezengard, R.; Newman, M.G. *Microbiologia Oral e Imunologia*. 2.ed. Guanabara Koogan. pp.309-330, Rio de Janeiro.

Pachaly, J.R. (2006) Odontoestomatologia. In: Cubas, Z.S.; Silva, J.C.R.; Catão-dias, Z.S. *Tratado de animais selvagens*. Editora Roca, pp. 1068-1091, São Paulo.

Picosse, M. (1987) *Anatomia dentária*. 4.ed. Sarvier, São Paulo.

Pieri, F.A. (2004) *Tratamento endodôntico em pequenos animais*. Faculdade de Medicina Veterinária da Universidade Federal Rural de Pernambuco, Recife. 33p.

Pieri, F.A. (2010) Clinical and microbiological effects of copaiba oil (Copaifera officinalis) on dental plaque forming bacteria in dogs. *Arquivo Brasileiro de Medicina Veterinária e Zootecnia*, Vol 62, No. 3, pp.578-585.

Pope, E.R. (1993) Periodontal and endodontic disease. In: Bojrab, M.J. *Disease Mechanisms in Small Animal Surgery*. 3ed. Lea Febiger, p.187-190, Philadelphia.

Prabhakar, A.R.; Vipin, A.; Basappa, N. (2009) Effect of curry leaves, garlic and tea tree oil on Streptococcus mutans and Lactobacilli in children. *Pesquisa Brasileira de Odontopediatria Clínica Integrada*, Vol.9, pp.259-263.

Puttarak, P.; Charoonratana, T. ; Panichayupakaranant, P. (2010) Antimicrobial activity and stability of rhinacanthins-rich Rhinacanthus nasutus extract. *Phytomedicine*, Vol.17, pp.323-327.

Riggio, M.P.; Lennon, A.; Taylor, D.J.; Bennett, D. (2011) Molecular identification of bacteria associated with canine periodontal disease. *Veterinary Microbiology*, Vol.150, No.3-4, pp. 394-400.

Robinson, J. (1995) Chlorhexidine Gluconate – the solution for dental problems. *Journal of Veterinary Dentistry*, Vol.12, pp.29-31.

Roman, F.S.; Cancio, S.; Cediel, R.; Garcia, P.; Sanches, M. (1995) Periodoncia. *Canis et felis*, Vol.16, pp.37-38.

Roza, M.R. (2004) *Odontologia em pequenos animais*. L.F. Livros de Veterinária, Rio de Janeiro.

Sans, M.; Newman, M.G. (1997) Placa dental e cálculo. In: Niezengard, R.J.; Newman, M.G. (1997) *Microbiologia Oral e Imunologia*. 2.ed. Guanabara Koogan, pp.275-292, Rio de Janeiro.

Senhorinho, G.N.A., Nakano, V., Liu, C., Song, Y., Finegold, S.M., Avila-Campos, M.J. (2011) Detection of Porphyromonas gulae from subgingival biofilms of dogs with and without periodontitis. *Anaerobe*, in press.

Simões, C.A. (2004) Brazilian Patent n°PI0404266-2. Instituto Nacional de Propriedade Industrial, Rio de Janeiro.

Slee, A.; O'Connor, J. (1983) In vitro activity of octenidine dihydrochloride (WIN 41464-2) against preformed plaques of selected oral plaque forming microorganisms. *Antimicrobial Agents and Chemotherapy*, Vol.23, pp.379-384.

Slee, A.; O'Connor, J.; Bailey, D. (1983) Relationship between structure and antiplaque and antimicrobial activities for a series of bispyridines. *Antimicrobial Agents and Chemotherapy*, Vol.23, pp.531-535.

Sudo, S.; Schotzko, N.K.; Floke, L.E. (1976) Use of hydroxyapatite-coated glass beads for preclinical testing of potential antiplaque agents. *Applied and Environmental Microbiology*, Vol.32, pp.428-432.

Swerts, M.S.; Costa, A.M.; Fiorini, J.E. (2005) Efeito da associação de clorexidina e própolis na inibição da aderência de *Streptococcus spp. Revista Internacional de Periodontia Clínica*, Vol.2, pp.10-16.

Tanzer, J.M.; Freedman M.L.; Fitzgerald, R.J.; Larson, R.H. (1974) Diminished virulence of glucan synthesis-defective of *Streptococcus mutans*. *Infection and Immunity*. Vol.16, pp.197-203.

Tanzer JM, Slee A, Kamay B ; Scheer E (1977) In vitro evaluation of three iodine-containing compounds as antiplaque agents. Antimicrobial Agents and Chemotherapy, 12:107-113.

Valdevite, L.M.; Leitão, D.P.; Leite, M.F.; Polizello, A.C.; Freitas, O.; Spadaro, A. (2007) Study of the in vitro effect of copaíba oil upon virulence factors of the cariogenic bacterium Streptococcus mutans. In: Anals of 10th IUBMB Conference e 36ª Reunião Anual da SBBq, Salvador, Brazil.

Wiggs, R.B.; Lobprise, H. (1997) *Veterinary dentistry principles and practice*. Lippincott-Raven, Philadelphia.

Wilderer, P.A.; Charaklis, W.G. (1989) *Structure and function of biofilms*. John Wiley, Chichester.

Yim, N.; Ha, D.; Trung, T.; Kim, J.; Lee, S.; Na, M.; Jung, H.; Kim, H.; Kim, Y.; Bae, K. (2010) The antimicrobial activity of compounds from the leaf and stem of Vitis amurensis against two oral pathogens. *Bioorganic & Medicinal Chemistry Letters*, Vol.20, pp.1165-1168

Zanini, A.C.; Basile, A.C.; Martin, M.I.; Oga, S. (1995) *Guia de Medicamentos*. Atheneu, São Paulo:

8

Continuous Electrocardiography in Dogs and Cats

Guilherme Albuquerque de Oliveira Cavalcanti
Federal University of Minas Gerais,
Brazil

1. Introduction

A new electrocardiogram (ECG) was started in 1961 when J. Norman Holter introduced a system to record the ECG of a patient during their activities for long periods of time. This method was identified as a method of continuous electrocardiography (CE), long-term electrocardiogram, dynamic electrocardiography, ambulatory electrocardiographic, or simply Holter. In subsequent years, the development of technology has introduced a great number of advances and improvements in the fidelity of the recording, size and weight of equipment, systems acquisition and data analysis. The intermittent recording capacity triggered by the owner or by the occurrence of arrhythmia, has become available. Systems to record and reproduce the CE continue to evolve and improvements in the capacity of analysis and editing of commercial systems have frequently been introduced.

The entry of the CE in veterinary medicine contributes to a better understanding of cardiac arrhythmias, to study the cardiac response to drugs and to diagnose heart disease. But before you do the examination, the classic electrocardiographic (ECG) should be performed, because this modality is able to observe the cardiac depolarization for more angles (leads) that the CE.

2. The continuous electrocardiographic in diagnosis support

The most appropriate method to evaluate the heart rate in dogs is the CE system. This test allows assessment of rhythm for 24 hours, while conventional electrocardiography can only do about 0.2% of this period. Thus, this method allows the recognition of rhythm with the animal in different types of activity (sleep, exercise, feeding) and, consequently, under different physiological states.

Currently this method is most widely using the following conditions: a) confirmation of an arrhythmia as the cause of symptoms that occur during daily activities, b) prediction of future cardiac events, c) evidence of therapeutic efficacy of antiarrhythmic agents, d) detection of myocardial ischemia (MacKie et al., 2010).

There are some arrhythmias that occur at intervals greater than 24 hours, in such cases it is recommended either to repeat the exam, or use of cardiac event recorders (CER). When the owner presses a button on the device of CER, for example in the moment when the clinical sign occurs, the device records the moments before, during and after the clinical signs which should be evaluated. The CER device is smaller and can be used for a week or more, but requires constant observation of the animal, although there are some devices that can function as EC conventionally or as CER at the same time.

In humans, medicine is defined in three classes of indications to perform CE: Class I - there is a consensus that the CE is a useful tool and reliable examination, class II - CE is useful and reliable, but there was no consensus, class III – there is consensus that the CE is unnecessary. In all situations in which the role of CE is discussed, it should be taken in account the history and the physical examination of the patient, and the review of the usefulness of the test. The decision to conduct a CE examination and interpretation of their results cannot be performed independently.

The major use of this examination in dogs and cats is to identify the type and degree of cardiac arrhythmias.

Being the main indications:

-   Animals that have unexplained episodes of syncope, collapse, transient weakness and ataxia, even without previous history of heart disease.
-   Prediction of dilated cardiomyopathy (DCM) in healthy adult dogs of the predisposed breeds (mostly Doberman and Boxer).
-   Animals with relatives who have sudden death with no identified cause or relatives who had DCM.
-   Identification of arrhythmias with sporadic or intermittent clinical signs.
-   The monitoring of the antiarrhythmic treatment.

In moments of bradycardia, usually myocytes specialized in electrical conduction, trigger stimulus that can result in repeated arrhythmias. Therefore, due to the fact that some arrhythmias begin in a moment of great parasympathetic stimulation, it is logical to think that in an examination that is performed for 24 hours, with the animal performing its daily activities, it would be superior to the classic ECG in which the animal is contained on a clinic table. However, the ECG provides a panoramic view of the heart in ten different views (leads), not being replaced by the CE examination.

3. Attaching the holter monitor

The Holter apparatus is a handheld device that runs tests and consists of an ECG recording unit that has conductors of electromagnetic waves coupled to the animal by adhesives or suction cups. The recording of the examination is decoded by a computer program that specifically allows the evaluation of cardiac rhythm throughout the recording period.

In order for the recorders to meet the standards required by the *American Heart Association*, they should be able to record undistorted signals of high and low frequency, between 0.05 and 100Hz. These systems are able to record the signal ST. The recording can be common on cassette or memory card (more usual today) that stores the fully digitized signals captured by the electrodes. The advantage of scanning equipment is to reduce the weight and size of the recorders and the elimination of mechanical parts such as motor and reduction system. The recording should be in two leads. Devices that record in three channels can replace the two channels monitors.

The systems analysis should always allow classification of the forms of waves and broad interaction with the device analyst for corrections and to eliminate possible artifacts.

The two channels apparatus have five electrodes and the three channels have seven. When using two channels device, the electrodes are fixed to the skin on the chest of the animal, according to the Ware scheme (1998):

Channel 1 - White electrode (negative): the sixth right intercostal space, two fingers above the costochondral articulation;

- Red lead (positive): the sixth right intercostal space, in the location of costochondral joint;
- Green lead (ground): the sixth right intercostal space near the sternum.

Channel 2 - Brown electrode (negative): the sixth left intercostal space, two fingers above the costochondral articulation;

- Black electrode (positive): the sixth left intercostal space toward intermediate between red and green electrodes positioned on the opposite side.

In equipment with four electrodes (Cardioflash® or Cardiolight®: www.cardios.com.br), the local standard ECG precordial examination can been adapted for CE as follows: position of red electrode in V2 place (sixth left intercostal space adjacent to the sternum), black in V4 (sixth left intercostal space in the costochondral junction location), orange electrode between black and red, and white electrode in the V1 position of conventional ECG (fifth right intercostal space near the sternum), as shown in figure 1.

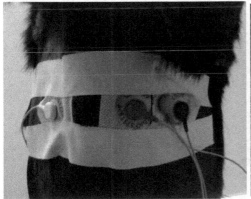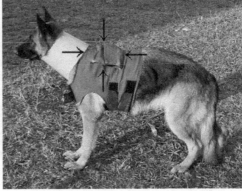

Fig. 1. Left side of the figure - Animal with electrodes attached to the chest for the conduct of examination by equipment with four electrodes (See the text for more details). Note the shaved area with the setting of adhesives and the coupling of electrodes. Right side of the figure – Dog using cervical collar and being subjected to examination. Note that the device is packed in the side pocket of its waistcoat (arrows).

In the thoracic region, where the adhesive electrodes are positioned, there must be ample shaving, cleaning of the area with alcohol to remove the hair and skin oils. After the gel electrodes are fixed with adhesive tape, dry the skin (Figure 1) and it should be held with a protective bandage to prevent the electrodes to come off.

Later, you put on a denim jacket or something similar, which will remain on the animal during the exam. The CE device will be packaged in the side pocket of the jacket and the cables will remain protected (Figure 1).

There is the possibility of performing the examination without the use of waistcoat only conditioning the device with bandage. After placing the recording monitor, cervical or Elizabethan collar should be used to prevent dog bites and damages to the unit. In the literature, the use of cervical or Elizabethan collars did not influence the heart rate in healthy dogs (Cavalcanti et al., 2007). However, it is clear that some dogs tolerate the use of cervical collar better than the Elizabethan one.

The weight of the device and the size of the vest should be compatible with the size of the animal; cats should use smaller devices

4. The result of the examination

Every animal should have a sheet of notes taken during the activities along the course of the recording. It should be noted that the starting time of the examination correlates with the observed daily heart rate (HR) and, possibly, arrhythmias. The report should contain the results of the exam starting time, duration of the examination, the level of recording quality, the maximum, average and minimum HR in each hour and the same HR data on the total examination time. Some supraventricular and ventricular premature complexes may occur in healthy dogs and cats, and in humans these premature complexes increased with age. Atrioventricular blocks of first or second degrees may also occur in healthy dogs. Variations and changes unique to the T wave are not considered diagnostic of CE in small animals.

4.1 Heart rate

Athlete human beings and athlete dogs have mean HR and maximum HR lower than sedentary individuals, the physical activity modulates the sinus node causing decrease of the average of these HR (Cavalcanti et al., 2009, Martinelli et al., 2005), and increasing HR variability and the average RR interval. Endurance exercise training has been established to alter autonomic nervous system activity, resulting in an apparent increase in cardiac parasympathetic tone coupled with decreases in sympathetic activity. For example, in both humans and animals, the heart rate at submaximal workloads was reduced in trained individuals compared with sedentary controls (Smith et al., 1989). A resting bradycardia is a well-established consequence of exercise training and is, in fact, used as a marker that the exercise-trained state has been achieved. Both acetylcholine content and cholineacetyl transferase were increased in the hearts of trained rats compared with control rats (DeSchryver and Mertens-Strythaggen, 1975).

The circadian variation in HR is similar to that illustrated in Figure 2. Obviously, the limits of the upper and lower HR should be calibrated in the software, according to the animal being studied.

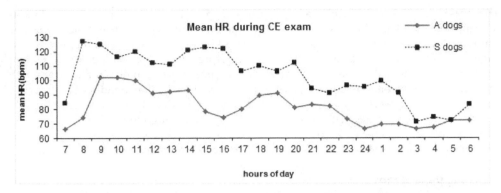

Fig. 2. Graphics show the average of the mean HR at different times of day, observed in sedentary (S) and athlete (A) dogs of the German shepherd breed. Note that the two groups of dog exhibit the same trend to increase and decrease in mean HR over 24 hours, and lower heart rates were observed from three to six hours of the morning.

4.2 Indication of the CE to evaluate clinical signs related to arrhythmias

Monitoring with the CE for 24 hours is especially useful because it provides details of the patient's heart rhythm, the total number and type of abnormal complexes, as well as the specific time of the day when they occurred. The clinician can assess the animal's activities in the period of recording and correlate exam results with clinical signs manifested at every moment.

The method of CE does the ECG recording for long periods and during the patient's daily activities. This allows us to observe spontaneous changes and those caused by activities or situations experienced by the patient's daily routine and, above all, make sure that the reported symptom related to whether or not an electrocardiographic changes. Symptoms that may be caused by changes in heart rhythm should occur often enough to be surprised while doing the recording of the ECG; however, the direct relationship is not always present and can have situations like:

a.   a) Without clinical signs and without arrhythmia
b.   b) Without clinical sign and with arrhythmia
c.   c) With clinical sign and without arrhythmia
d.   d) With clinical sign and with arrhythmia, but no correlation.

In the situation "a" it is impossible to establish any relationship and the examination should be repeated depending on the severity of the clinical suspicion, in "b", though symptoms do not occur, the type of arrhythmia observed may suggest a possible correlation with the sign mentioned above; in "c", discards the possibility of a relationship of symptoms with arrhythmia and another cause should be investigated, in "d", each case must be individualized, because we have patients that fall in both "b" and "c".

4.3 Supraventricular arrhythmias

The CE detects the same supraventricular arrhythmias than the ECG, however there are some considerations to be taken.

The presence of supraventricular arrhythmias is typically observed in less than 25% of healthy small animals within 24 hours. The evaluation of this type of arrhythmia should be cautious; the software which reads the tapes are calibrated to values of human waves and sinus arrhythmia of normal dogs may be misinterpreted as supraventricular premature complex, and even if there are trembling in the baseline sinus, arrhythmia associated with the software can be interpreted incorrectly, such as atrial fibrillation. Solid memory devices (e.g. Memory card) work similarly to cassette and offer the advantage to be programmed to work with range of values of dogs and cats ranges, minimizing the number of premature supraventricular complexes false positive in the exam. So when the reading is done, someone familiar with sinus arrhythmia of dogs must be present to review this arrhythmia.

4.4 Sinus Pauses (SP)

The long SP (more than 2 seconds) or in high quantity may be a factor in the initiation of arrhythmias. The SP generally occurs when the animal's FC is the lowest. Among the breeds studied: 40% of healthy German shepherd dogs had SP. All healthy Doberman and Boxer dogs and 70% of healthy dogs of the English cocker spaniel breed also presented it, so the frequency of SP varies among healthy individuals of different breeds. The median frequency of SP also varies among different breeds, English cocker spaniel, German shepherd, Boxer and Doberman dogs, showed median SP, respectively, 3, 32.5, 366 and 141 in 24 hours. The average of greater SP is more similar: 2.5, 2.87, 3.5 and 3.3, respectively. Therefore, these preliminary studies, the median of PS varies among breeds more than the average of greater SP. The SP occurs with a wide variation among the numbers of healthy individuals and may be higher than 5 seconds at times of low HR in normal dogs.

4.5 Ventricular arrhythmias

The EC detects the same changes of the ECG ventricular depolarization, but measured by a prolonged period and it identifies the different morphologies of normal and premature ventricular complexes (PVC) and is useful in predicting the DCM and in the identification of intermittent arrhythmias.

The presence of multiple PVC, single or repeated (mainly paroxysmal ventricular tachycardia) is associated with episodes of syncope or weakness. In more than half of the Boxer dogs who have syncope, the examination identifies at least 50 PVC in 24 hours.

Also, there is variation in the amount of PVC in dogs of different breeds; the occurrence is 26% for animals of the Beagle breed, 10% for the Doberman dogs, 20% in German shepherd and 40% in English cocker spaniel. However, between 50 and 70% of healthy Boxer dogs, have presented ventricular ectopic activity.

Doberman dogs that have more than 50 PVC in 24 hours have a higher risk of developing DCM, and it is considered abnormal if the presence of PVC is greater than 100 in 24 hours, especially if PVC are repeated or multiform. Based on studies a table was made (Table 1) for the evaluation of EC exams in Doberman pinschers. And Boxer dogs that present more than 91 PVC in 24 hours may have represented dogs with arrhythmogenic right ventricular cardiomyopathy or other disease processes that could have resulted in the development of ventricular arrhythmias (Stern et al., 2010).

Frequency of premature ventricular complexes in 24 hours	Interpretation
None	Annual reassessment of the CE, if the animal is of a predisposed family
Less than 50	May be the initial DCM, annual reassessment required.
Between 50 and 100	Suspect animal, revaluation every three to six months.
More than 100	Likely to be suffering from DCM, revaluation of 3 to 6 months.

Table 1. Recommendations for interpretation of CE exam in Doberman dogs (Goodwin, 1998).

Sudden death has been reported in young dogs of German shepherd breed, very similar to the illness of sudden death in human babies. Both are characterized by paroxysmal ventricular tachycardia at moments of parasympathetic influences, as in deep sleep and after exercise. Any animal displaying episodes of ventricular tachycardia has high risk of sudden death.

This familiar arrhythmia in German shepherd dogs usually decreases after seven months of age, but can be detected in animals older than 5 years and are considered affected, the animals showing more than 240 PVC during the examination. Death was observed in 15 to 20% of affected animals and usually occurs at the age of 4-8 months (Moise et al., 1997). In Brazil, there are no reports of this hereditary disease that has been observed in North America.

4.6 CE Indication for detection of myocardial ischemia

The study of myocardial ischemia by CE was made possible by technical advances in recording systems, with enhancements to the registry of the ST segment. As the ST as a sign of low frequency response, its correct detection and registration will depend on the frequency range of recorders, which should be between 0.05 and 100 Hz. The analysis system should be able to do it automatically, exposing the behavior of the ST segment graphically in time function, with the possibility of observation and interaction of events by the analyst. In general, the electrocardiogram is superior to CE in detecting myocardial ischemia due to greater number of variations of electrode placement.

In veterinary medicine, myocardial ischemia due to obstruction of large coronary vessels is uncommon and ST segment changes may occur in cases of hypertrophic left ventricle due to obstruction of small vessels. No healthy dogs of the Boxer, English cocker spaniel, Doberman and German shepherd breeds have shown significant change in the ST segment.

The ventricular arrhythmia is a common consequence of myocardial infarction and is easily identified and quantified in dogs with induced myocardial infarction and examined by CE. Moreover, it is known that at the time of greatest oxygen demand of the heart muscle (e.g. during exercise, stress ECG) ST changes are best identified in humans and the same occurs in dogs subjected to experimental infarction and evaluated by CE, moreover, the CE has a higher ability to detect small myocardial infarction in dogs than the resting ECG.

The ST segment analysis by electrocardiography is inadequate when there is left bundle branch block or Wolff-Parkinson-White syndrome or QRS complex with very low amplitude. Moreover, in large variations in the morphology of the QRS complex, the ST segment assessment should be undertaken with caution, even if it is caused by change of posture. It is noteworthy that a normal examination does not exclude ischemic heart disease, even by the natural variability of ischemic injury.

4.7 Evaluation of therapeutic procedures results

The diagnosis of cardiac arrhythmias and evaluation of therapeutic results requires prolonged observation of the ECG; in addition, the long-term ECG enables clarity of paroxysmal symptoms that may occur after a therapeutic procedure. The aggravation of preexisting arrhythmias or the emergence of new arrhythmias (proarrhythmia) is a phenomenon that can occur during treatment, especially the drug induced treatment, and the CE exam can provide information, even in asymptomatic cases. The CE should not be routinely done in the monitoring of patients with artificial pacemakers; however, it constitutes a powerful tool in the elucidation of paroxysmal symptoms in this group of patients.

In veterinary medicine, it is considered efficient the drug that causes a decrease of at least 70% in the number of premature supraventricular complexes. In dogs of the Doberman breed with DCM and treated with tocainamida, the total number of CVPs decreased between 70 and 80%, and the ventricular tachycardia 90%, which can be defined as therapeutic success in the treatment of DCM in PVC (Calvert et al., 1996).

4.8 Heart rate variability

Several types of analysis of the variability of intervals between R waves are provided by the examination. The RR variability is a way to evaluate the cardiac autonomic system functioning, and high variability of RR indicates a good heart function.

The analysis of HR variability is achieved through the study of parameters for time domain and frequency, provided directly by the computer analysis program. Although there are certain parameters in the time domain that can be analyzed by the ECG, the best method for this analysis is the CE, because this evaluation is made considering more data and obtains more consistent results.

The following variables are evaluated in the time domain: mean NN (mean of all normal RR intervals of the exam), SDNN (standard deviation of all normal sinus R-R intervals), SDANN (standard deviation of the averaged normal sinus R-R intervals for all 5-minute segments of the entire recording), SDNN index (mean of the standard deviations of all normal R-R intervals for all 5-minute segments of the entire recording), rMSSD (root mean square of the sum of squared difference of adjacent normal RR intervals throughout the exam) and pNN50 (the percentage of adjacent R-R intervals that varied by more than 50 ms).

In the frequency domain, the following variables are assessed: HF (high frequency), which comprises 0.15 to 0.4 Hz or 2.5 to 6.6 s / cycle; LF (low frequency), consisting of 0.0033 to 0.04 Hz or 5min/ciclo the 25s, ULF (ultra low frequency), which includes values less than 0.0033 Hz, and the ratio between the LF and HF components (LF / HF).

Human beings studies of HR variability in the spectral domain have shown that the spectral power contained in certain frequency bands reflects, in part, the sympathetic and parasympathetic modulation of sinus node activity. Studies using selective autonomic blockade have shown that power in the frequencies of HR variability > 0.15 Hz can be attributed to parasympathetic modulation, whereas power in frequencies < 0.15 Hz are related to both sympathetic and parasympathetic modulation, thus spectral analyses of HR variability have been used in a variety of settings and pathologies to assess autonomic modulation. Rapid changes in sympathovagal control are known to occur in the setting of exercise and recovery from exercise. Exercise is characterized by a decrease in parasympathetic tone and an increase in sympathetic tone, resulting in an increase in heart rate. During recovery from exercise, HR gradually decreases as parasympathetic tone returns and sympathetic tone withdraws.

In human medicine the variability of RR intervals provides useful information in defining patient prognosis after acute myocardial infarction, in the person with DCM, as well as to stratify the risk of sudden death in diabetic patients. it is known that the variability decreases in the presence of heart failure in dogs with chronic myxomatous mitral valve (Crosara et al., 2010) and in advanced DCM (Calvert and Wall, 2001), and a study of HR variability in cats has not been found yet. Perhaps with more studies, HR variability will be more used in Veterinary Medicine

5. References

Calvert, C. A.; Jacobs, G. J.; Smith, D. D.; Rathbun, S. L.; Pickus, C. W. Association between results of ambulatory electrocardiography and development of cardiomyopathy during long-term follow-up of Doberman pinchers. *Journal of the American Veterinary Association*, v.216, n. 1, p.34-39, 2000.

Calvert, C. A.; Pickus, C.W.; Jacobs, G. J. Efficacy and toxicity of tocainide for the treatment of ventricular tachyarrhythmias in Doberman pinschers with occult cardiomyopathy. *Journal of Veterinary Internal Medicine*, v.4, n. 10, p.235-240, 1996.

Calvert, C. A.; Wall, M. Effect of severity of myocardial failure on heart rate variability in Doberman pinschers with and without echocardiographic evidence of dilated cardiomyopathy. *Journal of the American Veterinary Medical Association*, v.219, n. 8, p.1084-1088, 2001.

Cavalcanti, G. A. de O.; Nogueira, R. B.; Gonçalves, R.S. ; Araujo, R. B. ; Muzzi, R. A. L.; Sampaio, G. R. Influência da utilização de colar elizabetano ou colar cervical em cães submetidos a eletrocardiografia contínua (Holter). *Revista Universidade Rural. Série Ciências da Vida*, v. 27, p. 461-463, 2007.

Cavalcanti, G. A. O.; Nogueira, R. B.; Sampaio, G. R.; Araujo, R. B.; Gonçalves, R.S. Avaliação por eletrocardiografia contínua (holter) em cães da raça Pastor Alemão praticantes de atividade física regular. *Arquivo Brasileiro de Medicina Veterinária e Zootecnia*, v. 61, p. 1446-1449, 2009.

Crosara, S.; Borgarelli, M.; Perego, M.; Häggström, J.; LA Rosa, G.; Tarducci, A.; Santilli, R. A. Holter monitoring in 36 dogs with myxomatous mitral valve disease. *Australian Veterinary Journal*, v. 88, n. 10, p. 386-392, 2010.

Dae, M. W.; Lee, R. J.; Ursell, P. C. ; Chin, M.C.; Stillson, C. A.; Moise, S. Heterogeneous Sympathetic Innervation in German Shepherd Dogs With Inherited Ventricular Arrhythmia and Sudden Cardiac Death. *Circulation*, v. 96, n. 4, p. 1337-1342, 1997.

Deschryver, C.; Mertens-Strythaggen, J. Heart tissue acetylcholine in chronically exercised rats. *Experientia*, v.31, p.316– 318, 1975.

Goodwin, J. CE monitoring and cardiac event recording. *Veterinary Clinics of North America: Small Animal Practice*, v. 28, n. 6, p. 1391-1407, 1998.

Mackie, B. A.; Stepien, R. L.; Kellihan, H. B. Retrospective analysis of an implantable loop recorder for evaluation of syncope, collapse, or intermittent weakness in 23 dogs (2004-2008). *Journal of Veterinary Cardiology*, v. 12, n. 1, p. 25-33, 2010.

Martinelli, F. S.; Chacon-Mikahil, M. P. T.; Martins, L. E. B.; Lima-Filho, E. C. ; Golfetti, R.; Paschoal, M. A.; Gallo-Junior, L. Heart rate variability in athletes and nonathletes at rest and during head-up tilt. *Brazilian Journal of Medical and Biological Research*, v. 38, n. 4, p. 639-647, 2005.

Möise, N.S.; Defrancesco, T. Twentyfour-hour ambulatory eletrocardiography (CE monitoring). In: BONAGURA, J.D. (Ed). KIRK'S current veterinary therapy. XII: Small animal practice. Philadelphia: W.B. Saunders, 1995. p.792-799.

Moïse, N. S.; Gilmour, R. F.; Riccio, M. L.; Flahive, W. S. Diagnosis of inherited ventricular tachycardia in German Shepherd dogs. *Journal of the American Veterinary Medical Association*, v.210, n. 3, p.403-410, 1997.

Nogueira, R. B.; Muzzi, R. A. L.; Herrera, D. S.; Falco, I. R.; CavalcantI, G. A. O. Avaliação do ritmo cardíaco em cães da raça boxer saudáveis por meio da eletrocardiografia contínua (CE). *Arquivo Brasileiro de Medicina Veterinária e Zootecnia*, v.58, n. 1, p.133-136, 2006.

Smith M. L.; Hudson, D. L.; Graitzer, H. M..; Raven, P. B. Exercise training bradycardia: the role of autonomic balance. *Medicine Science Sports Exercise*, v.21, p. 40–44, 1989.

Sosa, E. A.; Terzi, R.; Gruppi, S.; Brito, F. S.; Paola, A. A. V.; Pimenta, J.; Lorga, A. M.; Maia, I. G.; Gizi, J. C.; Solimene, M. C.; Camargo, S. P. A. B.; Albanezi-Filho, F. Consenso SOCESP-SBC sobre Eletrocardiografia pelo Sistema CE. *Arquivo Brasileiro de Cardiologia*, v.65, n. 5, p.447-450, 1995.

Stepien, R. L.; Hinchcliff, K. W.; Constable, P. D.; Olson, J. Effect of endurance training on cardiac morphology in Alaskan sled dog. *Journal of Applied Physiology*, v. 85, n. 4, p. 1368-1375, 1998.

Stern, J. A.; Meurs, K. M.; Spier, A. W.; Koplitz, S. L.; Baumwart, R. D. Ambulatory electrocardiography evaluation of clinically normal adult Boxers. *Journal of American Veterinary Medical Association*, v. 236, n. 4, p. 430-433, 2010.

Tilley, L.P. *Essentials of canine and feline electrocardiography interpretation and treatment*. 3.ed. Philadelphia: Lea & Febiger, 1992. 470p.

Yamada, M.; Tokuriki, M. Effects of a canine Elizabethan collar on ambulatory electrocardiogram recorded by a CE recording system and spontaneous activities measured continuously by an accelerometer in beagle dogs. *Journal of Veterinary Medical Science*, v.62, n. 5, p. 549-552, 2000.

Ware, W. A. Practical use of CE monitoring. Compendium on Continuing Education for the Practicing Veterinarian, v.20, n. 2, p.167-177, 1998.

9

Atresia Ani in Dogs and Cats

Lysimachos G. Papazoglou[1] and Gary W. Ellison[2]

[1]Department of Clinical Sciences, Faculty of Veterinary Medicine,
Aristotle University of Thessaloniki,
[2]Department of Small Animal Clinical Sciences, Health Science Center,
University of Florida Gainesville,
[1]Greece
[2]USA

1. Introduction

Congenital deformities of the anorectum are rarely encountered in small animals with atresia ani being the most common one. Atresia ani is a congenital defect of the anorectum, resulting in anal canal closure and /or abnormal routing of feces (Bright & Bauer, 1994). Among large animals congenital atresia ani most often occurs in pigs and calves and is considered hereditary. In these species atresia may be seen as a separate entity or in conjunction with other malformations of the distal vertebral column, urogenital tract and sometimes with intestinal atresia or colonic agenesis (Kilic & Sariepler, 2004; Maxie, 2007). In pigs atresia is associated with a high mortality rate but selective breeding decreased its occurrence (Partlow et al., 1993; Viana &Tobias, 2005).

2. Epidemiology

Atresia ani is uncommonly described in dogs and it is even less frequently reported in cats; the true incidence of this abnormality is difficult to determine and may be greater than reported because many newborn puppies and kittens are euthanatized before being evaluated based on the hypothesis that surgical correction is unsuccessful; additionally unpublished data may hide true prevalence as complications associated with surgical correction of these deformities are common (Prassinos et al.,. 2003; Mahler & Williams, 2005; Viana & Tobias, 2005). According to a review of Veterinary Medical Database atresia ani in dogs accounts for 0.0007 with females more likely to be affected than males (female/male =1.79/1) [Viana & Tobias, 2005]. Canine breeds overpresented include Finish spitz, Boston teriers, Maltese, chow chow, German shorthair pointer, toy poodle and miniature schnauzer (Viana & Tobias, 2005). In cats females are more commonly affected than males (Suess et al., 1992; van de Broek et al., 1988; Tsioli et al., 2009, Tomsa et al., 2011).

3. Normal and abnormal embryologic development

The embryologic development of the canine and feline anorectum resembles that of the human development (Greiner, 1972; Amand, 1974; Suess et al., 1992; Sadler, 1995; Viana &

Tobias, 2005). The cloaca is a common route for gastrointestinal and urogenital tracts in the canine and feline embryo. Retention of the cloaca occurs in vertebrate animals other than placental mammals; in higher mammals the cloaca separates during embryologic development. By the seventh to eighth week of development the urorectal fold, which located between the allantois and the hindgut openings in the cloaca, initially divides the cloaca into the dorsal part called the rectum and the ventral part called the urogenital sinus (Figures 1 &2). The urogenital sinus is further differentiated into the urethra and the urinary bladder. The terminal end of the hindgut forms the cranial anal canal and the anus is formed at a later time by ectodermal ingrowth of the perineum. A breakdown in physiological embryologic differentiation of the cloacal region may lead to a variety of congenital malformations of the anorectum. Failure of the urorectal fold to divide the cloaca completely or failure of the anal membrane to rupture after anal creation results in atresia ani.

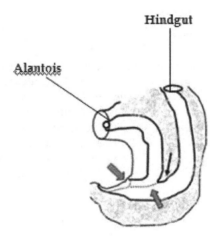

Fig. 1. Urorectal fold (arrows) located between the alantois and hindgut by 7th to 8th week of development.

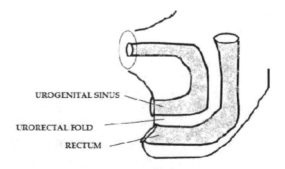

Fig. 2. The cloaca is divided into urorectal sinus and rectum.

4. Classification

Four anatomic types of atresia ani have been described in dogs and cats (Aronson, 2003; Viana &Tobias, 2005; Ellison & Papazoglou, 2011) [Figures 3-7].

External anal sphincter and anal sacs are usually develop normally in type II anomalies (Seim, 1986; Ellison & Papazoglou, 2011), while agenesis of the external anal sphincter, anal sacs or tail are reported in type III anomalies (Rawlings & Capps, 1971; Knecht & Westerfield, 1971; Loug & van Schouwenburg, 1982; Ellison & Papazoglou, 2011). Occasionally dogs and more rarely cats with type II and more uncommonly with type III atresia ani may be associated with rectovaginal, rectovestibular or urethrorectal fistulas (Holt, 1985; van den Broek et al., 1988; Chandler & MacPhail, 2001; Aronson, 2003; Ellison & Papazoglou, 2011). Animals with type III atresia ani associated with rectovaginal fistula are also reported as having an ectopic anus (Prassinos et al., 2003). However, it is unclear if type IV atresia ani has ever been reported in dogs and cats (Ellison & Papazoglou, 2011).

Atresia Type	Anomaly
Type I	Congenital stenosis of a patent anus
Type II	Persistence of a complete anal membrane alone or a combination of an anal membrane with the rectum ending as a blind pouch cranial to the membrane.
Type III	Presence of an imperforate anus with the rectum terminating further cranially.
Type IV	Normal ending of the terminal rectum and anus while the cranial rectum terminates as a blind pouch within the pelvis.

Table 1. Anatomic types of atresia ani in dogs and cats

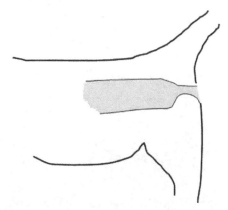

Fig. 3. Schematic representation of type I atresia ani.

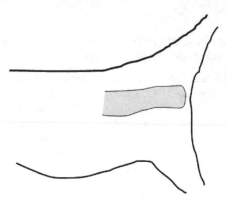

Fig. 4. Schematic representation of type II atresia ani.

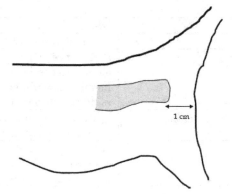

Fig. 5. Schematic representation of type III atresia ani. The blind rectal pouch is more than 1 cm away from the anal dimple.

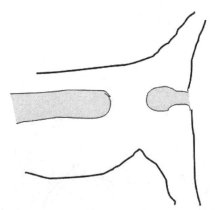

Fig. 6. Schematic representation of type III atresia ani. It is not clear if this type of atresia has been reported in small animals.

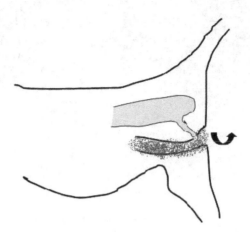

Fig. 7. Schematic representation of type II atresia ani combined with rectovaginal fistula.

5. History and clinical signs

A history of absence of defecation, which sometimes may go unnoticed, is reported. Clinical signs of atresia ani are usually evident within a few weeks of birth and depend on the type of atresia (Aronson, 2003; Viana &Tobias, 2005; Ellison & Papazoglou, 2011). Animals with type I atresia ani may exhibit constipation and tenesmus soon after weaning (Figure 8). A stenosed anal opening is evident on digital rectal palpation. Puppies and kittens belonging to types II, III and IV are clinically normal for the first 2 to 4 weeks of birth. A history of anorexia, depression, absence of defecation, tenesmus and abdominal distention are reported to follow this time frame (Figure 9). Physical examination may also reveal a dimple at the site of the closed anal opening (Figures 10 &11), abdominal enlargement, discomfort on abdominal palpation and perineal swelling depending on the type of anomaly. Abdominal enlargement may be attributed to colonic distention with feces or gas, fecal impaction or even megacolon. Longstanding cases may develop vomiting and dehydration. Animals with rectovaginal or rectourethral communications often show passage of watery to formed feces through the vagina or urethra; these animals may be in better physical condition that others with no rectovaginal or rectourethral communications (Prassinos et al., 2003; Rahal et al., 2007) [Figure 12]. Multiple congenital anomalies such as umbilical hernias, cleft palates, open fontanels, hypospadias, tail agenesis and deafness in dogs and sacrocaudal dysgenesis and hydrocepahalus in kittens may accompany atresia ani and should not escape a thorough physical or other diagnostic examination (Suess et al., 1992; Aronson, 2003; Prassinos et al., 2003; Rahal et al., 2007; Ellison & Papazoglou, 2011) [Figure 13]. Rectocutaneous fistulas associated with type II atresia ani have been recently reported in a cat (Tsioli et al., 2009) [Figure 14].

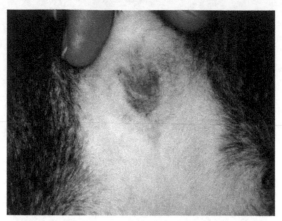

Fig. 8. Atresia ani type I in a mixed breed puppy.

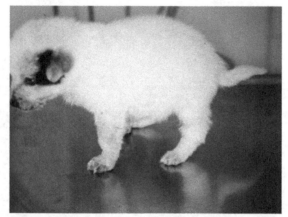

Fig. 9. A mixed breed puppy with abdominal distention associated with type II atresia ani.

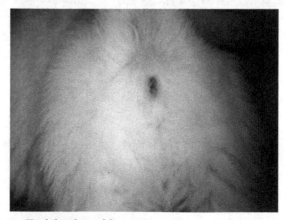

Fig. 10. Atresia ani type II of the dog of figure 9.

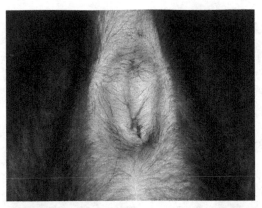

Fig. 11. An anal dimple associated with type II atresia ani in a dog.

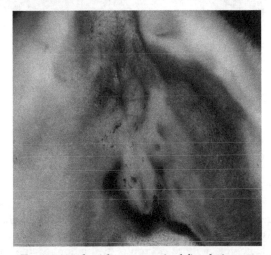

Fig. 12. Atresia ani type II associated with rectovaginal fistula in a puppy.

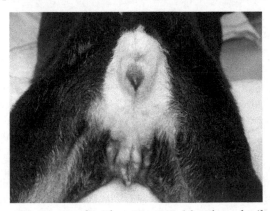

Fig. 13. Atresia ani type III associated with rectovaginal fistula and tail agenesis in a puppy.

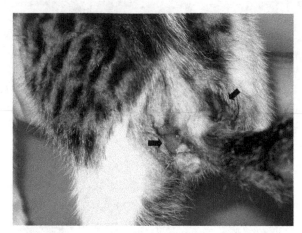

Fig. 14. Rectocutaneous fistulas ventral and lateral to the tail (arrows) in a cat with type II atresia ani

6. Diagnosis

Diagnosis of atresia ani is based in clinical signs, physical examination findings and confirmed with radiographic examination. Evaluation of external anal sphincter muscle presence and function is important for prognostic purposes.

6.1 Diagnostic tests

Penile bulb or vulva pinching may result in an anal wink (bulbourethral reflex) [Chambers, 1986; Hosgood & Hoskins, 1998]. Electro stimulation of perineal muscles using electrocautery at surgery or nerve stimulators may also be used to check for a strong anal response (Mahler & Williams, 2005). Electromyography for external anal sphincter muscle may be used if available for a more accurate evaluation of the anal tone (Ellison & Papazoglou, 2011).

6.2 Radiographic examination

Abdominal radiography is useful in atresia ani anatomic typing and ruling out colonic distention, which may lead in megacolon that affects management and prognosis (Figures 15-18). Gas accumulation in colon and rectum, as visualized in plain radiographs, may help in determining the position of the terminal rectum. Horizontal beam abdominal radiographs with the animal suspended upside down and pressure around the abdomen may help to visualize gas accumulation migrating to the terminal colon and rectum and outlining the borders of the rectal pouch (Greiner, 1972; Bright & Bauer, 1994). Additionally, a coin is placed at the anal dimple to help outline the anus (Greiner et al., 1984). In case of rectovaginal or urethrorectal fistulation positive contrast vaginography or urethrography may help determine fistula and terminal rectum location (Aronson, 2003; Prassinos et al., 2003; Viana &Tobias, 2005; Rahal et al., 2007; Ellison & Papazoglou, 2011).

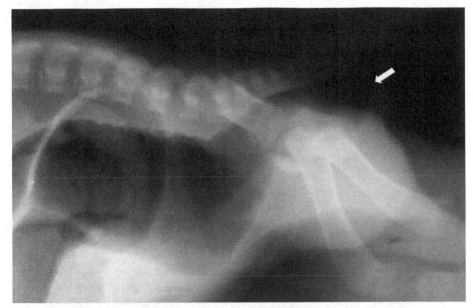

Fig. 15. Abdominal radiograph of a dog visualizing gas accumulation in the colon and rectum. The location of the terminal rectum is also shown (arrow) [Courtesy Dr. M.N. Patsikas, Aristotle University of Thessaloniki].

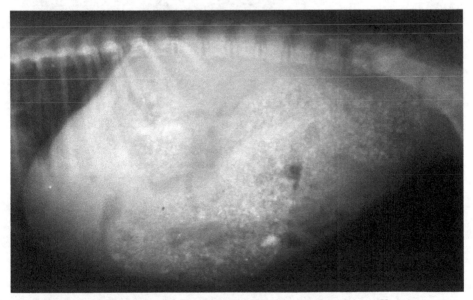

Fig. 16. Abdominal radiograph showing megacolon associated with type II atresia ani in a dog (Courtesy Dr. M.N. Patsikas, Aristotle University of Thessaloniki).

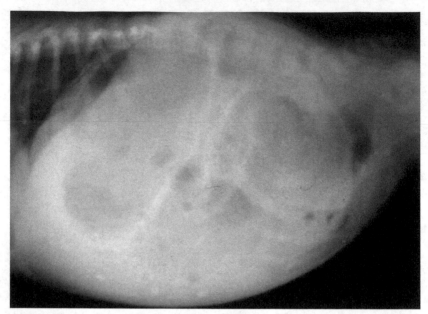

Fig. 17. Abdominal radiograph of a boxer puppy depicting colonic gas distention associated with type II atresia ani (Courtesy Dr. M.N. Patsikas, Aristotle University of Thessaloniki).

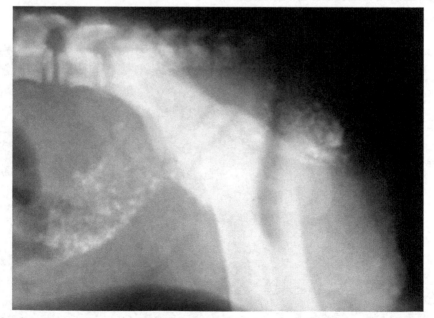

Fig. 18. Abdominal radiograph of a female rottweiler cross puppy with type III atresia ani and rectovaginal fistula showing fecal material in the colon, terminal rectum and over the vagina level. (Courtesy Dr. M.N. Patsikas, Aristotle University of Thessaloniki).

7. Treatment

Surgical correction is considered the only treatment for atresia ani. Anatomical typing of atresia ani should be performed to help determining the type of surgical correction for each case (Ellison & Papazoglou, 2011). However, non surgical management may also be applied for type I cases (Tomsa et al., 2011; Ellison & Papazoglou, 2011). Numerous case reports have appeared in the literature reporting surgical treatment of atresia ani in dogs and cats. Currently there are only 3 small and 1 larger case series reporting surgical treatment in dogs (Prassinos et al., 2003; Vianna & Tobias, 2005; Rahal et al., 2007) and 2 small case series in cats describing surgical or medical management of atresia ani (Suess et al., 1992; Tomsa et al., 2011). Anoplasty is the most common procedure performed. The aim of surgery is to restore anorectal continuity, to preserve the external anal sphincter, to preserve or restore colonic function and to eliminate any rectovaginal or urethrorectal communication. Surgical treatment should be prompt and performed before colonic atony or megacolon associated with chronic and prolonged distention or possible urinary tract infection ensues (Prassinos et al., 2003). Animals with atresia ani type II and III that are unable to defecate if not treated surgically will die because of bowel stasis. End-on temporary colostomy may be considered as an option for the treatment of cats with rectocutaneous fistulas associated with atresia ani (Tsioli et al., 2009). The perineal approach is used for all surgical corrections of atresia types I-III. Prophylactic antibiotics (cefoxitin 20 mg/kg) are administered intravenously at anesthetic induction.

7.1 Type I atresia ani

Animals with this type of atresia ani are placed in ventral decumbency and treated with resection of the strictured portion of the rectum through a 360^0 anoplasty. After excision of the stricture the rectal mucosa is brought distally so as mucosa to skin apposition is achieved with simple interrupted sutures using synthetic non absorbable monofilament 4/0-5/0 suture material (Figure 19). Care is taken during dissection to preserve the external anal

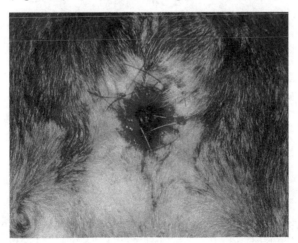

Fig. 19. Anoplasty in the dog of figure 8 with atresia ani type I.

sphincter and anal sacs (Hosgood & Hoskins, 1998; Aronson, 2003; Prassinos et al., 2003; Ellison & Papazoglou, 2011). Type I atresia ani may also be treated with bougienage or balloon dilatation in a single or multiple treatments; however, failures are not uncommon (Hosgood & Hoskins, 1998; Webb et al., 2007; Tomsa et al., 2011; Ellison & Papazoglou, 2011). Recently, a single balloon dilatation procedure alone or combined with intralesional triamcinolone injection was used to successfully treat type I atresia ani in 5 kittens and two dogs (Webb et al., 2007; Tomsa et al., 2011). Prospective studies are needed to evaluate balloon dilatation for the treatment of congenital anorectal strictures in small animals.

7.2 Type II & III atresia ani

For animals with type II or III atresia ventral recumbency is used and a cruciate, vertical or vertical elliptical incision is made over the anal dimple and medial to the ducts of the anal sacs. The triangular flaps or elliptical skin created are excised. The external sphincter and distal rectal pouch are identified and dissection is continued medial to the sphincter using fine scissors. The rectum is mobilized through the sphincter by using stay sutures, opened and sutured to the subcutaneous tissue and skin with 4/0-5/0 monofilament absorbable or non absorbable suture material respectively (Figures 20-22). In some animals with Type III atresia ani the rectal pouch is located more than 1 cm away from the anal dimple dissection for identification and mobilization of the rectum is achieved through rectal pull through procedure. The colon and rectum should be evacuated from feces before recovery, while the animal is still in anesthesia, to promote normal intestinal function (Hosgood & Hoskins, 1998; Aronson, 2003; Prassinos et al., 2006; Ellison & Papazoglou, 2011).

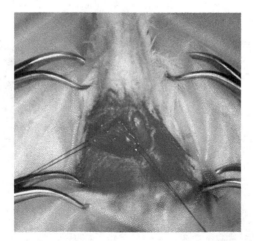

Fig. 20. The rectal pouch was identified through a cruciate incision made over the anal dimple in a puppy of figure 9. Two stay sutures were placed in the rectum to allow easy handling.

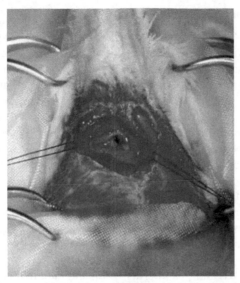

Fig. 21. The rectum of the dog of figure 9 was mobilized and opened to allow an anoplasty procedure.

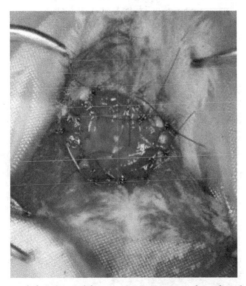

Fig. 22. The rectal mucosa of the dog of figure 9 was sutured to the skin with simple interrupted nylon sutures to complete the anoplasty.

7.3 Type IV atresia ani

Animals with this type of atresia may need an abdominal approach to isolate, mobilize and anastomose the cranial colon with the distal colon and rectum usually through a pubic symphisiotomy procedure (Hosgood & Hoskins, 1998; Aronson, 2003).

7.4 Types II-III atresia ani with rectovaginal fistula

Three surgical techniques are used for the correction of rectovaginal fistula in dogs and cats. Initial approach is through a vertical midline perineal incision extending from the ventral anus to the vulva. In one technique the fistula is isolated, excised and the rectal and vulvar lumens are ligated or oversewn separately with 3/0 -4/0 monofilament absorbable suture material or hemostatic clips followed by closure of the vertical perineal incision; An anoplasty procedure for atresia correction as previously described is performed afterwards (Chambers, 1986; Hosgood & Hoskins, 1998; Aronson, 2003; Prassinos et al., 2003; Viana &Tobias, 2005; Rahal et al., 2007; Ellison & Papazoglou, 2011). Fistula obliteration by performing numerous purse-string sutures placed along its length was also described in a dog (Louw & van Schouwenburg, 1982). According to another technique, used in 3 cats and 1 dog, the rectum is transected cranial to the fistulous opening, the affected rectal portion is excised and the terminal part of the rectum is sutured to the anus (Rawlings & Capps, 1971; Suess et al., 1992; Aronson, 2003). In the third technique the fistulous tract is preserved, isolated, mobilized through the anus and sutured to the skin at the level of the external anal sphincter; this technique was used for anal reconstruction in 2 dogs (Prassinos et al., 2003; Ellison & Papazoglou, 2011) and 1 cat (Bornet, 1990) and modified to be performed in 2 dogs through an episiotomy approach (Mahler &Williams, 2005) [Figures 23-25]. With this technique the preserved fistulus tract is considered the terminal part of the rectum and thus function of the internal anal sphincter is maintained (Prassinos et al., 2003; Mahler & Williams, 2005).

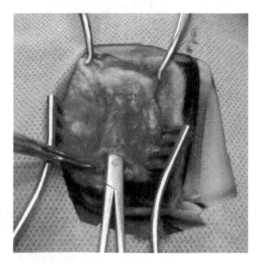

Fig. 23. Atresia ani type III associated with a rectovaginal fistula. The fistulous tract of the dog of figure 12 was isolated through a vertical midline perineal incision extending from the anus to the vulva. A pair of closed needle holders was inserted through the tract.

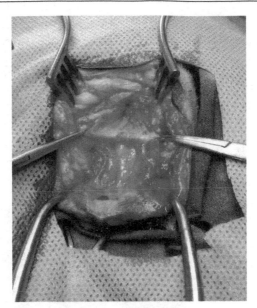

Fig. 24. Atresia ani type III associated with a rectovaginal fistula. The fistulous tract grasped with mosquito hemostats was dissected from the vagina.

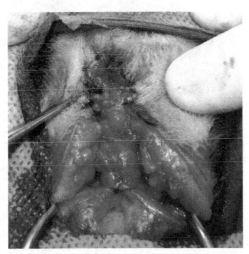

Fig. 25. Atresia ani type III associated with a rectovaginal fistula. The fistulous tract was sutured to the external anal sphincter and the vaginal mucosa was closed with simple interrupted sutures.

7.5 Temporary end-on colostomy for the management of cats with rectocutaneous fistulas associated with type II atresia ani

Temporary incontinent end-on colostomy may be performed initially for fecal diversion to help eliminate rectocutaneous fistulas. Colostomy is located in the lateroventral abdominal wall. Soon after colostomy and following resolution of fistulas a second surgery is performed for colostomy closure and reconstruction of the atresia ani by performing anoplasty (Tsioli et al., 2009) [Figures 26 & 27].

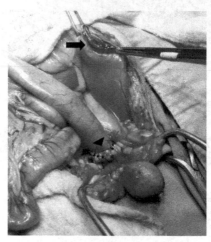

Fig. 26. Following resolution of fistulas the colostomy was closed (arrow) and an end to end colocolonic anastomosis was performed (arrowhead) through a ventral midline celiotomy in a cat.

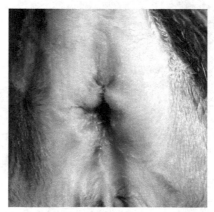

Fig. 27. Atresia ani reconstruction through anoplasty was performed following colostomy closure in a cat.

8. Postoperative care

Postoperatively analgesia through opioid administration for a week's time, cisapride to promote colonic motility and stool softeners as lactulose to combat constipation are provided. Fecal impaction may be relieved manually and multiple enemas should be avoided. Many animals start to defecate soon after surgery (Prassinos et al., 2003; Rahal et al., 2007; Ellison & Papazoglou, 2011).

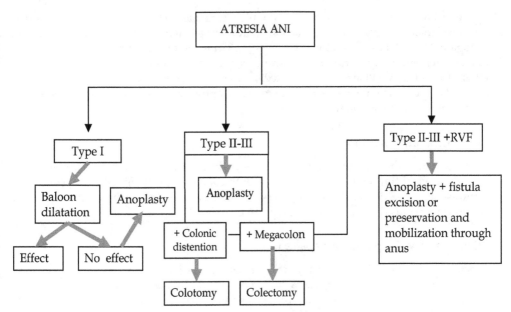

Table 2. Algorithm for atresia ani treatment methods in dogs and cats. RVF : rectovaginal fistula

9. Complications

Postoperative complications may include tenesmus, fecal incontinence, wound dehiscence, stricture of the anoplasty, colonic atony or megacolon and rectal prolapse (Suess et al., 1992; Prassinos et al., 2003; Vian & Tobias, 2005; Rahal et al., 2007; Ellison & Papazoglou, 2011). Fecal incontinence, a common complication after surgery, may be transient (Prassinos et al., 2003; Viana & Tobias, 2005, Rahal et al., 2007), intermittent or permanent (Suess et al., 1992; Ellison & Papazoglou, 2011) and related to a congenital absence of functional external anal sphincter or surgical trauma to the sphincter muscle innervation during dissection (Aronson, 2003; Prassinos et al., 2003; Viana & Tobias, 2005; Ellison & Papazoglou, 2011). Fecal incontinence secondary to surgical intervention in dogs may resolve several weeks to a year after surgery (Prassinos et al., 2003; Viana & Tobias, 2005; Rahal et al., 2007). Semitendinosus muscle flap application was proposed as an option to improve anal tone in a dog with atresia ani and rectovaginal fistula (Chambers & Rawlings, 1991). Wound dehiscence may be related to tension on the anastomosis and fecal contamination of the surgical site (Suess et al., 1992) and may be prevented by meticulous surgical technique. Stricure of the anoplasty site and fecal retention associated with colonic atony or megacolon are two common complications requiring a second surgery such as revision anoplasty, subtotal colectomy or colotomy (Viana & Tobias, 2005, Ellison & Papazoglou, 2011). Animals with stricture of the anoplasty site may develop tenesmus, constipation and fecal impaction. This complication may need a revision anoplasty or baloon dilatation to resolve. In a recent study with 12 cases of dogs and cats with atresia ani having surgical management, 5 animals with type II-III atresia ani, 4 of which combined with rectovaginal fistula, developed postoperative stricture and had initially balloon dilatation, which failed in all but one case.

Of these failures 5 had revision anoplasty which was successful in 4 animals and 3 had concurrent colotomy for fecal impaction removal, all with good results (Ellison & Papazoglou 2011). Subtotal colectomy that was performed in one dog with type II atresia ani 2 weeks after anoplasty continued to show constipation associated with megacolon 9 months after surgery (Viana & Tobias, 2005). Colotomy or subtotal colectomy might be performed at the same time with anoplasty to help improve colonic function in animals with colonic dilatation or megacolon.

10. Outcome and prognosis

In the larger study reported to date 10 of 12 dogs with type I and II atresia ani survived long term with survival times ranged from 12-96 months and 6 of the 8 animals were continent. In contrast 2 of the 3 animals having type III atresia ani were euthanized because of continuous tenesmus (Ellison & Papazoglou, 2011).

11. Comparative aspects of atresia ani

Anorectal malformations represent a wide spesctrum of disorders in boys and girls associated with urogenital tract, sacral or spinal defects. These defects are grouped in anatomic categories sharing similar prognosis and management. Treatment of these anorectal malformations aims at anatomical reconstruction, diagnosis and treatment of any associated defects and provides patients with good quality of life by addressing the functional sequelae of these malformations (Pena & Hong, 2000). The most common defect in males include imperforate anus with rectourethral fistula; some of these fistulas are associated with good quality muscles, well developed sacrum and anal dimple whereas some others are related with poor quality muscles, abnormally developed sacrum and hardly visible dimple. The most common defect in females is rectovestibular fistula and this anomaly has excellent functional prognosis (Levitt & Penna, 2005). About 75% of the patients with anorectal malformations will pass voluntary bowel motions and enjoy a good quality of life postoperatively, while constipation urinary and fecal incontinence are common complications following anorectal reconstruction (Pena & Hong, 2000).

12. References

Amand, W. (1974). Nonneurogenic disorders of the anus and rectum. *Veterinary Clinics of North America*, Vol. 4, No. 3,   (August 1974), pp. 535-550

Aronson, L. (2003). Rectum and Anus, In: Textbook of Small Animal Surgery, D. Slatter, (Ed), 682-708, Saunders, ISBN 0721686079, Philadelphia, USA

Bornet, J. (1990). Fistule recto-vaginale et imporforation anale chez une chatte: traitment chirurgical. *Bulletin de l'Academie Veterinaire de France*, Vol. 63, No. 1, (January-March 1990), pp. 53-65

Bright, R. & Bauer M. (1994). Surgery of the digestive system, In: The Cat Diseases and Clinical Management, R. Sherding, (Ed), 1353-1401, Churchill Livingstone, ISBN 0443088799, New York, USA

Brown, C., Baker, D. & Barker, I. (2007). Alimentary system, In: Jubb, Kennedy and Palmer's Pathology of Domestic Animals, M. Maxie (Ed), ISBN 13978070202785, Saunders, Edinburgh, UK

Chambers, J. (1986). Surgical diseases of the anorectum, In: Canine and Feline Gastroenterology, B. Jones (Ed), 279-294, Saunders, ISBN 0721652069, Philadelphia, USA

Chandler, J. & MacPhail, C. (2001). Congenital urethrorectal fistulas. *Compendium on Continuing Education for the Practicing Veterinarian*, Vol. 23, No. 11, (November 2001), pp. 995-1002

Ellison, G. & Papazoglou, L. (2011). Long-term results of surgery for atresia ani in small animals-12 cases. *Journal of the American Veterinary Medical Association*, n.d.

Greiner, T. (1972). Surgery of the rectum and anus. *Veterinary Clinics of North America*, Vol. 2, No. 1, (January 1972), pp. 167-180

Holt, P. (1985). Anal and perianal surgery in dogs and cats. *In Practice*, Vol. 7, No. 3, (May 1985), pp. 82- 89

Hosgood, G. & Hoskins, J. (1998). Abdominal cavity and gastrointestinal disorders, In: Small Animal Paediatric Medicine and Surgery, G. Hosgood & J. Hoskins (Eds), 68-114, Butterworth Heinemann, ISBN 0750635991, Woburn, USA

Kilic, N. & Sarierler, M. (2004). Congenital intestinal atresia in calves. *Revue de Medecine Veterinaire*, Vol. 155, No. 7 (July 2004), pp. 381-384

Knecht, C. & Westerfield, C. (1971). Anorecto-urogenital anomalies in a dog. *Journal of the American Veterinary Medical Association*, Vol. 159, No. 1 (July 1971), pp. 91-92

Levitt, M. & Pena, A. (2005). Outcomes from the correction of anorectal malformations. *Current Opinion in Pediatrics*, Vol. 17, No.3, (June 2005), pp. 394-401

Louw, G. & van Schouwenburg, J. (1982). The surgical repair of atresia ani in a dobermann bitch. *Journal of the South African Veterinary Association*, vol. 53, No. 2, (June 1982), pp. 119-120

Mahler, S. & Williams, G. (2005). Preservation of the fistula for reconstruction of the anal canal and the anus in atresia ani and rectovestibular fistula in 2 dogs. *Veterinary Surgery*, Vol.34, No. 2, (March-April 2005), pp. 148-152

Partlow, G., Fisher, K., Page, P., MacMilan, K. & Walker, A. (1993). Prevalence and types of birth defects in Ontario swine determined by mail survey. *Canadian Journal of Veterinary Research*, Vol. 57, No. 2, (April 1993), pp. 67-73

Pena, A. & Hong, A. (2000). Advances in the management of anorectal malformations. *The American Journal of Surgery*, Vol. 180, No. 11, (November 2000), pp. 370-376

Prassinos, N., Papazoglou,L., Adamama-Moraitou, K., Galatos, A., Gouletsou, P. & Rallis, T. (2003). Congenital anorectal abnormalities in six dogs. *Veterinary Record*, Vol.153, No. 3, (July 2003), pp. 81-85

Rahal, S., Vicente, C., Mortari, A., Mamprim, M. & Caporalli, E. (2007). Rectovaginal fistula with atresia ani in 5 dogs. *Canadian Veterinary Journal*, Vol. 48, No. 8, (August 2007), pp. 827-830

Rawlings, C. & Capps, W. (1971). Rectovaginal fistula and imperforate anus in a dog. *Journal of the American Veterinary Medical Association*, Vol. 159, No. 3, (August 1971), pp. 320-326

Sadler, T. (1995). Digestive system, In: Langman's Medical Embryology, T. Sandler (Ed), 242-271, Williams and Wilkins, ISBN 068307489X, Baltimore, USA

Suess, R., Martin, R., Moon, M. & Dallman, M. (1982). Rectovaginal fistula with atresia ani in three kittens. *Cornell Vet*, Vol. 82, No. 2, (April 1992), pp. 141-153

Tomsa, K. , Major, A. & Galus , T. (2011). Treatment of atresia ani type I by balloon dilatation in 5 kittens and one puppy. *Schweizer Archiv fur Tierheilkunde*, Vol. 153, No. 6, (June 2011), pp. 277 -280

Tsioli, V., Papazoglou, L., Anagnostou, T., Kouti, V. & Papadopoulou, P. (2009). Use of a temporary incontinent end-on colostomy in a cat for the management of rectocutaneous fistulas associated with atresia ani. *Journal of Feline Medicine and Surgery*, Vol. 11, No. 12, (Dec 2009), pp. 1011-1014

Van den Broek, A., Else, R. & Hunter, M. (1988). Atresia ani and urethrorectal fistula in a kitten. *Journal of Small Animal Practice*, Vol. 29, No. 2, (February 1988), pp. 91-94

Vianna, M. & Tobias, K. (2005). Atresia ani in the dog: a retrospective study. *Journal of the American Animal Hospital Association*, Vol. 41, No. 5. (September-October 2005), pp. 317-322

Webb, G., McCord, K. & Twedt, D. (2007). Rectal stricture in 19 dogs: 1997-2005. *Journal of the American Animal Hospital Association*, Vol. 43, No. 6, (November-December 2007), pp. 332-336

10

Arthroscopic Follow-Up After Rupture of the Cranial Cruciateligament

Cleuza Maria de Faria Rezende,
Eliane Gonçalves de Melo and Natalie Ferreira Borges
Escola de Veterinária – UFMG,
Brazil

1. Introduction

The femoro-patellar-tibial joint is one of the most complex, with different structures that, altogether, keep the joint stability and functionality (Cook, 2010; de Rooster et al., 2010, Pozzi & Kim, 2010). Due to its big functional demand, the cranial cruciate ligament (CrCL) is the structure most frequently injured. The rupture of this ligament is of the most common causes of lameness in the dog and the resulting instability leads to the development of degenerative joint disease (DJD). Still today, the search for the ideal technique to treat CrCL rupture, with joint stabilization and prevention or minimization of DJD, persists. However, would joint stabilization be the only factor to be considered for the treatment of CrCL rupture and its sequels? Won't the effects of instability on the other structures deserve more investigation? Would the inflammatory response mediators be responsible for the looseness of the intra-articular graft or is it exclusively due to improper fixation or inadequate post-operatory?

According to literature, the joint degeneration process starts as soon as seven days after CrCL rupture and, at Day 21, signals suggesting osteoarthritis can be radiographically examined. In arthroscopic evaluation, however, lesions are already significant and characteristic in this period.

Arthroscopy is a minimally invasive exam, with minimal morbidity, which allows complete visualization of structures with magnification of images and precise diagnosis of the articular condition in its natural environment. The minimal morbidity enables periodic joint evaluations (Van Ryssen & Van Bree, 1998; Hulse et al., 2010; Goldhammer et al., 2010), what permits to monitor the lesion (Borges, 2006; Bleedorn et al., 2011) and the treatment evolution (Case et al., 2008), allowing the articular function prognosis (Ljungvall & Ronéus, 2011).

Arthroscopy can be employed for evaluating and defining the DJD staging. It gives the surgeon a better understanding of the joint degeneration process, the most prevailing condition among all diseases in the dog.

The arthroscopy had a significant impact especially in our clinical practice in what concerns diagnosis and treatment of articular alterations in the dog. Non-specific arthritis, hemarthrosis, meniscus lesions, ligament partial ruptures, femoral condyle osteochondrosis, and presence of loose cartilaginous bodies not diagnosed by the radiographic exam are examples of clinical situations that nowadays are promptly diagnosed and treated through arthroscopy.

The arthroscopic monitoring of the femoro-patellar-tibial joint after CrCL rupture changed the procedures by which such condition is treated in our routine, and its stabilization began to be considered as a condition that must be treated the most precociously possible and through arthroscopy. The main challenge is the development of efficient therapies for the osteoarthritis control. The association of articular stabilization with cell therapy (stem cells, growth factors) is one of the alternatives under study at the moment. The purpose of this chapter is, in the meanwhile, presenting the articular findings, under arthroscopic vision, 21 days after arthroscope-guided CrCL rupture, taking as reference the parameters found in the arthroscopic exam right before rupture.

The rupture of the cranial cruciate ligament (CrCL) is one of the most frequent orthopedic affections in the dog (Johnston, 1997; Beale & Hulse, 2010; Van Bree et al., 2010). After rupture, the CrCL does not regenerate, leading to lost of joint stability. The resulting instability leads to the development of degenerative joint disease (DJD) (Innes, 2010), and treatment is still challenging. The unavoidable DJD progression (Vasseur & Berry, 1992; Lazar et al., 2005) is caused by enzymatic degradation of the articular cartilage (Bennett & May, 1997). As the alterations in the cartilage progress, reduction in the content of proteoglycans, hyalunoric acid, and collagen (in minor proportion) occur due to the action of catabolic enzymes released by the DJD. Once the cartilaginous lesion is installed, the subchondral bone is exposed to the synovial fluid and, when subjected to abnormal pressures and tensions, reacts forming osteophytes and subchondral sclerosis (Johnston, 1997). Periarticular osteophytes indicate articular instability and are one of the most evident radiographic signs of DJD (Schrader, 1995; Innes et al., 2004). Osteophytes are bone projections located at the peripheral region of the joint, most frequently at the osseous insertion of the synovial membrane, the perichondrium, and the periosteum, though it may occur at the central region of the joint (Johnston, 1997). As the DJD evolves, after CrCL rupture, formation of osteophytes occurs first at the osteochondral margin of the lateral and medial trochlear ridges, then at the proximal region of the tibia and the proximal and distal borders of the patella (Lewis et al., 1987; Moore & Read, 1996). Some studies attribute to the synovitis and the consequent release of inflammatory mediators by the synoviocytes the triggering factors for DJD (Lipowitz et al., 1985;). In DJD, the synovial villi are hypertrophied, with augmented mature and immature collagen in the subsynovial tissue (Jonhston, 1997). McIlwraith & Fessler (1978) classified morphologically the villi in filamentous, thin, interlaced, short, and in the shapes of polyp, staff, fringe, bush, fan, and cauliflower. In normal joints, the thin polyp-shaped, and the short, rounded, membranous and staff-shaped villi are commonly observed (McIlwraith & Fessler, 1978; Kurosaka et al., 1991), while bigger and reddish villi, with petechial hemorrhages, and in the shapes of fan, cauliflower, fringe and bush are frequently found in joints with synovitis (McIlwraith & Fessler, 1978). The follow-up of the degenerative process evolution, as well as its treatment response, is constantly challenging. Among the methods routinely used in DJD diagnosis are the clinical evaluation (which is subjective) and the radiographic and ultrasonographic examination (which rely on the evaluator's experience). The arthroscopy is another diagnostic method that, despite being an invasive procedure and requiring anesthesia, it allows direct and magnified evaluation of the articular structures, and enables serial evaluations, once tissue invasion and morbidity are minimal (Van Ryssen & Van Bree, 1998; Frizziero & Ronchetti, 2002; Arias et al., 2003; Beale et al., 2003; Melo et al., 2003; Borges, 2006; Rezende et al., 2006; Hulse, et al., 2010; Bleedorn et al., 2011). In CrCL rupture, arthroscopy offers more than a precise diagnosis of the affection, it allows evaluation through magnified visualization of degenerative alterations of the joint such as fibrillation, cartilage erosion, synovial membrane proliferation, and neovascularization, osteophytes formation, besides detecting lesions in the menisci (Siemering & Eilert, 1986; Adamiak, 2002; Borges, 2006; Case et al., 2008; Goldhammer et al., 2010; Hulse et al., 2010; Bleedorn et al., 2011.

Arthroscopy in dogs, initially employed for diagnostic purpose, has become a surgical alternative to many articular affections (Rochat, 2001) and has revolutionized the treatment of joint disease in human beings and animals (Beale & Hulse, 2010). The magnifying of the structures allows the surgeon to recognize and treat lesions that could not be distinguished through arthrotomy (Van Ryssen & Van Bree, 1998; Sams, 2000; Borges, 2006; Beale & Hulse, 2010; Hulse et al, 2010; Bleedorn et al., 2011).

2. Materials and methods

This study was submitted to and approved by the UFMG committee for ethics in research, under protocol number 14/02.

Eighteen mixed breed, adult healthy dogs (9 males and 9 females), with 18 to 25kg of body mass were used in this work. The animals were sheltered in individual cages and fed with commercial pet food and water *ad libitum*. Bilateral radiographic examination of the stifle joint was performed in craniocaudal and mediolateral incidences to confirm the radiographic normality of these joints in both hind limbs. Blood samples were collected for serum biochemical analysis, hemogram, and coagulogram. After 15 days of adaptation period, the first arthroscopy was performed to articular evaluation and CrCL section, and the second, for articular evaluation 21 days later. The animals were premedicated with atropine sulfate (0.044mg/kg), subcutaneously, and xylazine chlorhydrate (1mg/kg), intramuscularly. Anesthesia was induced with sodium thiopental (12.5mg/kg), intravenously, and maintained with isoflurane in semi-open circuit. Antibiotic prophylaxis was performed with cefalotin (30mg/kg), intravenously, 30 minutes before surgery. All animals received tramadol chlorhydrate (2mg/kg), intramuscularly, in the immediate post-operative period and during 24 hours for pain management.

The animals were submitted to arthroscopic evaluation and subsequent CrCL section. The animals were prepared for aseptic surgery and positioned in dorsal recumbence over a metal gutter. Synovial fluid was collected in heparinized syringe and the joint cavity was distended with 10 to 15 ml of Ringer's lactate solution thereafter. A 5 mm cutaneous incision was performed in the lateral parapatellar region, and the articular capsule was incisioned with a scalpel blade No. 11 for introducing the arthroscopic sheath guided by atraumatic trocar. The irrigation system was attached to the arthroscopic sheath while the atraumatic trocar was removed and replaced by a 2.7mm, 30° arthroscope, connected to the camera. Arthroscopic evaluation was conducted based on the articular compartments, as suggested by Person (1985). Articular structures were inspected: the lateral compartment with visualization of the synovial membrane, the lateral femur condyle, the long digital extensor tendon, the intercondylar fossa, the tibial plateau, the menisci, the intermeniscal and cruciate ligaments, the medial compartment, the medial femur condyle, the femoropatellar joint (articular surfaces of femur and patella, trochlear ridges), and the suprapatellar pouch. A second cutaneous and capsular incision was performed in the medial parapatellar region for introducing the arthroscopic scissor, as mentioned above. The CrCL was sectioned, remaining the intra-articular stumps. The CrCL section was confirmed by direct visualization by arthroscopy, and by the test of cranially dislocating the tibia in relation to the femur. The animals were kept in individual 4.5m^2 cages, for 21 days, and, after that period, submitted to new arthroscopic examination. Synovial fluid was collected, and the joint cavity was distented as described above. The intra-articular structures were systematically evaluated, as previously described, and the alterations found in the soft and in the hard tissues were documented . The images were analyzed based on the arthroscopic findings on Day 0, when the first arthroscopy was performed followed by the CrCL rupture, and at Day 21, when a new arthroscopy was conducted for evaluating the articular lesions. The structures were also individually evaluated, and abnormalities were registered. According to their quantity and aspect, villi were classified (Tab.1) from 1 to 4; grade 1 represented absence of lesion and 4, severe lesion. The villi were also morphologically classified as: filamentous, thin, interlaced, short, and as polyp, staff, fringe, bush, fan, and cauliflower shapes. In addition, they were categorized in respect to their localization: lateral and medial compartments, patellar ligament, and patellar tendon. The presence or absence of intra-articular fibrous cords was taken into account. Additionally, the articular cartilage was evaluated by area: patella, suprapatellar pouch, trochlear surface, intercondylar fossa, medial and lateral femur condyles, trochlear ridges of the femur, and surface of the tibia condyles. Likewise, the presence of osteophytes was classified according to the scores in Table 2.

Villi of the synovial membrane

Score	Description
1	Absent.
2	Mild: thin, filamentous, and short villi; white or rosy.
3	Moderate: thin, filamentous, short, in the shapes of polyp, fan, bush, and staff villi; reddish.
4	Severe: numerous villi, dense in the shapes of cauliflower, fringe, located mainly at the lateral and medial compartments; with hemorrhagic aspect and reddish color.

Vascularization of the synovial membrane

Score	Description
1	Absent.
2	Mild: discrete presence of ingurgitated vessel in up to two regions.
3	Moderate: vascularization, apparent hyperemia at the lateral and medial compartments, cruciate ligaments, and menisci.
4	Severe: hypervascularization, hyperemia of the lateral and medial compartments, menisci, and ligaments; articular hemorrhage.

Table 1. Scores system for the synovial membrane characteristics evaluated by stifle joint arthroscopy on Days 0 and 21 after section of the cranial cruciate ligament (CrCL).

Score	Description
1	Absent: smooth articular surface.
2	Mild: low projection irregularities.
3	Moderate: remarkable low projection irregularities, countable bone neoformation with individualized contour.
4	Severe: remarkable irregularity, neoformations with high projection individualized contour, present all over the periarticular region, including the suprapatellar pouch, the tibial plateau, and the intercondylar fossa.

Table 2. Score system for the presence of osteophytes evaluated by stifle joint arthroscopy on Days 0 and 21 after section of the cranial cruciate ligament (CrCL).

The lateral and medial menisci were evaluated according to the presence or absence of lesion. For the cruciate ligaments, the presence or absence of alterations was determined, according to neovascularization, looseness, and fiber rupture. The long digital extensor tendon was evaluated according to the presence or absence of neovascularization and villi at the insertion of the femur condyle. The variables of this study are the lesions that might have arisen or evolved, after the ligament rupture, evaluated on Day 21 by arthroscopy. The Wilcoxon test was employed for paired samples for all variables (lesions), except osteophytes, for which a unilateral test was used. For comparisons, significance was set at $P < 0.05$.

3. Results and discussion

The arthroscopic examination was possible in both evaluation moments, and, as described by Person (1985), systematic examination of the joint allowed the ordering of the results (Tables 3 and 4). All structures that were visualized on Day 0 were also seen on Day 21, when it was possible to detect, in 100% of the joints, alterations in relation to Day 0, fact that was expected given the joint instability, however, statistical significance was noticed in 83.3% (Table 5). The parapatellar approach was adequate for evaluating all the articular structures or regions in this study, as well as for sectioning the CrCL. The positioning of the animal allowed flexion, extension, *varus* and *valgus* movements, and rotation of the joint during the procedure, facilitating the detailed arthroscopic examination, as reported in literature (Van Ryssen & Van Bree, 1998; Arias et al., 2003; Beale et al., 2003; Melo et al., 2003; Rezende et al., 2006, Borges, 2006).

Structure	Region	Alteration	Wilcoxon	P-value
Synovial membrane	Lateral and medial compartments, suprapatellar region, and insertion of the patellar ligament and tendon	Villi	136.0	0.000
		Vascularization	120.0	0.001
		Fibrous cord		No variability[1]
Articular cartilage	Patella	Erosion		No variability[1]
		Fibrillation	10.00	0.100
		Vascularization	1.00	1.000

Structure	Region	Alteration	Wilcoxon	P-value
Patellar pouch		Erosion		No variability[1]
		Fibrillation	10.00	0.100
		Vascularization	45.00	0.009
Trochlea		Erosion		No variability[1]
		Fibrillation	6.00	0.181
		Vascularization	3.00	0.371
Intercondy-lar fossa		Erosion		No variability[1]
		Fibrillation	3.00	0.371
		Vascularization	10.00	0.100
Lateral femoral condyle		Erosion		No variability[1]
		Fibrillation	55.00	0.006
		Vascularization	36.00	0.014
Medial femoral condyle		Erosion		No variability[1]
		Fibrillation	21.00	0.036
		Vascularization	21.00	0.036
Tibia		Erosion		No variability[1]
		Fibrillation		
		Vascularization		No variability[2]
Lateral trochlear ridge		Erosion		No variability[1]
		Fibrillation	10.00	0.100
		Vascularization	1.000	1.000
Medial trochlear ridge		Erosion		No variability[1]
		Fibrillation	6.00	0.181
		Vascularization	1.00	1.000
Medial meniscus			10.00	0.100
Lateral meniscus				No variability[1]
Cranial cruciate ligament		Vascularization	10.00	0.100

Structure	Region	Alteration	Wilcoxon	P-value
Caudal cruciate ligament		Vascularization	6.00	0.181
Long digital extensor tendon		Neovascularization	6.00	0.181
		Villi		No variability[3]

[1] All the evaluated differences were equal to 0, thus no lesion was observed on Days 0 and 21.
[2] All the evaluated differences were equal to 0, thus no lesion was observed on Days 0 and 21, except one dog, which already presented lesion before the rupture that persisted after the 21-day period.
[3] All the evaluated differences were equal to 0, thus no lesion was observed on Days 0 and 21, except one dog, which already presented lesion before the rupture that persisted after the 21-day period.

Table 3. Wilcoxon test for the different lesions, observed between Days 0 and 21, at the stifle joint of dogs submitted to arthroscope-guided section of the cranial cruciate ligament (CrCL).

Structure	Region	Wilcoxon	P-value
Articular cartilage	Patella	1.00	0.500
	Suprapatellar pouch	10.00	0.050
	Trochlea	No variability[1]	
	Intercondylar fossa	No variability[1]	
	Lateral femoral condyle	1.00	1.000
	Medialfemoral condyle	No variability[1]	
	Tibia	No variability[1]	
	Lateral trochlear ridge	45.00	0.005
	Medial trochlear ridge	13.00	0.089

[1]All the observed differences were equal to 0, thus no lesion was observed on Days 0 and 21.

Table 4. Wilcoxon test for osteophyte presence, observed on Days 0 and 21, at the stifle joint of dogs submitted to arthroscope-guided section of the cranial cruciate ligament (CrCL).

Dog	1	2	3	4	5	6	7	8	9
Wilcoxon	120	3	113	15	105	66	66	21	21
P-value	0.001	0.371	0.003	0.059	0.001	0.004	0.004	0.036	0.036
Dog	10	11	12	13	14	15	16	17	18
Wilcoxon	28	21	91	91	105	66	10	15	55
P-value	0.022	0.036	0.002	0.002	0.001	0.004	0.100	0.059	0.006

Table 5. Individual analysis of the intra-articular lesions of dogs, evaluated on Days 0 and 21, after arthroscope-guided section of the cranial cruciate ligament (CrCL).

It was possible to precisely evaluate the menisci, the intermeniscal ligament, the synovial membrane, the articular cartilage, the cruciate ligaments, and the long digital extensor tendon by arthroscopy, as described in the literature (Van Ryssen & Van Bree, 1998; Adamiak, 2002; Beale et al., 2003; Borges, 2006). The precision offered by the arthroscopic examination is reported by distinct authors (Sams, 2000; Adamiak, 2002; Arias et al., 2003; Beale et al., 2003; Melo et al., 2003; Rezende et al., 2006; Beale & Hulse, 2010). Subcutaneous infiltration of liquid was not observed. Depending on the intensity of infiltration, capsule distension is impaired, and the examination becomes unviable (Van Ryssen et al., 1993). The arthroscopy showed itself as an effective method for evaluating the degenerative alterations after experimental CrCL section. According to Lipowitz et al. (1985) and Lewis et al. (1987), the CrCL section is accepted as the best model for the experimental induction of degenerative lesions. This result was observed in this study, with the additional advantage of direct visualization and magnification of image by arthroscopy, which allowed the evaluation of joint instability, as already reported by others (Lipowitz et al., 1985; Johnson & Johnson, 1993; Glyde et al., 2002; Hulse et al., 2010; Bleedorn et al., 2011). According to Arnoczcky & Marshall (1977), the degenerative process begins one week after CrCL rupture; thus, the articular evaluation on Day 21 is able to identify macroscopic lesions precociously, as observed in this study.

Signs of articular degeneration and inflammation could be noticed at the arthroscopic examination. According to Bennett & May (1997) and Vaughan-Scott & Taylor (1997), the unavoidable DJD progression can be mostly attributed to the enzymatic degradation of the articular cartilage.

For each dog, 14 areas or structures were evaluated by arthroscopy, in a total of 504 individual evaluations. On the day of the CrCL section, 17 dogs (94.4%) presented shining and smooth surfaces of femur and patella, without periarticular osteophytes (Fig. 1.1). Only in one animal (5.6%), irregularities at the trochlear ridge were detected.

From 18 evaluated joints, eight (44.4%) had villous proliferation of thin and filamentous types (Fig. 1.2), considered normal according to McIlwraith & Fessler (1978) and Lewis et al. (1987). In one animal, these villi were hyperemic, and, in nine, the synovial membrane was smooth, without villi. In all the cases, the villi were located at the medial compartment. McIlwraith & Fessler (1978) reported that, in normal articulations, the thin, filamentous, and polyp-shaped villi are commonly observed in equines. Similar findings were reported in dogs (Lewis et al., 1987). Joint with normal villi, but with evident hyperemia suggests inflammatory process, and once the villous type is considered normal, it is possible to infer that the process is at an initial phase.

Discrete hyperemia of the synovial membrane was observed in 17 (94.4%) dogs on Day 0 (Fig. 1.3), during the procedure that lasted 15 minutes on average. Due to the absence of dense fibrous tissue in the synovial membrane, increased local irrigation with congestion and swelling can develop during prolonged arthroscopic procedure (Lewis et al., 1987; Kurosaka et al., 1991), what may explain the findings of this work, not being, necessarily, synovial inflammation. In 14 dogs, the presence of blood vessels (Fig. 1.4) was observed along the CrCL. Despite these alterations in vascularization, the CrCL was intact and shining on Day 0, as well as the caudal cruciate ligament, the meniscofemoral ligament (Fig.1.5), and the long digital extensor tendon (Fig. 1.6). The origin of the popliteus muscle tendon was visualized in two animals (Fig. 1.7), and presented no alteration.

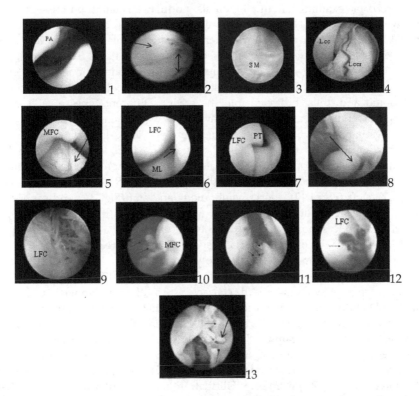

Fig. 1. Arthroscopic images of the stifle joint of dogs submitted to experimental section of the cranial cruciate ligament (Days 0 and 21) guided by arthroscopy. 1) Articular surfaces of the patella (PA) and trochlea (TC) of the femur without alterations; 2) Synovial membrane of the lateral compartment with filamentous villi (arrow), lateral condyle of the femur (arrow); 3) Synovial membrane (MS) with discrete hyperemia at the medial compartment; 4) Blood vessel along of the cranial cruciate ligament (LCCr), caudal cruciate ligament(LCCd); 5) Meniscofemoral ligament (arrow); 6) Lateral compartment showing the lateral femoral condyle (LFC), long digital extensor tendon (arrow) and lateral meniscus (LM) 7) Origin of the popliteus muscle tendon(PT); 8) Intercondylar fossa with thin villi, stump of the cranial cruciate ligament showing nodular formation on the end of the torn ligament (arrow); 9) Villi in the shape of filamentous at the lateral compartiment; 10) Villi in the shape of polyp (arrows) at the medial compartment, medial femoral condyle (MFC); 11) Villus in the shape of fringe(arrows), lateral femoral condyle (LFC); 12) Villus in the shape of fan (arrow), lateral femoral condyle (CLF); 13) Lateral compartment showing villi in the shape of staff (arrow).

On Day 21 after CrCL section, at the arthroscopic examination, alterations suggesting articular degenerative process came to evidence. The arthroscopy, as mentioned by Adamiak (2002), is effective in precisely diagnosing the CrCL rupture and evaluating the evolution of the degenerative lesions of the joint, fact that was verified in this study.

At the arthroscopic examination, in all animals, nodular formation on the end of the torn ligament were observed in the remaining stump of the CrCL on Day 21 (Fig. 1.8). In all animals, villous proliferation and synovial membrane hyperemia were observed, suggesting synovitis. As already reported by Van Ryssen & Van Bree (1998), Sams (2000), Adamiak (2002), and Beale & Hulse (2010), arthroscopy is an ideal diagnostic mean for evaluating macroscopically the synovial membrane, since the villi are kept in suspension in the irrigation liquid and, thus, projected into the cavity. Different types of villi, as well as different grades of hyperemia and vascularization were identified in detail (Table 1). Increase in the quantity of villi and new shapes were verified. Also, villous proliferations in all articular compartments were evidenced, suggesting DJD, as described in literature (Lewis et al., 1987; Kurosaka et al., 1991; Beale et al, 2003; Borges, 2006). Filamentous and thin (Fig 1.9), short, interlaced, as well as in the shape of polyp (Fig. 1.10), fringe (Fig. 1.11), fan (Fig. 1.12), staff (Fig. 1.13), short, membranous and staff(Fig. 2.1) and cauliflower villi were identified. In 21.8% of the joints, there were only short, thin, and filamentous villi, characterizing discrete synovitis. These three types of villi were found in bigger quantity and in all joints. In 55.5% of the animals, associated to the already mentioned villi, there were also those in the shape of bush, fan, polyp, and interlaced, characterizing moderate synovitis. In 22.7%, villi in the shape of fringe and cauliflower were also found, characterizing severe synovitis. Such characteristics of the synovial membrane are associated to DJD. In humans, the arthroscopic examination of the synovial membrane is employed for characterizing and diagnosing different types of pathological articular processes, as, for instance, traumatic, suppurative, tubercular, and rheumatoid arthritis (Kurosaka et al., 1991). At the insertion of the long digital extensor tendon, neovascularization was noticed in three animals (Fig. 2.2), while, in two, thin and apparently normal-colored villi (Fig. 2.3) were seen. Fibrillation in the articular cartilage and absence of erosion in the articular surfaces were verified in all evaluated animals. Fibrillation, according to Johnston (1997), is the initial microscopic finding of DJD. It may be observed as soon as one week after CrCL rupture (Johnson and Johnson, 1993), while erosive lesions are late findings, which occur with, at least, 60 days of joint instability. Statistically, fibrillation was predominant (Table 3) at the medial and lateral condyles (Fig. 2.4). Areas of fibrillation at the articular surface of the patella, the trochlear ridges of the femur, and the intercondylar fossa were also observed (Fig. 2.5). Fibrillation of the articular surface was arthroscopically evidenced as filaments from the cartilage into the articular space. In arthroscopy, the visualization of fibrillation is possible due to the amplified image and the liquid environment. By arthrotomy, it is only possible to detect areas that are apparently thickened, rugose, and opaque, corresponding to fibrillation (Sams, 2000; Adamiak, 2002). There was also fibrin at the lateral (66.%) and medial (34%) compartments (Fig. 2.6 and 2.7, respectively), and at the suprapatellar pouch (27.7%; Fig. 2.8), as well as osteophytes at the trochlear ridges, distal extremity of the patella, and suprapatellar pouch. Osteophytosis was statistically significant (Table 4) at the lateral trochlear ridge (Fig. 2.9). Muzzi (2003) detected radiographically the formation of osteophytes with, at least, 30 days of CrCL rupture. The arthroscopic findings concerning the presence of osteophytes, 21 days after articular destabilization were similar to those reported by Lewis et al. (1987). The presence of periarticular osteophytes is one of the signs of DJD (Elkins et al., 1991; Moore & Read, 1996). Thirteen animals presented vascularization of the articular cartilage, evidenced at the insertion of the patellar ligament and quadriceps tendon (Fig. 2.10 and 2.11), at the suprapatellar pouch towards the trochlea (Fig. 2.12), at the femoral condyles (2.13), and at the intercondylar fossa towards the condyles. This was statistically significant for the region of the femoral condyles. Such a finding corresponds not to the cartilage vascularization itself, but to the synovial membrane vascularization that invades the cartilage.

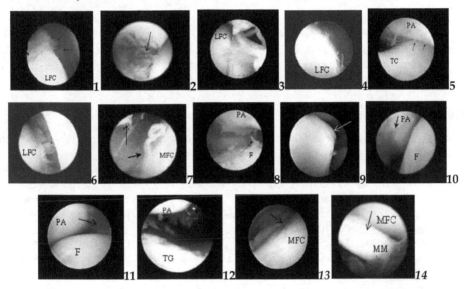

Fig. 2. Arthroscopic images of the stifle joint of dogs submitted to experimental section of the cranial cruciate ligament (Days 0 and 21) guided by arthroscopy. 1) Lateral compartment showing villi short, membranous and in the shape of staff (arrows); 2) Visualization of the long digital extensor tendon, vascularization (arrow), 3) Thin villi at the long digital extensor tendon (arrow), lateral femoral condyle (LFC), 4) Fibrillation at the lateral femoral condyle (LFC); 5) Fibrillation (arrows) and fibrin at the surface of the patella (PA), proximal trochlear groove (TC); 6) Fibrin attached to the lateral femoral condyle (LFC) (arrows); 7) Fibrin at the medial femoral condyle (arrow) and patella; 8) Supratellar pouch with vascularization and fibrin (arrow); 9) Lateral femoral condyle (LFC) with mild osteophytes (irregularities: arrow); 10) Vascularization at the insertion of the patellar ligament (arrow); 11) patellar tendon (arrow); 12) suprapatellar pouch 13); and at the medial trochlear ridge of the femoral condyle (arrow) 14) Prolapse of the caudal horn of the medial meniscus (MM).

Statistically, the results regarding the lesion in the menisci were not significant; nevertheless, prolapse of the caudal horn of medial meniscus (Fig. 2.14) was visualized in four animals (22.2%). In one of them, on Day 0, there were alterations compatible with synovitis, like hyperemia and increased synovial membrane villi. Three of them presented, on Day 21, meniscus lesion and periarticular irregularities. The medial meniscus is more susceptive to lesions due to its capsule fixation (Moore & Read, 1996). It is reported that meniscus lesions occur about the seventh week of articular instability by CrCL rupture (Johnson & Johnson, 1993). In this work, the precocious occurrence of this kind of lesion may be attributed to the eventual excited behavior of the patients. Concerning the DJD, the body mass of the animals, which ranged from 18 to 25 kg, must also be considered for this study. According to Bennett et al. (1988), the CrCL rupture in dogs with body mass under 15 kg usually causes degenerative alterations that are less severe than in heavier dogs.

4. Conclusions

As a valuable instrument for macroscopic evaluation of articular tissues, arthroscopy is a safe method for diagnosing and following-up the alterations in the stifle joint of dogs. The technique allows tracking the evolution of the degenerative lesions, as well as classifying the synovitis according to the villi shape and synovial membrane hyperemia.

5. References

Adamiak, Z. (2002). Arthroscopy in dogs with cranial cruciate ligament injuries.*Indian Vet. J.* vol.79, n° 2, pp.177-178, ISSN 0019-6479

Arias, S.A., Rezende, C.M.F., Melo, E.G.,Nunes, V.A. & Correa, J.C (2003). Radiological, arthroscopical evaluation and synovial membrane histology of the knee of dogs treated with chondroitin sulphate- sodium hialuronate association after experimental degenerative joint disease. *Brasilian J. Vet. Res. Anim. Sci.*, vol.55, n°4, pp. 421-429, ISSN 0102-0935

Arnoczky, S.P. & Marshall, J.L. (1977). The cruciate ligaments of the canine stifle: An anatomical and funcional analysis. *Am. J. Vet. Res.*, vol.38, n° 11, pp.1807-1814, ISSN 0002-9645

Beale, B. S., Hulse, D. A., Schulz, K. S.,Whitney, W. O. (2003). Arthroscopically assisted surgery of the stifle joint, In: *Small Animal arthroscopy*, 117-157, Saunders, ISBN 0-7216-8969-8, Philadelphia, Pennsylvania

Beale, B. S. & Hulse, D. A.(2010). Arthroscopy versus arthrotomy for surgical treatment, In: *Advances in the canine cranial cruciate ligament*, P. Muir,(Ed.), 145-158, Wiley-Blackwell, ISBN 978-0-8138-1852-8, Ames, Iowa

Bennett, D. & May, C. (1997). Joint diseases of dogs and cats. In: *Textbook of Veterinary Internal Medicine.* 4.ed., S.J. Ettinger & E.C. Feldman (Eds.), pp. 2032-2077, Saunders, ISBN 0721634273, Philadelphia, Pensylvania.

Bennett, D. Tennant, B. Lewis, D.G. Baughan, J. May, C. & Carter, S. (1988). A re-appraisal of anterior cruciate ligament disease in the dog. *J. Small Anim. Pract.*, vol. 29, n°5, pp.275-297, ISSN 0022-4510

Bleedorn, J. A, Greuel, E. N., Manley, P. A., Schaefer, S. L., Markel, M. D., Holzman, G., Muir, P. (2011). Synovitis in dogs with stable stifle joints and incipient cranial cruciate ligament rupture: a cross-sectional study. Vet. Surg. vol 40, n° 5, pp. 531-543, ISSN 0161-3499

Borges, N.F. (2006).*Videoarthroscopy of the femorotibiopatellar joint in dogs before and 21 daysafter cranial cruciate ligament rupture (experimental study).* 40pp. Dissertation) Escola de Veterinária, Universidade Federal de Minas Gerais, Belo Horizonte, Brazil

Case, J. B., Hulse, D. Kerwin, S. C., Peycke, L. E. (2008). Meniscal injury following initialcranial cruciate ligament stabilization surgery in 26 dogs (29 stifles). *Vet. Comp.Orthop. Traumatol.*, vol. 21, n° 4, pp. 365-367, ISSN 0932-0814

Cook, J. L. (2010). Cranial cruciate ligament disease in dogs: biology versus biomechanics.Vet. Surg. vol. 39, n° 3, pp. 270-277, ISSN 0161-3499

de Rooster, H., de Bruin,T., Van Bree, H. (2010). Morphology and function of the cruciate ligaments, In: *Advances in the canine cranial cruciate ligament*, P. Muir,(Ed.), 5-12, Wiley-Blackwell, ISBN 978-0-8138-1852-8, Ames, Iowa

Elkins, A.D., Pechman, R. & Kearney, M.T. (1991). A retrospective study evaluating the degree of degenerative joint disease in the stifle joint of dogs following surgical repair of anterior cruciate ligament rupture. *J. Am. Anim. Hosp. Assoc.*, vol.27, September/October, pp.533-540, ISSN 0587-2871

Frizziero,L. & Ronchetti, I.P.(2002). Intra-articular treatment of osteoarthritis of the knee: an Anthroscopic and clinical comparison between sodium hyaluronate (500-730 kDa) and methilprednisolone acetate. *J.Orthopaed. Traumatol.*, vol. 3, n°2, pp.89-96, ISSN 1590-9921

Glyde, M.R. Wong, W.T., Lidbetter, D. Parry, B. & Middleton, D. (2002). Partial rupture of the cranial cruciate ligament in 13 dogs: Clinical, radiological, clinicopathological and histhopathological features. *Ir. Vet. J.*, vol. 55, n°6, pp. 271-276, ISSN 0368-0762

Goldhammer,M.A., Smith, S. H., Fitzpatrick, N., Clements, D. N. (2010). A comparison of radiographic, arthroscopic and histological measures of articular pathology in the canine elbow joint. *The Vet. Journal*, vol.186, n° 1, pp. 96-103, ISSN 1090-0233

Hulse, D., Beale, B., Kerwin, S. (2010). Second look arthroscopic findings after tibial plateauLeveling osteotomy. *Vet. Surg.* vol. 39, n° 3, pp. 350-354, ISSN 0161-3499

Innes, J. F., Costello ,M., Barr, F. J., Rudorf, H., Barry, A. R. S.(2004). *Vet. Radiol. Ultrasound*,vol. 45, n° 2, pp.143-148, ISSN 1058-8183

Innes, J. F.(2010). Progression of arthritis after stifle stabilization, In: *Advances in the caninecranial cruciate ligament*, P. Muir,(Ed.), 229-232, Wiley-Blackwell, ISBN 978-0-8138 -1852-8, Ames, Iowa

Johnson, J.M. & Johnson, A.L. (1993). Cranial cruciate ligament rupture: pathogenesis, diagnosis, and postoperative rehabilitation. *Vet. Clin. North Am.: Small Anim. Pract.*, vol.23 n°4, pp.717-733, ISSN 0195-5616

Johnston, A.S. (1997). Ostearthritis: joint anatomy, physiology and pathobiology. *Vet. Clin. North. Am.:Small Anim. Pract.*, vol.27, n°4, pp. 699-719, ISSN 0195-5616

Kurosaka, M., Ohno, O.& Hirorat, A.K.(1991). Arthroscopic evaluation of synovitis in the knee joints. *Arthroscopy*, vol.7, n° 2, pp.162-170, ISSN 0749-8063

Lazar, T. P., Berry, C. R., de Haan, J. J., Peck,J. N. Correoa, M.(2005). Long-term radio-graphic comparison of tibial plateau leveling osteotomy versus extra-capsular stabilization for cranial cruciate ligament rupture in the dog. *Vet. Surg.*, vol.34, n° 2, pp. 133-141, ISSN 0161-3499

Lewis, D.D.; Goring, R.L.; Parker, R.B. & Curasi, P.A. (1987). A comparison of diagnostic methods used in the evaluation of early degenerative joint disease in the dog. *J. Am. Anim. Hosp. Assoc.*, vol.23, May/June, pp. 305-315, ISSN 0587-2871

Lipowitz, A.J.; Wong, P.L.; Stevens, J.B. (1985). Synovial membrane changes after experimental transecction of the cranial cruciate ligament in dogs. *Am. J. Vet. Res.*, vol. 46, n° 5, pp.1166-1170, ISSN 0002-9645

Ljungvall, K. & Ronéus, B. (2011). Arthroscopic surgery of the middle carpal joint in trotting Standardbreds: findings and outcome. Vet. Comp. Orthop. Traumatol. , vol. 24, N° 5, PMID 21792476, DOI: 10.3415/VCOT-10-12-0161, ISSN 0932-0814

McIlwraith, C.W.& Fessler, J.F. (1978). Arthroscopy in the diagnosis of equine joint disease. *J. Am. Vet. Med. Assoc.*, vol.172, n° 3, p.263-268, ISSN 0003-1488

Melo, E.G., Rezende, C.M.F., Gomes, M.G., Freitas, P.M., Arias, S.A.S. (2003) .Chondroitin sulfate and sodium hialuronate in treatment of the degenerative joint disease in dogs. Clinical and radiological aspects. *Brasilian J. Vet. Res. Anim. Sci.* vol. 55, n° 1, pp.35-43, ISSN 0102-0935

Moore, K.W. & Read, R.A. (1996). Rupture of the cranial cruciate ligament in dogs. Part I. *Compend. Cont. Educ. Pract. Vet.*, vol.18, n°3, p.223-234, ISSN 0193-1903

Muzzi, L.A.L. (2003). *Physiotherapie and temporary immobilization after arthroscopic repair of the cranial cruciate ligament in dogs.* 79pp. (Thesis) - Escola de Veterinária, Universidade Federal de Minas Gerais, Belo Horizonte, Brazil

Person, M.W. (1985). A procedure for arthroscopic examination of the canine stifle joint. *J. Am. Anim. Hosp. Assoc.*, vol.21, March/April, pp.179-186, ISSN 0587-2871

Pozzi, A. & Kim, S. E.(2010). Biomechanics of the normal and cranial cruciate ligament-deficient stifle, In: *Advances in the canine cranial cruciate ligament*, P. Muir,(Ed.), 37-42, Wiley-Blackwell, ISBN 978-0-8138-1852-8, Ames, Iowa

Rezende, C.M.F., Melo, E.G., Madureira, N.G., Freitas, P. M. (2006). Arthroscopy of the stifle joint in dogs. *Brasilian J.Vet.Res.Anim. Sci.* vol. 58, n° 5, pp. 841-848, ISSN 0102-0935

Rochat, M.C. Arthroscopy. (2001).*Vet. Clin. North. Am.:Small Anim. Pract.*, vol.31, pp.761-787, ISSN 0195-5616

Sams, A.E. (2000). Canine elbow joint arthroscopy: introduction and description of technique. *Comp. cont. Educ. Pract.Vet.* vol. 22. n° 2, pp.135-144, ISSN 0193-1903

Schrader, S.C. (1995). Joint diseases of the dog and cat. In: *Small animal orthopedics*, M.L. Olmstead, (Ed.), pp.437-471, Mosby, ISBN 0-8016-5874-8, St. Louis, Missouri

Siemering, G.B. & Eilert, R.E. (1986). Arthroscopy study of cranial cruciate ligament and medial meniscal lesions in the dog. *Vet. Surg.* vol.15, n° 3,pp.265-269, ISSN 0161-3499

Van Bree, H., de Rooster, H., Gielen, I. (2010). Stress radiography of the stifle,In: *Advances in the canine cranial cruciate ligament*, P. Muir,(Ed.), 113-116,Wiley-Blackwell, ISBN 978-0-8138-1852-8, Ames, Iowa

Van Ryssen, B., Van Bree, H. & Missinne, S. (1993).Successfull arthroscopy treatment of shoulder osteochondrosis in the dog. *J. Small Anim. Pract.*, vol.34, n° 10, pp.521-528, ISSN 0022-4510

Van Ryssen, B. & Van Bree, H. (1998). Diagnostic and surgical arthroscopy in small animals, In: *Canine Sports Medicine and Surgery*, M.S. Bloomberg, J.F.Dee & R. A.Taylor,(Eds.), pp.250-254, Saunders, ISBN 0-7216-5022-8, Philadelphia, Pennsylvania

Vasseur, P. B. & Berry, C. R.(1992). Progression of stifle osteoarthrosis followingreconstruction of the cranial cruciate ligament in 21 dogs. J. Am. Anim. Hosp.Assoc., vol. 28, March/april, pp.129-136, ISSN 0587-2871

Vaughan-Scott, T. & Taylor, J.H. (1997).The pathophysiology and medical management of canine osteoarthrtitis. *J. S. Afr. Vet. Assoc.*, vol.68, n° 1, pp.21-25,ISSN 0038-2809

11

Congenital Aplasia of the Uterine-Vaginal Segment in Dogs

Bruno Colaço, Maria dos Anjos Pires
and Rita Payan-Carreira
CECAV, Univ. of Trás-os-Montes and Alto Douro,
Portugal

1. Introduction

Müllerian duct abnormalities consist of a set of structural malformations that include diverse situations of agenesis or aplasia, which may evolve according to three distinct patterns: a failure of the paramesonephric ducts (Müllerian ducts) to develop in the whole or in part (uterus unicornis and segmental aplasia of uterine horn, respectively), the failure of caudal part of the paramesonephric ducts to the fuse and to form one single lumen (leading to situations such as uterus didelphus and the cranial vagina septation) and the failure of the fused caudal paramesonephric ducts to fuse with the urogenital sinus with consequent absence of anatomic continuity between the cranial vagina and the vestibule (originating an imperforate hymen or the vaginal stenosis).

Prevalence of these anomalies ranges from 0.02 to 0.05% in the canine population (Roberts, 1971; McIntyre et al., 2010). The relative frequency of the different abnormalities varies upon the region and the year of publication (Roberts, 1971; Ortega & Pacheco, 2007; McIntyre et al., 2010), and the clinical descriptions are insufficient to establish epidemiology of the defects.

In dogs, the uterine and vaginal segments can show developmental abnormalities ranging in severity from hypoplasia to complete agenesis (Romagnoli & Schlafer, 2006; McIntyre et al., 2010), and the severity of the defect influences the reproductive outcome and the existence of clinical side effects. The mildest form is the vagino-vestibular stricture, where secretions are collected in the cranial vagina and uterus, while in the more extreme form the uterus may be partially or in the whole reduced to a string, fibrous structure.

Although not uncommonly found during elective ovariohysterectomy, often they are detected co-existing with increased dimensions of the uterus and signs of mucometra or pyometra. There is a complete obstruction to fluid drainage from the uterus (as in vaginal or cervical atresia) and the owner may complaints that the female does not evidence the expected estrus vulvar discharge. With time, in obstructive diseases of the uterus or vagina, it is also possible to observe dysuria, cystitis, pyometra and renal failure (Kyles et al, 1996). However, in unicornuate uterus this is seldom the case and often the main complaint is infertility or sterility (Romagnoli & Schlafer, 2006; McIntyre et al., 2010). The animal may have been breed with success previous to the diagnosis, albeit the number of puppies in the litter is usually remarkably small comparing to the normal for the breed (Romagnoli & Schlafer, 2006; McIntyre et al., 2010). Sporadically, vulvar discharge, excessive vulvar licking and attraction of the male have been described (Kyles et al, 1996; Tsumagari et al., 2001).

The aim of this study was to discuss embryology, the gross anatomic features, clinical signs and implications, and available diagnostic approaches in cases of Müllerian duct anomalies.

2. Classification

Non-development or non-fusion (partial or complete) of Müllerian ducts may result in a variety of anomalies ranging from complete agenesis to duplication of female reproductive organs (Moore & Persaud, 2008).

In different clinical reports, a tendency for the use of different classifications for a common defect was found. Also, it is frequently found similar defects named distinctly for different species, in which develop with different patterns. These are indicative of the necessity of adopting a more uniform nomenclature. In an attempt to clarify the nomenclature used in this review, and to allow the easy identification of underlying major causes for a given defect, table 1 presents the classification for the anatomical congenital defects of the uterine-vaginal segment in dogs.

Main cause	Malformation	Classification	
Failure in organogenesis	Failure of segments of Müllerian ducts to develop	Complete	Uterus unicornis
		Incomplete	Segmental aplasia of the uterus (uni or bilateral)
Failure in fusion	Failure of the caudal parts of the two Müllerian ducts to fuse appropriately and develop a single lumen	Segmental aplasia of the body or the cervix	
		Longitudinal septation of the uterine body* Uterus didelphus*	
	Failure of caudal ends of the Müllerian ducts to fuse with invaginated urogenital sinus thus impairing the establishment of anatomical continuity	Segmental stenosis or aplasia of the vagina (Also named vestibulo-vaginal constriction)	
		Longitudinal septum in the cranial vagina* Imperforate hymen*	

* Out of the scope of this review

Table 1. Classification of developmental abnormalities of the uterine-vaginal segment in dogs according to underlying malformations.

Congenital aplasia of the uterus or vagina may occur in two variants: showing the normal development of muscular and serosal external layers, but without development of the mucosa, originating the atresia of the more internal layers; or may result from failure in development of all the layers in a more or less extended segment, which is reduced to a fibrous cordiform remnant. The former gives origin to a dense fibrous transverse partition in middle to caudal vagina, while in the later the agenesis segment miss from the normal anatomy (Gee et al., 1977; Moore & Persaud, 2008; McIntyre et al., 2010).

3. Physiopathology

Many vertebrates share a common genetic system for embryonic patterning that includes the reproductive tract. To better understand the uterus and vagina congenital anomalies we will first discuss the normal tubular genitalia development.

Normal development of the female reproductive tract involves a series of highly orchestrated, complex interactions that direct differentiation of the Müllerian ducts and urogenital sinus to form the internal female reproductive tract. This dynamic process is completed throughout mechanisms of differentiation, migration, fusion, and canalization. In the indifferent stage both male and female embryos have 2 sets of paired genital ducts (Mcgeady et al., 2006): Wolffian (mesonephric) and the Müllerian (paramesonephric). Differentiation of the Wolffian ducts occurs earlier in the male embryo, and persists after the mesonephros disintegrates (Noden & de Lahunta, 1985; Moore & Persaud, 2008). The female differentiation occurs in a later gestational age, and is characterized by regression of the Wolffian ducts due to absence of masculinisation influences from the gonads, and by stabilization of the Müllerian ducts, which is estrogen sensitive in a precise window of time (Moore & Persaud, 2008). Estrogens block the development of the Müllerian ducts if applied before the differentiation began, or cause hypertrophy of the differentiated portion and prevented further differentiation of the ducts in more caudal regions, when applied afterwards (Dood & Wibbels, 2008).

The funnel-shaped cranial region of each paramesonephric duct remains open (communicating with the coelomic cavity) and will form the uterine tube. Postnatally the communication persists from the peritoneal cavity to the exterior (exclusively in females). Caudal to this, each duct develops into an uterine horn. The bilateral paramesonephric ducts caudal portion shift medially and fuse into a single tube. The paired Müllerian ducts, initially separated by a septum, fuse and form a single Y-shaped tubular structure, the uterovaginal primordium (UVP). UVP becomes the uterine body, uterine cervix, and the cranial third of the vagina. Uterine morphology varies significantly in mammals, due to different degrees of fusion of the distinct Müllerian ducts (Noden & de Lahunta, 1985; Moore & Persaud, 2008).

Normal vaginal development requires the fusion of components that derive from 2 embryologic structures: the mesodermal Müllerian ducts and the endodermal urogenital sinus (UGS). To achieve this fusion the bilateral blind ending paramesonephric ducts enter in contact with UGS. This contact promotes the cellular proliferation of the endoderm from the urogenital sinus and the formation of the vaginal plate. The vagina is derived from both the vaginal plate and the fused ends of paramesonephric ducts (Mcgeady et al., 2006). The cranial one-third comes from fused paramesonephric ducts and the caudal two-thirds originate from the vaginal plate. Degeneration of the center of the vaginal plate creates the vaginal lumen. A hymen may persist where the vagina joins urogenital sinus although in most domestic species it tend to disappear before puberty. The urogenital sinus forms the vestibule (Noden & de Lahunta, 1985; Moore & Persaud, 2008).

Apart from some remnants of the excretory tubes and a small portion of the mesonephric duct, with varying importance according to the species, all the female mesonephric derivates atrophies (Moore & Persaud, 2008).

The cause and heritability of congenital abnormalities in dogs remain undetermined (McIntyre et al., 2010). With exception for the situations accompanying intersex conditions, the karyotype is normal. We are unaware if the condition develops in consequence of genetic, endocrine, or environmental influences. Neither it is known if it might be associated to failure of the gonad or the mesonephros development (which absence may co-exist with the *uterus unicornis*), to failure in local gene expression or, in the case of a segmental aplasia, if it might be determined by disruption of the blood supply to the affected segment (Ribeiro et al., 2009; McIntyre et al., 2010).

A *unilateral uterine aplasia* (also termed unicornuate uterus) develops when one paramesonephric duct fails to develop; this results in a uterus with one uterine horn (Moore & Persaud, 2008). The kidney and the paramesonephric ducts have the same embryologic origin therefore this anomaly is usually associated with ipsilateral kidney absence (Chang et al., 2008). Unilateral uterine aplasia has been reported in dogs and cats (Schulman & Bolton, 1997; Pinto Filho et al., 2001; Güvenç et al., 2006). However, the ovary is of a separate embryological origin and is usually present (Moore & Persaud, 2008; Thode & Johnston, 2009).

Development defects of the Müllerian duct system may cause *segmental aplasia* in several portions of the Müllerian duct system. Partial or complete fusion or occlusion of one uterine horn, of the body of the uterus, or of the most caudal segments, such as the cervix and cranial vagina, may cause fluid accumulation cranially to the occlusion (McEntee, 1990; Oh et al., 2005; Romagnoli & Schlafer, 2006; Almeida et al., 2010; McIntyre et al., 2010). Failure of canalization of the vaginal plate results in atresia (blockage) of the vagina, originating a *transverse vaginal stenosis* or a segmental aplasia, which is found between the middle and the caudal third of the vagina (Schlafer & Miller, 2007). Isolated vaginal atresia is an extremely rare finding.

Given the many variables that are involved in the female genital tract differentiation and growth, the pathogenesis for each anomaly may be multifactorial and hence of difficult identification (McIntyre et al., 2010).

4. Gross morphology

The gross morphological signs vary according to the defect and also the co-existence of secondary diseases or other concomitant uterine or vaginal disease.

4.1 Unilateral uterine aplasia (Unicornuate uterus)

In unicornuate uterus situations, aplasia of one uterine horn is the major finding, as it is reduced to a fibrous threadlike structure (Figure 1A and 1B), composed of fibrous tissue with some muscle strands (McIntyre et al., 2010) that frequently fail to present a lumen. As the contralateral uterine horn and the other genital segments retain patency, fluid accumulation does not occur unless the female develop cystic endometrial hyperplasia (CEH)/pyometra or other situations of segmental aplasia in the contralateral uterine horn are present (Figure 1A). The non-patent uterine horn may induce fluid accumulation in the oviducts that distend (Figure 1C).

Due to a common embryologic origin, this malformation might co-exist with ipsilateral tubal and renal agenesis (Chang et al., 2008). Although this situation is described with more frequency in cats than in dogs, on its survey McIntyre et al. (2010) found a relative lower frequency of 28% in cats than 45.5% in dogs. Co-existence of renal agenesis appears also on older reports on *uterus unicornis* in female beagles in research colonies (Höfliger, 1971, cited by McEntee, 1990). As those animals were euthanized after the end of the experiments (they integrated the control groups), at young ages, clinical signs were absent. Often the abnormality is detected only at necropsy or surprises the surgeon during the surgery. In contrast, due to a different embryologic origin, most frequently both ovaries are found (Romagnoli & Schlafer, 2006; McIntyre et al., 2010). Other congenital defects besides kidney agenesis were found in animals bearing unicornuate uterus: ectopic contralateral ureter, absent ipsilateral suspensory ligament and umbilical hernia (McIntyre et al., 2010).

Acquired diseases found in described conditions of unicornuate uterus include CEH of the contralateral uterine horn and polycystic ovaries. According to the descriptions, the later could correspond to cystic proliferation of the rete or the cranial uterine tube (Güvenc et al., 2006).

4.2 Segmental aplasia of the uterus

In cases of segmental aplasia, whether its location may be at the uterine horns, body or cervix, frequently the anomalies are grossly visible as missing segments or strictures that interrupt the normal anatomy of the uterine-vaginal segment, and that correspond to failure of the development of all the layers of that segment, which are often reduced to a streak cord-like rudiment. However, in few situations the external layers of the Müllerian duct derivates (serosal and muscle layers) are properly differentiated, but the inner layers (mucosal and sub-mucosal layers) do not differentiate (Moore & Persaud, 2008). This is more often found in the vagina than the uterus. In practical terms, the potential deleterious effects over the reproductive potential and the occurrence of secondary diseases are similar in the two situations.

As the situation usually remains undiagnosed in young animals that maintain regular reproductive activity, the normally developed portion cranial to the atresia is distended due to fluid accumulation (Figure 1D to 1H). Distension of the uterine tube (Figure 1F) is possible (McIntyre et al., 2010). Primary lesions at the endometrium are rarely reported, but CEH may develop in older animals. However, due to excessive mucous fluid pressure of the ongoing mucometra, with time reduction in the thickness of the uterine walls and compression and attenuation of the endometrial glands is commonly found (McIntyre et al., 2010).

Segmental aplasia of the uterine horns may develop at any point of the structure (Figure 1A, 1C and 1G) (Schlafer & Miller, 2007; McIntyre et al., 2010), with segmental agenesis being irregularly distributed for different segments of the uterine horns.

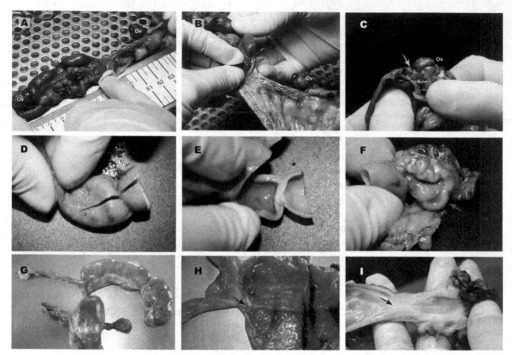

Fig. 1. Canine congenital aplasia of the uterine-vaginal segment: **A**: The external morphological evaluation showed the complete agenesis of the right uterine horn (unicornuate uterus) co-existing with segmental aplasia of the contralateral uterine horn. Both ovaries (Ov) were present. Arrows indicate areas of agenesis. **B**: Closer inspection showed that the caudal segment of the left uterine horn is patent, while the right uterine horn is reduced to a threadlike structure parallel to the uterine vessels. The ipsilateral ovary (Ov) was present, within the ovarian bursa. Arrows indicate areas of agenesis. **C**: Dilatation of the uterine tube (cyan arrow) ipsilateral to the non-developed uterine horn. **D**: Externally, segmental aplasia of the uterine horn may appear as a marked constriction of the organ. **E**: When opened, those areas showed the absence of fusion between adjacent segments, which fail to communicate. Outside undeveloped areas the uterus maintain its normal morphology. **F**: The ipsilateral uterine tube is distended (arrow), due to fluid pressure. **G**: Segmental aplasia at the basis of the right uterine horn in a 15 years-old bitch (distension of the vagina was due to a fibroma). **H**: The arrow points to the area of aplasia. Long-term effects of the secondary fluid accumulation induced a reduction in the thickness of the walls. **I**: Segmental stenosis of the vagina: the arrow points to the obstruction.

In animals with segmental aplasia of the uterine body or cervix, as communication between the two uterine horns is possible, equivalent and bilateral uterine horn distension is found (McEntee, 1990; McIntyre et al., 2010). Undeveloped segments are usually reduced to cord-like remnants. In cases of cervical aplasia, the uterine body ends blindly in a pouch, a membranous tissue separating the uterus from the vagina (McEntee, 1990).

4.3 Segmental stenosis of the vagina

Vaginal stenosis has been described as occurring as a complete misdevelopment of all the layers of the vagina, which may be reduced to an atretic segment with variable importance (Figure 1I) (Gee et al., 1977; Viehoff & Sjollema, 2003; Romagnoli & Schlafer, 2006) or as originating from the absence of internal canalization with normal developmental of the external layers (Wadsword et al., 1978). The existence of a vaginal cyst cranial to the occlusion has been referred, which has been attributed to incomplete canalization of the embryonic derivate, hence allowing the development of intermediary segments between missing portions (Gee et al., 1977; McEntee, 1990). The undeveloped segment is usually located near the vestibulo-vaginal junction (Gee et al., 1977; Kyles et al., 1996; Viehoff & Sjollema, 2003) and on gross evaluation morphology of the anatomical region may share some resemblances with imperforate hymen. The missing segment may present variable extension.

Similarly to the findings for segmental aplasia of the uterine body or cervix, fluid accumulation above the agenesis induces uterine dilatation, but contrasting to those malformations, fluid accumulation also occurs on the remainder cranial segment of the vagina.

Vaginal cysts near the point of stenosis have been described (Gee et al., 1977). It has been proposed to correspond to incomplete canalization of atrectic segments (Gee et al., 1977; McIntyre et al., 2010). Impairment of fluid drainage induces fluid accumulation above the obstruction and consequently distension of cranial reproductive tract (Gee et al., 1977; Viehoff & Sjollema, 2003; McIntyre et al., 2010). In contrast to the observed in the previously described situations, fluid accumulates within the uterus (mucometra) and the vagina (hydrocolpos). As vaginal walls are thinner than those of the uterus they distend more easily, thus reaching higher increases in size comparatively to the uterine distension. These morphological features are not exclusive for the segmental stenosis of the vagina. Imperforate hymen shares similar gross appearance (Tsumagari et al., 2001; Schlafer & Miller, 2007), except that the transverse partition is thinner in the later than in the segmental stenosis.

5. Clinical signs

Congenital abnormalities of the uterine-vaginal segment in dogs are seldom detected before puberty. Furthermore, in a large number of cases remains unnoticed until secondary diseases develop or until unsuccessful attempts for breeding the female alert the owner to the need for a detailed reproductive examination of the infertile animal. Early diagnosis of those conditions would avoid owners to maintain a bitch with severe congenital diseases in the reproductive stock. Also, the correct identification of the disease and evaluation of the importance of the defect would allow proper counselling on the therapeutic approach and establish a prognosis for a specific condition. Further, it will permit to anticipate the occurrence of secondary, associated diseases that can develop if the primary condition is not treated and that may threaten the health of the female.

5.1 Unilateral uterine aplasia (Unicornuate uterus)

The occurrence of unicornuate uterus is rare, but results from different surveys report different relative frequencies. Ortega and Pacheco (2007) in tropical regions reported a frequency of 0.3% (1:300 lesions of the genital tract) whilst McIntyre et al. (2010) found 73.3% (11:15 of the canine uterus disorders found). It is possible that the genetics of the population surveyed may have influenced, in particular the proportion of purebred and crossbred females, as well as the analysed segments of the genital tract.

Most often, in cases of complete aplasia of one uterine horn the female usually presents regular oestrous cycles (Pinto Filho et al., 2001; Güvenç et al., 2006; Almeida et al., 2010), and often the animal history include the reference to successful pregnancy and parturition, although with a smaller litter size than the expected for the breed (Romagnoli &Schlafer, 2006; McIntyre et al., 2010). It is also possible the reference to the existence of a reduced intensity in the vaginal discharge accompanying estrus, but this is not usually reported in any of the cited literature. Individuals with agenesis of one uterine horn may also have an increased incidence of premature delivery (Seyrek-Intas et al., 2004). Usually, in young dogs clinical signs other than sub-fertility are absent, the condition being detected at the necropsy or during a convenience OVH. That was the case in one of the situations we had: a small Poodle dog of 2 years of age with regular estrous cycles that was submitted to convenience OVH. The uterine defect was found during surgical procedure, in the absence of symptoms. The owner only reported the existence of a vulvar discharge of decreased intensity when compared to that of her mother. Pinto Filho et al. (2001) described a similar situation in a Poodle female with 2 years of age, without clinical signs, that was submitted to elective surgery.

However, older animals may present signs of disease located in the uterus (such as CEH or pyometra), as in the report by Güvenç et al. (2006). Nevertheless, one should be aware that those are generally of independent occurrence, as CEH/pyometra frequently develops in the uterus of old intact females. Güvenç et al. (2006), report in a 12 years-old Cocker Spaniel, the existence of a serous sanguineous vulvar discharge persisting for 5 weeks, in the absence of other clinical symptoms, which was the main reason for the consultation. However, at surgery polycystic ovaries were found. Thus it cannot be excluded that the discharge might rather be associated to the ovarian disease than to the uterine defect.

The bilateral agenesis of the uterine horns is extremely rare in dogs (Schlafer and Miller, 2007).

5.2 Segmental aplasia of the uterine(s) horn(s)

Partial or complete agenesis of a more or less extended segment of the uterine horns (segmental aplasia) is relatively common in dogs; in the survey by McIntyre and colleagues (2010) it accounted for 20% of the congenital anomalies of the uterus. Most frequently it is an unilateral condition, but some descriptions referred to bilateral situations (McIntyre et al., 2010), in which segmental agenesis was irregularly distributed for different segments of both uterine horns. This was also observed in one of our cases, in middle aged Poodle crossbred female. The agenesic segment may develop at any point of the uterine horns (McEntee, 1990; Romagnoli & Schlafer, 2006; McIntyre et al., 2010). The moment for the onset of clinical signs detection partly depends on its location and extension. Whenever it exists an obstruction to the normal outflow of the endometrial secretions, accumulation of a sterile fluid with distension of uterine walls (Figure 1 D and 1G) is the main outcome

(McEntee, 1990; Romagnoli & Schlafer, 2006; McIntyre et al., 2010). As consequence of the excessive pressure, the female may present mild signs of uterine disease (such as abdominal distension, tenesmus or dysuria) albeit usually haematological exams and clinical biochemistry are within or close to normal values. In one of the situations we had, in a Rottweiler female with 5 years of age, signs of cystic endometrial hyperplasia co-existed in the remainder segments of the uterus. Though these are unrelated conditions, as already mentioned, the uterine segment retaining patency may develop a pyometra, which may completely change the clinical scenario for the patient. In this particular case, the segmental aplasia was diagnosed after surgery.

Whenever a segmental aplasia of the cranial part of the uterine horn is found, it may also be found a distended uterine tube. This situation has been described for cats and rabbits (Thode & Johnston, 2009), but was not mentioned in the reports on dogs we have accessed. However, non-mention may also mean that the structure was not evaluated. In our Rottweiler case, gross evaluation of the excised genitalia fail to evidence distension of the uterine tubes; however, a muco-purulent fluid was found in the ovarian bursa suggesting the flow of the uterine content through the oviducts. Also in two other situations, oviductal dilatation was found during histopathological evaluation (Figures 1C and 1F).

5.3 Segmental aplasia of the uterine body and cervix

Although rare, sporadic reports on the agenesis of the uterine body have been published for the dog (Oh et al., 2005; McIntyre et al., 2010). The aplasia of the canine cervix was seldom described (McEntee, 1990).

Both conditions allow communication between the two uterine horns and completely impair fluid drainage from the uterus. Consequently, one of the main symptoms may be the existence of estrus signs (swollen vulva and male attraction) in the absence of the characteristic vulvar discharge (non-technically described as "dry" estrus). Furthermore, as none of the endometrial secretions drain from the genital tract, as the female retains her cyclicity, signs secondary to excessive fluid accumulation may develop earlier when compared to segmental aplasia, and the abdominal distension is usually noticed earlier. Uterine distension, in this situation, is bilateral and symmetric (Oh et al., 2005; McIntyre et al., 2010).

5.4 Segmental stenosis of the vagina

Animals presenting segmental stenosis of the vagina, as do those showing aplasia of the uterus or of the cervix, do not present the typical estrus vulvar discharge, despite the existence of regular cyclicity (Viehoff & Sjollema, 2003). However, chronicle, intermittent vaginitis is the most frequently described clinical symptom and the common to all the reports on segmental stenosis of the vagina (Gee et al., 1977; Kyles et al., 1996; Viehoff & Sjollema, 2003). It usually induces a more or less intense vulvar discharge, excessive licking of the vagina and dysuria. Recurrent cystitis was also found in such conditions (Kyles et al., 1996). Due to common symptoms, differential diagnosis between segmental stenosis of the vagina (Viehoff & Sjollema, 2003) and the imperforate hymen (Tsumagari et al., 2001) on the basis of the symptoms is difficult.

6. Diagnosis

Diagnosis of aplasia of the uterine-vaginal segment in dog before puberty or in young non-breeding dogs is seldom achieved, as clinical evidences are absent. Also, since the ovaries are present in congenital aplasia of the uterine-vaginal segment, normal cyclicity after puberty does not allow suspecting the existence of a defect.

Thus congenital aplasia of the uterine-vaginal is frequently asymptomatic and often missed during routine gynaecological examination, unless side effects associated to failure of genital patency develop in more severe or more prolonged situations. Further, due to unspecific and limited clinical symptoms described, congenital aplasia often requires more than one diagnostic approach to assure success.

Clinical signs or mild illness appears in older bitches, usually associated with fluid retention within the uterus or with other age-related diseases of the genital tract. The later is not taken into consideration herein when describing the diagnostic approach.

In *unilateral uterine aplasia*, few clinical signs develop even in older animals that may be related to the defect. The owner may complain on the female low prolificacy (Romagnoli & Schlafer, 2006; McIntyre et al., 2010) or on the tendency of recurrent abortion in the absence of microbiological or parasitic agents. Vaginoscopy or digital manipulation fails to evidence the primary defect. On ultrasound, the inability to find one uterine horn or the finding of a fibrous threadlike structure on its normal location are the expected findings. Both ovaries are found. Simple X-rays are not useful for diagnosis unless hysterosalpingography (a contrast X-ray) is performed. This would reveal that diffusion of the contrast is limited to one of the uterine horns, particular when using dorso-ventral projections.

A similar situation is found in the *segmental aplasia of the uterine horns*. Unless fluid accumulation in the uterine segment above the atresia becomes important and may be suspected during routine abdominal palpation or ultrasound, the defect remains undetectable in routine consultations. Complains on the female sub-fertility in the presence of regular estrous cycles may exist. The vaginoscopy and digital manipulation are not useful to evidence the primary defect. On ultrasound, segments of the uterus may show uterine distension, uterine walls of variable thickness and areas where the uterus is absent or reduced to a cord-like fibrous structure. However, often the image resembles that of a mucometra/pyometra, except that uterine distension may be limited to one portion of the uterus. On simple X-ray it may be observed dense, non-continuous masses in the normal location of the uterus, frequently in one side of the body, while the remainder parts of the genital tract are not visible. Comparison of these X-rays with those obtained by hysterosalpingography will allow to visualise the occlusion and the existence of a dense pouch cranially.

In the *segmental aplasia of the uterine body and cervix*, the most important symptom for diagnosis is the absence of the typical estrus vulvar discharge in a regularly cycling female (Oh et al., 2005; McIntyre et al., 2010). With time, also abdominal distension associated to uterine distension due to mucometra is found. During abdominal palpation, a uterus increased in size is detected. The vaginoscopy and digital manipulation fail to evidence the primary defect. On ultrasound, bilateral distension of the uterus, thin uterine walls and anechoic or hypoechoic uterine content are commonly found. The distension of the body of the uterus may be found when cervical agenesis exists. The thickness of the uterine walls is equivalent in the uterine horns and body. Radiographic signs are similar to those of mucometra or pyometra. Hysterosalpingography allows to identify the local of occlusion.

In case of *segmental stenosis of the vagina*, the major symptom is also the absence of the estrus vulvar discharge in a regularly cycling female. However, a large number of females also present clinical history of intermittent, chronic vaginitis or of recurrent, chronic lower urinary tract infection (Kyles et al, 1996; McIntyre et al., 2010), which have not being reported in the aplasia of the uterine body or cervix. Abdominal palpation shows increased size of the uterus that prolongs caudally into the pelvic brim (cranial segment of the vagina). As the vagina dilates more than the uterine body, it can appear as being more ballooned. Also transrectal digital palpation shows the distension of the vagina, that appears as a balloon at the entrance of the pelvic vault. Digital manipulation of the vagina or vaginoscopy usually allows detecting the defect (Kyles et al., 1996; Viehoff & Sjollema, 2003). On the ultrasound bilateral distension of the uterus is observed, as in the segmental aplasia of the uterine body or cervix, which is prolonged beneath the urinary bladder into the pelvic brim. The bladder may be dislocated from its normal position. Ultrasound scans allow to distinguish between the uterine and the vaginal segment, the latter having thinner walls and usually increased dilatation. On simple X-rays cranioventral displacement of the bladder and increased dimensions of the uterus, extending into the vaginal position, are observed. Hysterosalpingography allows the localization of the occlusion.

For the defects originating in the cervix or the vagina, endoscopic visualization of the vaginal cavity and of the cervical morphology may be useful in diagnosis. Furthermore, three-dimension ultrasonography and the magnetic resonance imaging may give useful information on the development of the genital structures even when secondary diseases are absent. However, these techniques are not easy to develop in the current veterinary clinics.

On table 2 we condensed the most relevant information to reach diagnosis.

7. Therapeutic management

To propose a treatment for any of the different conditions of congenital aplasia of the uterine-vaginal segment in dogs is a difficult task. For unicornuate uterus no direct negative effects arise from the defect by itself, and there are no additional risks for the health of the bitch other than those associated with age in intact females.

For the different segmental aplasia of the uterus (concerning the uterine horns, body or cervix) no effective therapeutic approach is available, and ovariohysterectomy remains the solution to avoid future health problems for the bitch, associated to fluid retention in the uterus with posterior inflammation.

In the case of segmental stenosis of the vagina, the treatment of the defect may be attempt to maintain the breeding status of the bitch, unless a large segment of the vagina is missing, which could bring potential problems during mating and delivery (Viehoff & Sjollema, 2003). Anastomosis of the vagina and vestibule may be attempt through episiotomy (Kyles et al., 1996; Viehoff & Sjollema, 2003). The success of the technique has yet to be ascertained in more severe cases of agenesis of the vaginal segment.

Defect	Unicornuate uterus	Segmental aplasia of the uterine horns	Segmental aplasia of the uterine body or cervix	Segmental vaginal stenosis
Main clinical sign	Sub-fertility (low prolificity) in the presence of regular estrous cycles		Absence of vulvar discharge at estrus ("Dry" estrus)	
Other symptoms	None, unless uterine or ovarian concurrent diseases	Uterine distension as "in pouches" None, unless uterine or ovarian concurrent diseases	Mucometra Bilateral uterine distension Abdominal distension	Intermittent, chronic vaginitis or cystitis Bilateral mucometra and hydrocolpos Abdominal distension
Physical examination	Without results	Areas of uterine dilatation alternating with areas where the uterus is not perceived or appear as a fibrous cord.	Increased dimensions of the uterus during abdominal palpation	Digital manipulation and vaginoscopy shows occlusion Increased dimensions of the uterus during abdominal palpation
Simple X-rays	Not useful	Dense, non-continuous masses in the normal location of the uterus	Visualization of bilateral increased dimensions of the uterus (similar to mucometra or pyometra)	Cranioventral displacement of the bladder and increased dimension of the uterus and cranial vagina
Ultrasound	Only one uterine horn usually detected; presence of both ovaries	Uterine wall distension similar to the observed in mucometra or pyometra	Visualization of bilateral increased dimensions of the uterus (similar to mucometra or pyometra) The distension is limited to the horns or body; image of the uterine body below the bladder	Bilateral enlargement of the uterus and vagina. Differences in the thickness of the walls may distinguish between uterus and vagina
Other complementary exams	Hysterosalpingography		Vagino-uretrocystography: the existence of an occlusion hampers the passage to the contrast medium	

Table 2. Resumed guidelines for reach a diagnosis in congenital segmental agenesis of the uterine-vaginal segment in dogs.

8. Conclusions

Congenital agenesis of the uterine-vaginal segment in dogs consists of a wide range of defects that usually progress undetected until development of associated side effects of the defect, such as mucometra and hydrocolpos, or recurrent cystitis or chronic vaginitis. Surgical correction of the congenital abnormality is seldom possible. Thus it is important to be aware of the most adequate approaches for its early diagnosis, allowing to exclude the affected animals from the reproductive stock.

9. Aknowledgements

This work was supported by the project from CECAV/UTAD with the reference PEst-OE/AGR/UI0772/2011, by the Portuguese Science and Technology Foundation.

10. References

Almeida, M.V.; Rezende, E.P.; Lamounier, A.R.; Rachid, M.A.; Nascimento, E.F.; Santos, R.L. & Valle, G.R. (2010) Aplasia segmentar de corpo uterino em cadela sem raça definida: relato de caso. *Arq. Bras. Med. Vet. Zootec.*, Vol. 62, N°4, pp.794-800.

Chang, J.; Jung, J.H.; Yoon, J.; Choi, M.C.; Park, J.H.; Seo, K.M. & Jeong, S.M. (2008) Segmental aplasia of the uterine horn with ipsilateral renal agenesis in a cat. *J. Vet. Med. Sci.*, Vol. 70, pp. 641-643.

Dood, K.L. & Wibbels, T. (2008) Estrogen inhibits caudal progression but stimulates proliferation of developing müllerian ducts in a turtle with temperature-dependent sex determination. *Comp. Biochem. Physiol.*, Vol.150, N°3,pp. 315-9

Gee, B.R.; Pharr, J.W. & Fuerneaux R.W. (1977) Segmental aplasia of Müllerian duct system in a dog. *Can. Vet. J.*, Vol. 18, pp. 281-286.

Güvenç, K.; Toydemir, F.S.; Sontaş, H.B. & Şenünver, A. (2006) A Cocker Spaniel bitch with uterus unicornis (unilateral cornual agenesis). *J. Fac. Vet. Med. Istanbul Univ.*, Vol. 32, n°3, 69-73.

Kyles, A.E.; Vaden,S.; Hardie, EM & Stone, E.A. (1996) Vestibulo-vaginal stenosis in dogs:18 cases[1987-1995]. *J. Am.Vet.Med. Assoc.*, Vol. 209, pp. 1889-93.

McEntee K. (1990) Reproductive pathology of domestic mammals, 1st ed. Academic Press, San Diego, CA.

Mcgeady, T.A.; Quinn, P.J.; Fitzpatrick, E.S. & Ryan, M.T. (2006) Veterinary embryology. Blackwell Publishing, Oxford.

McIntyre, R.L.; Levy, J.K.; Roberts, J.F. & Reep, R.L. (2010) Developmental uterine anomalies in cats and dogs undergoing elective ovariohysterectomy. *J. Am. Vet. Med. Assoc.*,Vol. 237, pp. 542-546

Moore, K.L. & Persaud, T.V. (2008) The urogenital system. In: The developing human clinically oriented embryology.8th ed. Saunders&Elsevier, Philadelphia, PA., pp. 243-269

Noden D.M. & de Lahunta A. (1985) The embryology of domestic animals,1st ed. Williams &Wilkins, Baltimore, MD.

Oh, K.S.; Son, C.H.; Kim, B.S.; Hwang, S.S.; Kim, Y.J.; Park, S.J.; Jeong, J.H.; Jeong, C.; Park, S.H. & Cho, K.O. (2005) Segmental aplasia of uterine body in an adult mixed breed dog. *J. Vet. Diag. Invest.*, Vol. 17, pp. 490-492

Ortega-Pacheco, A.; Segura-Correa, J.C.; Jimenez-Coello, M. & Forsberg, C.L.(2007) Reproductive patterns and reproductive pathologies of stray bitches in the tropics. *Theriogenology*, Vol. 67, pp. 382-390.

Pinto Filho, S.T.; Cunha, O.; Raiser, A.G.; Barbosa, G.S.;Portella, L.C. & Irigoyen, L.F. (2001) Unilateral uterine agenesis in a bitch- A case report. *Arq. Ciên. Vet. Zool. UNIPAR*, Vol. 4, N°1, pp.77-79.

Ribeiro, S.C.; Tormena, R.A.; Peterson, T.V.; Gonzáles, M.O.; Serrano, P.G.; Almeida, J.A. & Baracat, E.C. (2009) Müllerian duct anomalies:review of current management. *Sao Paulo Med. J.*, Vol. 127, n°2, pp. 92-6

Roberts, S.J. (1971). *Veterinary Obstetrics and Genital Diseases.* Woodstock, VT: Self published; First edition.

Romagnoli, S. & Schlafer, D.H. (2006) Disorders of sexual differentiation in puppies and kittens: a diagnostic and clinical approach. *Vet. Clin. North Am. Small Anim. Pract.*, Vol. 36, pp. 573-606.

Schlafer, D.H. & Miller, R.B. (2007) Female genital system. In: MAXIE, M.G. (Ed). Jubb, Kennedy, and Palmer's Pathology of Domestic Animals. 4th ed. Philadelphia: Elsevier Saunders:429-564.

Schulman, M.L. & Bolton, L.A. (1997) Uterine horn aplasia with complications in two mixed-breed bitches. *J.S. Afr. Vet. Assoc.*, Vol. 68, pp.150-153

Seyrek-Intaş, K.; Wehrend, A.; Nak, Y.; Tek, H.B.; Yilmazbaş, G.; Gökhan, T. & Bostedt, H. (2004) Unilateral hysterectomy (cornuectomy) in the bitch and its effect on subsequent fertility. *Theriogenology*, Vol. 61, pp.1713-1717

Thode,H.P. & Johnston, M.S. (2009) Probable congenital uterine developmental abnormalities in two domestic rabbits. *Vet. Rec.*, Vol. 164, pp.242-244

Tsumagari, S.; Takagi, S.; Takeishi, M. & Memon, M.A. (2001) A case of a bitch with imperforate hymen and hydrocolpos. *J.Vet. Med.Sci.* Vol. 63, N°4, pp. 475-477.

Viehoff, F.W & Sjollema, B.E. (2003) Hydrocolpus in dogs: surgical treatment in two cases. *J. Small Anim. Pract.* Vol. 44, pp. 404-407

Wadsworth, P.F.; Hall, J.C. & Prentice, D.E. (1978) Segmental aplasia of the vagina in the beagle bitch. *Lab. Anim.*, Vol. 12, pp.165-166.

12

Prospective Study of Tumor Markers as Prognostic Factors in the Histopathological Differential Diagnosis of Mammary Gland Neoplasms in Female Canines

Anna M. Badowska-Kozakiewicz
Department of Biophysics and Human Physiology,
Medical University of Warsaw,
Poland

1. Introduction

Cancer constitutes a major problem in animal pathology and is a subject of intensive research. The aim of this study was to gain comprehensive knowledge of cancer biology. Some animal tumors are also considered good research models in comparative oncology. Literature and own studies show that dogs often suffer from skin cancer and mammary gland tumors (Moulton, 1990). The incidence of mammary gland tumors in female canines is second only to skin cancer (Misdorp & Meuten, 2002; Ramalho et al, 2006). They most commonly appear between 6 and 10 years of age (Misdorp & Meuten, 2002; Hampe & Misdorp, 1974; Kubiak, 200). There are also documented cases of such tumors as early as at the age of two years and, very rarely, in males (Moulton, 1990). Histopathological examination in about 40-50% of cases shows malignant tumors, most of which are of epithelial origin (Rutteman, 2001). These cancers originate from epithelial follicles or ducts and take forms of papillary adenocarcinomas, simple or complex tubular and solid cancers (Misdorp & Meuten, 2002). There are also tumors derived from myoepithelial cells and mesenchymal tissue. In veterinary medicine there is a constant search for prognostic factors and predictors that allow for proper evaluation of the disease state, survival, susceptibility to treatment and risk of relapse. Recognized factors are: age of the animal, sentinel lymph node status, histological type of tumor and a histological grade of differentiation of malignancy. Beside the fundamental method in cancer diagnosis, which is the histopathological examination, additional information useful in this regard is provided by research on cancer biology, including, among others, the study of tumor markers. In histological examination of a tumor, markers of proliferative activity such as mitotic index, thymidine labeling index, percentage of cells in the S phase of cell cycle, expression of nuclear antigen Ki-67 and proliferating cells nuclear antigen (PCNA) are also taken into account. The following factors are also examined: expression of estrogen receptors, growth factor receptors such as: epidermal growth factor receptor (EGFR), insulin growth factor receptor (IGFR), growth hormone (GH),markers of high risk of metastasis: plasminogen activator and cathepsin D, oncogenes and tumor suppressor genes: c -erbB-2, c-myc, p53,

BRCA-1, BRCA-2, markers of tumor angiogenesis, and heat shock proteins (Koda et al, 2004; Niwińska, 1995; Olszewski, 1994). Diagnosis of neoplasms of the mammary gland in canines does not usually pose a problem, but in some cases there may be difficulties. Targeted diagnostic immunohistochemistry using a panel of antibodies makes it easier to determine the correct diagnosis. Difficulties encountered during routine diagnosis of neoplasms of the mammary gland in female dogs relate to assessing the origin of the tumor and its biology. Immunophenotyping can be helpful in the diagnostic process and tumor markers (expression of nuclear antigen Ki-67 and expression of estrogen receptors and the p53 protein) carry useful information, but determination of malignancy is still based on morphological criteria, such as mitotic index, which together with the histopathological criteria are the most important factors differentiating benign tumors from those of malignant nature;. In veterinary oncology there is a constant search for new tumor markers that could aid in differential diagnosis of mammary gland neoplasms in female canines. The aim of research on the mammary gland neoplasms in female dogs is to extend the panel of tumor markers by addition of new markers such as COX-2, P-gp, Hsp90 and Hsp70 and to incorporate them into routine diagnostics. Occurrence of mammary tumors in females as well as potential to use canine models in comparative pathology of these tumors makes it an interesting research material. It is known that the degree of malignancy is positively correlated with proliferative activity. Relationship between the expression of estrogen receptors and the degree of malignancy is not entirely clear, although most authors believe that expression of these receptors is greater in benign tumors. COX-2 is expressed in many canine tumors such as canine kidney, bladder, prostate, and mammary gland cancers, but there is no data on the relationship between expression of COX-2 and other markers, even though such relation would seem logical because the expression of COX-2 may be related to prognosis by indirect immunosuppressive effect and inhibition of apoptosis. Literature on the expression of heat shock protein or glycoprotein - P in breast cancer is very scarce. There is evidence of Hsp27, Hsp70 and Hsp90, as well as glycoprotein – P expression, which may influence susceptibility to therapy. One would expect a correlation between proliferative activity, degree of malignancy and expression of estrogen receptors, but no data is available on such relationship. The aim of the study was to analyze the role of classical and new tumor markers in the histopathological differential diagnosis of mammary gland neoplasms in female dogs. The objective of the present study was to investigate the expression of cyclooxygenase - 2 and heat shock proteins in canine mammary gland tumors and their correlations with histological type of tumor, degree of its histological malignancy, proliferative activity, estrogen receptor expression, infiltration by cells, as well as P-gp and p53 protein expression.

2. Materials, methods and results

2.1 Materials

Material for the investigation comprised 133 tumor samples of the mammary gland collected from female canines during surgical procedures performed at Warsaw Veterinary Clinics and Small Animal Clinic of the Department of Clinical Sciences, Faculty of Vetrinary Medicine, Warsaw University of Life Sciences – SGGW. Tumor samples were fixed in 8% formalin buffered with phosphates. After 24h fixing, material was dehydrated in a series of increasing concentrations of alcohol and embedded in paraffin. Paraffin blocks were cut into serial sections of 4µm in thickness.

2.2 Methods

Then, they were stained using proper methods. In sections stained with the routine H&E method, the following determinations were carried out: type of neoplasm (Misdorp et al, 1999), tumor grade including tubule formation, intensity of division and the degree of neoplastic cell differentiation (Misdorp & Meuten, 2002), mitotic index defined as a mean number of mitoses in neoplastic cells counted in 10 fields of vision at the lens magnification of 400x (surface field $0.17mm^2$). Paraffin sections on slides covered with 2% saline solution in acetone, at the temperature of 42^0C were used for immunohistochemical methods. In immunohistochemical reactions, the following antibodies, properly diluted in 1% BSA (Sigma), were used: mouse monoclonal antibody against human nuclear antigen Ki-67 (Dako) diluted 1:75 (Nieto et al, 2000), mouse monoclonal antibodies against p53 (Dako) human protein, diluted at a ratio 1:25 (Gamblin et al, 1994; Rodo, 2007), mouse monoclonal antibodies against alpha (Dako) human estrogen receptor, diluted at a ratio 1:35 (Mulas et al, 2005), mouse monoclonal antibodies against COX-2 (Dako) human receptor, diluted at a ratio 1:100 (Queiroga et al, 2007; Doré et al, 2003; Soslow et al, 2000), mouse monoclonal antibodies against Hsp70 (Novocastra) human heat shock proteins, diluted at a ratio 1:40 (Romanucci et al, 2006), mouse monoclonal antibodies against Hsp90 (Novocastra) human heat shock proteins, diluted at a ratio 1:40 (Romanucci et al, 2006) and mouse monoclonal antibodies against P-glycoprotein (Sigma), diluted at a ratio 1:100 (Petterino et al, 2006). Sections were deparafinized in xylene and rehydrated in increasing concentrations of alcohol. Then, they were placed in a buffer with a pH of 6 (Dako). In order to uncover the antigen epitope, sections were warmed up in a microwave oven (1x5 min at 600 W, 2x5 min at 300 W). Then, they were cooled for 20 min. After two washings in distilled water (5 min), slides were washed in TRIS-buffered saline with pH of 8 (Sigma) and incubated with the primary antibody for 1h at room temperature. Then, the preparations were washed with TRIS buffer for 10 min. The En Vision + TM System (Dako) was used for visualization. After 30 min of incubation with reagent, the slides were washed with TRIS buffer and a solution of diaminobenzidine (DAB, Dako), prepared according to the procedure supplied by the producer, was put on slides. The degree of slide staining was controlled. They were washed in tap water and stained with Ehrlich hematoxylin for 5 min, contrasted in 1% acid alcohol and washed again in tap water. Then, slides were dehydrated in graded alcohol concentrations, passed through xylene and fixed in DPX mounting medium (Gurr®). Computer image analysis and Lucia v. 4.21 software were used for interpretation of the results of Ki-67, ER, p53, COX-2, Hsp70, Hsp90 expression; using those facilities we could count the number of neoplastic cells featuring stained cytoplasm per 1,000 neoplastic cells. Results were analyzed using the SPSS 12.0 program. To determine whether differences for a few independent traits were significant, Kruskal-Wallis test was used. This test is an equivalent to the test of variance for traits without normal distribution. Two-sided correlations were performed using Spearman correlation test. The differences were deemed statistically significant at $P \leq 0.05$.

2.3 Results

Investigated material contained 14 adenomas (Fig.1), 66 complex carcinomas (adenocarcinomas), 47 simple carcinomas (adenocarcinomas) (Fig. 2, Fig. 3) and 6 solid carcinomas. The number of cancers with a defined grade amounted to, respectively, 1st grade – 48, 2nd grade – 39 and 3rd grade – 32. Mammary gland neoplasms were excised from female dogs belonging to 18 breeds in the ages between 3 and 16 years.

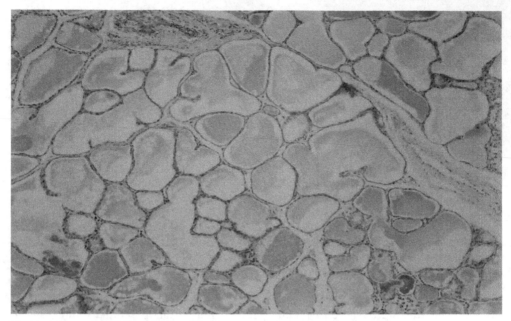

Fig. 1. Adenoma, H&E method x 20

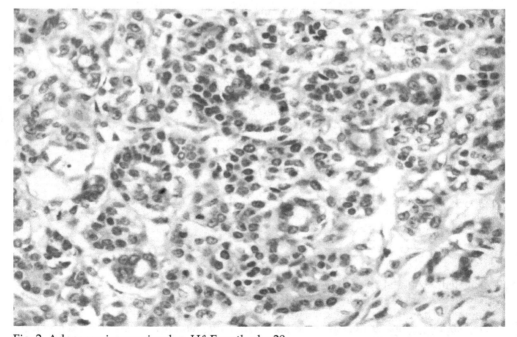

Fig. 2. Adenocarcinoma simplex, H&E method x 20

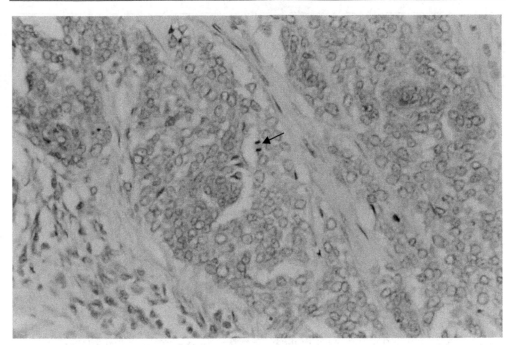

Fig. 3. Adenocarcinoma simplex, H&E (40x). The following mature tissues are visible:
pathologic mitotic figures

2.3.1 Relationship between age of bitches and the grade of malignancy and histological type of tumor of epithelial origin

Dogs were divided into three age groups: <8 years, 8 -12 years and >12 years. In the group of bitches below the age of 8, majority (61.1%) consisted of tumors with the lowest histological grade of malignancy (1st). In the oldest group, 1st and 2nd grade tumors in the 1st and 2nd accounted for 77.8%. In the entire pool of studied tumors in all age groups, the largest share consisted of tumors with the lowest degree of histological malignancy (40.4%) (Table 1). Assessment of the contribution of individual types of tumors at different ages showed that in bitches younger than 8 years the most common findings were adenomas (21.7%) and complex carcinomas (56.5%) and in those over 12 years simple carcinomas occurred most often (55.0%) (Table 2).

Age of bitches	Tumor grade			Total
	I°	II°	III°	
<8 lat (n=18)	11 (61,1%)	3 (16,7%)	4 (22,2%)	18
8-12 lat (n=83)	30 (36,0%)	29 (35,0%)	24 (29,0%)	83
>12 (n=18)	7 (38,9%)	7 (38,9%)	4 (22,2%)	18
total (n=119)	48 (40,4%)	39 (32,8%)	32 (26,8%)	119

Table 1. Incidence of malignancies of various grades in bitches in different age groups

Age of bitches	Types of tumors				Total
	Adenoma	Carcinoma solidum	Adenocarcinoma simplex	Adenocarcinoma complex	
<8 lat	5 (21,7%)	1 (4,3%)	4 (17,4%)	13 (56,5%)	23
8-12 lat	7 (7,8%)	4 (4,4%)	32 (35,6%)	47 (52,2%)	90
>12 lat	2 (10,0%)	1 (5,0%)	11 (55,0%)	6 (30,0%)	20
Total	14 (10,5%)	6 (4,5%)	47 (35,3%)	66 (49,6%)	133

Table 2. Occurrence of individual types of epithelial neoplasms in different age groups in bitches

2.3.2 Results of proliferative activity

The value of mitotic index differed significantly between types of tumors. The lowest proliferative activity was observed in adenomas, the highest in simple and solid carcinomas. The highest proliferative activity was found in tumors in the 3rd grade of malignancy, the lowest in the tumors in the 1st grade (Fig.4). Expression of Ki-67 protein was observed in the nuclei of neoplastic cells that have undergone division (Fig.5). Statistical analysis shows significant differences between particular types of tumors. The lowest number of cells exhibiting Ki-67 protein expression was observed in adenomas, the highest in the solid and simple carcinomas and in tumors with the highest histological grade of malignancy (3rd).

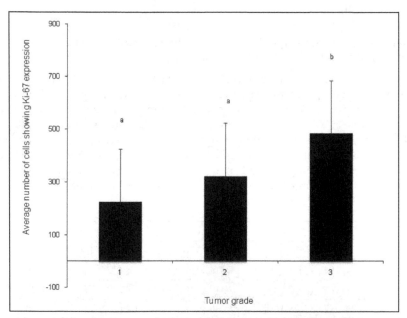

Fig. 4. Average number of cells showing Ki-67 expression depending on the tumor grade. Letters (a, b, c) above the columns show that the differences between mean values were statistically significant (P≤0.05).

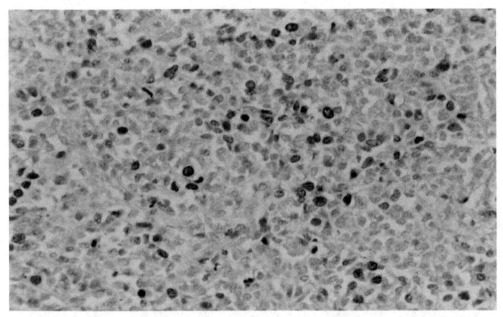

Fig. 5. Adenocarcinoma simplex, expression of Ki-67, immunohistochemical method. (40x)

2.3.3 Results of cellular infiltration in tumors of epithelial origin

In most cases, infiltrates were located predominantly in the stroma at the periphery of the tumor, and, in rare cases, occurred in the glandular alveoli. Inflammatory infiltrates consisted of lymphocytes, neutrophils and macrophages. The intensity of cellular infiltration was assessed on a four-level scale:: -/+; +; ++; +++. Statistical analysis indicates no correlation between the age of the dog and the intensity of cellular infiltration in the tumor. It is worth noting that, in bitches between the ages of 8 to 12 years, most tumors exhibited the intensity of infiltration at the first (+) level , which constituted 50% of tumors in this age group. A significant relationship was found between the intensity of cellular infiltration and the type of tumor. In 50% of solid cancers, there was no cellular infiltration. Only 33% of these tumors exhibited the presence of cellular infiltration at the first level (+), and 16.7% on the second level (++). Among the complex cancers, the largest group consisted of those, in which cellular infiltration was found at the first (+) and the second (++) level. The highest average intensity of cellular infiltration was found in complex carcinomas, followed by simple carcinomas, adenomas and solid carcinomas. Specific differences were seen between adenomas and complex carcinomas (P=0.007) and between solid carcinomas and complex carcinomas (P=0.005). While examining the relationship between intensity of cellular infiltration and histological grade of malignancy, no significant differences were revealed. But it may be noted that among tumors of all histological grades of malignancy, the largest group consisted of cancers with the first level of cellular infiltration. While analyzing the average intensity of cellular infiltration in tumors with various histological grades of malignancy no significant differences were found between groups with the exception of the tumors in the 3rd grade, where a significant difference was observed (P=0.023).

2.3.4 Results of p53 expression in neoplasms of mammary gland

Expression of p53 protein was observed in the nuclei of cancer cells (Fig.6). Positive reaction of p53 protein was observed in 70 (52.6%) of all tumors. Expression of p53 protein was found in 4 adenomas. The largest group of tumors positive for p53 protein were complex and simple cancers. Solid cancers belonged to a group, which rarely exhibited a positive reaction for nuclear p53. Analysis of the average number of cells with a positive reaction for p53 showed its highest expression in the case of complex cancers, as well as in 1st and 2nd grade tumors (Fig.7). The lowest level of expression of p53 protein was found in adenomas.

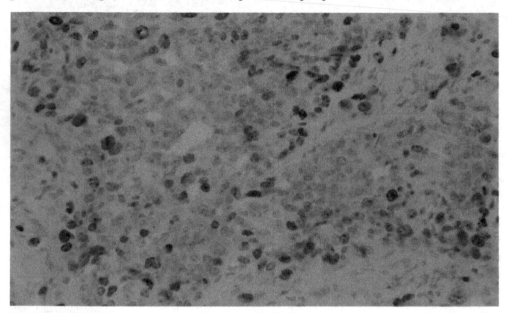

Fig. 6. Adenocarcinoma simplex, expression of p53, immunohistochemical method. (40x)

No statistically significant differences were shown between the examined groups. Comparing the ages of bitches, the highest average number of cells expressing p53 protein was found in tumors excised from younger dogs. However, there were no statistically significant differences among the age groups.

2.3.5 Results of estrogen receptor expression in neoplasms of mammary gland

Estrogen receptor expression was detected in the nuclei of tumor cells, but it was also seen in the cytoplasm. Cytoplasmic reaction was considered to be nonspecific. Among all tumors of epithelial origin, expression of estrogen receptors was found in 54 (40.6%) , and no reaction was noted in 79 (59.4%). Expression of estrogen receptors was most commonly found in complex cancers (43.9%) (Fig.8) , followed by simple cancers (42.6%) (Fig.9, Fig.10) and adenomas (28.6%), while solid cancers rarely expressed them (16.7%). The highest expression of estrogen receptors was found in simple carcinomas as well as in 3rd grade tumors, but no statistically significant differences were found between study groups (Fig. 11). Analysis of the average number of cells showing positive expression of estrogen receptors reveals that the level of expression increases with the histological grade of malignancy. It was also found that most tumors expressing estrogen receptors came from dogs younger than 8 years. A positive correlation was found between mitotic index and expression of estrogen receptors in specific types of cancer and statistically significant differences between tumor characteristics were demonstrated (P=0.042).

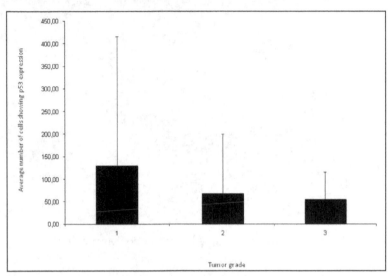

Fig. 7. Average number of cells showing p53 expression depending on the tumor grade.

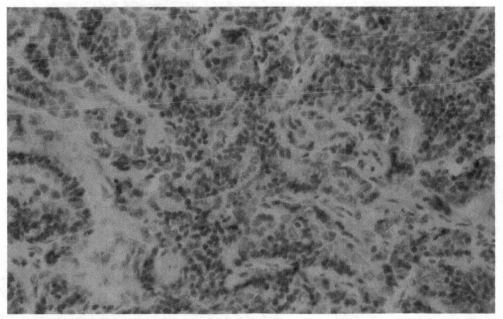

Fig. 8. Adenocarcinoma complex, expression of ER, immunohistochemical method. (40x)

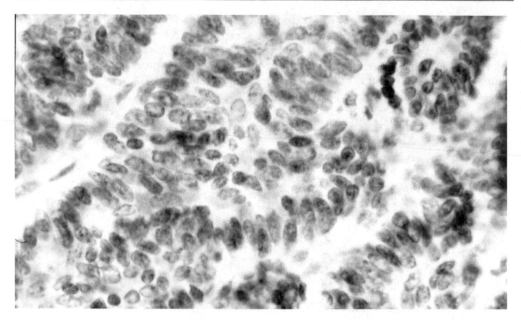

Fig. 9. Adenocarcinoma simplex, expression of ER, immunohistochemical method. (100x)

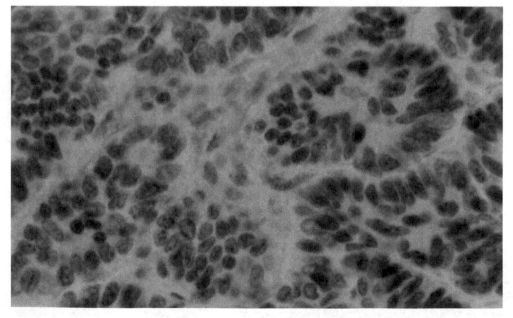

Fig. 10. Adenocarcinoma simplex, expression of ER, immunohistochemical method. (100x)

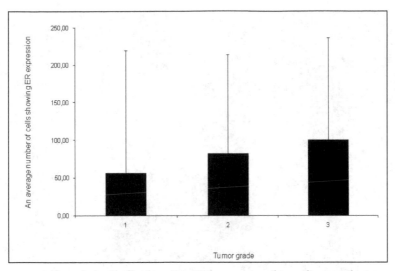

Fig. 11. An average number of cells showing ER expression depending on the tumor grade

2.3.6 Results of cyclooxygenase-2 expression in neoplasms of mammary gland

Expression of cyclooxygenase – 2 was observed in the neoplastic cell cytoplasm. It was confirmed in 13 of 14 adenomas. Similar results were obtained in solid cancers (5 of 6) (Fig. 12). Positive COX–2 reaction was found in 36.9% of simple carcinomas (Fig.13). Of all tumors, which exhibited a positive response (122), complex tumors demonstrated the highest percentage (48.4%). Statistical analysis, however, failed to demonstrate any significant differences regarding the COX–2 expression between the individual types of carcinoma (P = 0.978). According to the analysis of histological malignancy grades, the highest expression was found in 3rd grade cancers and statistical significance was confirmed for the individual histological malignancy grades (P = 0.047) (Fig. 14, Fig. 15). Furthermore, higher COX-2 expression level was demonstrated in carcinomas with higher mitotic index; statistical analysis demonstrated highly significant differences between neoplasms with high versus low mitotic index (P = 0.009) (Fig.16). The investigation into the relationship between expression of Ki-67 nuclear antigen and the COX-2 expression level did not reveal statistical significance (P = 0.614) (Fig. 17). Analysis of the relationship between the p53 protein expression and COX-2 expression level demonstrated a statistically significant correlation between these features (P = 0.034) (Fig. 18). An average number of cells expressing p53 protein was higher in carcinomas with higher COX-2 expression. In addition, experiments explored the relationship between Hsp70 protein and cyclooxygenase – 2 expression levels. The study proved a statistically high correlation between the investigated neoplastic characteristics (P = 0.006). The lowest Hsp70 protein expression was found in carcinomas exhibiting second degree COX-2 expression (Fig. 19). Analysis of the relationship between representative neoplastic features demonstrated statistically significant, positive correlations between COX-2 expression, mitotic index (P = 0.009) and p53 protein expression (P = 0.003); on the other hand, no correlation was found with regard to the Ki-67 nuclear antigen expression (P = 0.686). There was no correlation between the estrogen receptor expression and the above mentioned parameters. The highest expression of estrogen receptors was found in simple cancer types.

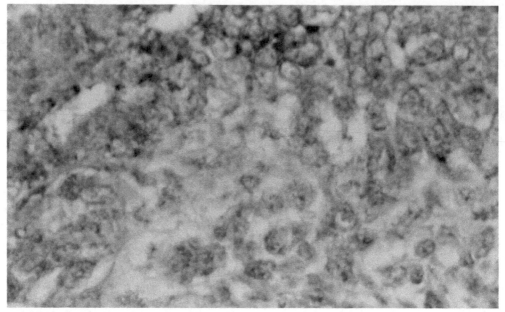

Fig. 12. Carcinoma solidum, expression of COX–2, immunohistochemical method. (100x)

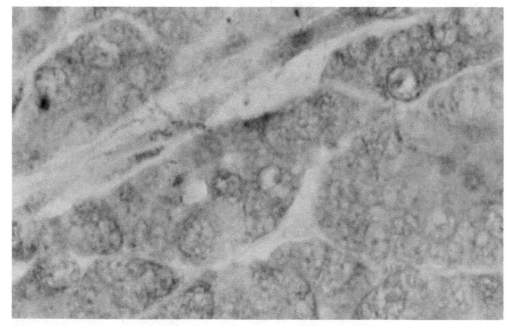

Fig. 13. Adenocarcinoma simplex, expression of COX–2, immunohistochemical method. (100x)

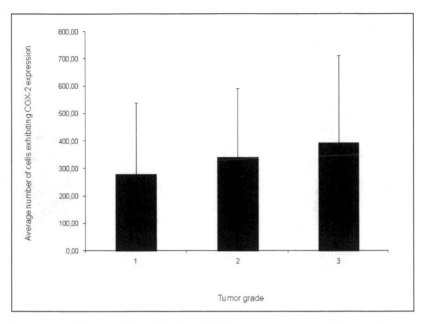

Fig. 14. Average number of cells exhibiting COX-2 expression depending on the tumor grade.

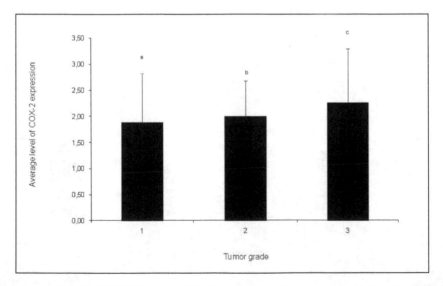

Fig. 15. Average level of COX-2 expression depending on tumor grade. Letters (a, b, c) above the columns show that the difference between means was statistically significant ($P \leq 0.05$).

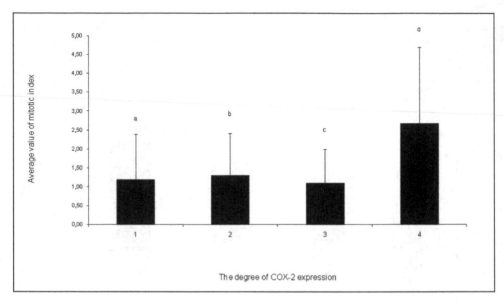

Fig. 16. Average value of mitotic index in tumors with different degrees of expression of cyclooxygenase – 2. Letters (a, b, c, d) above the columns show that the difference between means was statistically significant (P≤0.05).

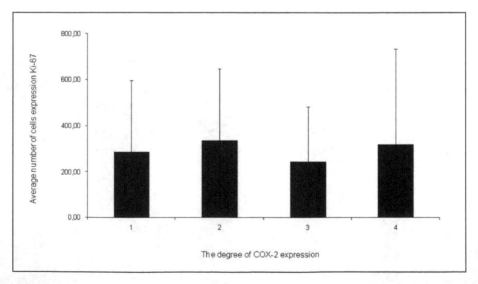

Fig. 17. Average number of cells expressing Ki-67, depending on the degree of expression of cyclooxygenase – 2.

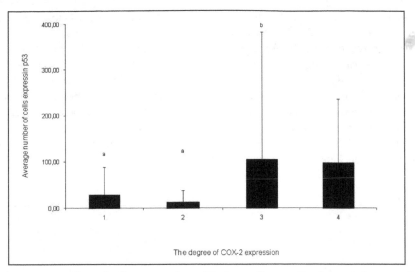

Fig. 18. Average number of cells expressing p53, depending on the degree of expression of cyclooxygenase – 2. Letters (a, b) above the columns show that the difference between means was statistically significant (P≤0.05).

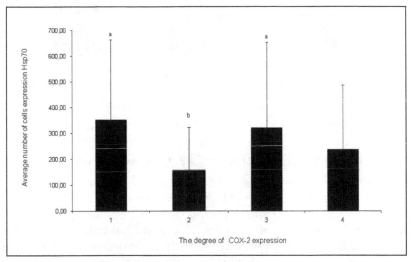

Fig. 19. Average number of cells expressing Hsp70, depending on the degree of expression of cyclooxygenase – 2. Letters (a, b) above the columns show that the difference between means was statistically significant (P≤0.05).

2.3.7 Results of P-glycoprotein expression in neoplasms of the mammary gland

Expression of P-glycoprotein was identified in cytoplasm and cell membranes of neoplastic cells. Positive reaction was found in 76% of all neoplasms. Complex carcinomas were the biggest group among cancer types, which demonstrated positive reaction to P-gp. In terms of histological malignancy grade, the most numerous were cancers featuring the lowest grade of malignancy (Fig. 20). In female canines aged 9 through 12 years, cancers exhibiting a positive P-gp reaction constituted the most numerous group (63.2%); on the other hand, this cancer type barely appeared in the oldest group (10.5%). Analysis of the average P - glycoprotein expression in different types of carcinomas did not reveal any significant differences. Correspondingly, evaluation of malignancy grade showed no statistical significance between examined features. Among different cancer types, the highest P-gp expression was demonstrated in solid carcinomas and cancers featuring the highest histological grade of malignancy. Positive correlation between investigated cancer features was found in the analysis of the relationship between cyclooxygenase-2 and P-gp expression, where P value was equal to 0.021.

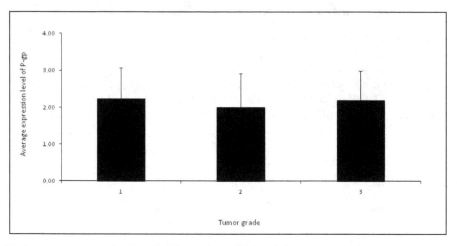

Fig. 20. Average expression level of P–gp depending on the tumor grade.

2.3.8 Results of heat shock protein expression in neoplasms of mammary gland

Heat shock proteins were found in the cytoplasm and nuclei of cancer cells (Fig. 21, Fig. 22, Fig. 23, Fig. 24). The largest group of tumors exhibiting Hsp70 and Hsp90 expression included simple and complex cancers, whereas solid tumors were the least numerous group. Grade 1 and 2 cancers constituted the largest group expressing both Hsp70 and Hsp90 (Fig. 25, Fig. 26) . Immunohistochemical analysis showed high expression of Hsp90 in simple and complex cancers, but no statistically significant differences were found between investigated types of tumors (P=0.443). High expression of Hsp90 was confirmed in solid cancers and, in this particular group, significant differences were found between types of tumor (P=0.032). As far as grading was concerned, no statistically significant differences were found between the mean number of cells exhibiting Hsp70 and Hsp90 protein expression and malignancy grade. When comparing the expression of Hsp70 to the expression of Hsp90 in particular types of cancers, we found a highly significant statistical difference (P=0.005) between the expression of both proteins. Results of a study on the expression of heat shock proteins (Hsp70 and Hsp90) were compared to nuclear antigen Ki-67 expression. It was found that the expression of nuclear antigen Ki-67 was most pronounced in solid tumors, as was the expression of Hsp90. Also, in neoplasms of the highest grade, expression of nuclear antigen Ki-67 and protein Hsp90 was the highest. High expression of Hsp70 was found in tumors with grade 1 and 3 of cyclooxygenase-2 expression, whereas the lowest Hsp70 expression was observed in tumors with grade 2 of cyclooxygenase-2 expression. Statistical significance was found between the investigated features of neoplasms (P=0.009). Increased expression of cyclooxygenase-2 was observed in tumors with a low mean number of cells showing positive immunohistochemical reaction for protein Hsp90. The highest level of expression of this protein was confirmed in tumors with grade 1 of cyclooxygenase-2 expression (Fig. 27). Between the mean number of cells showing positive Hsp90 reaction and cyclooxygenase-2 expression, there was a statistical significance observed for grade 1 and 2 of cyclooxygenase-2 expression (P=0.039). Statistical analysis proved a correlation between Hsp70 and p53 protein expression in tumors of epithelial origin. High statistical significance was shown for investigated neoplastic features (P = 0.002). Taking into account the type of tumor, expression of both proteins was highest in complex carcinomas and tumors with the lowest histological grade. High expression levels of Hsp90 protein and Ki-67 nuclear antigen was shown in cases of solid carcinomas and in carcinomas exhibiting 3rd histological grade of malignancy, described by a low apoptotic index.

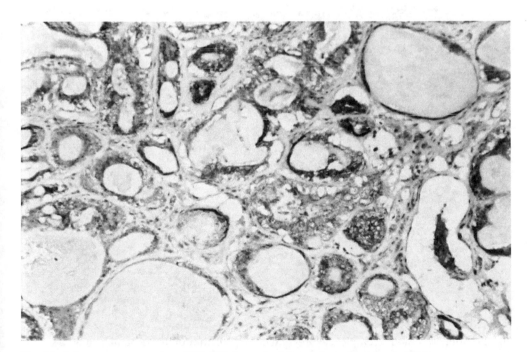

Fig. 21. Adenoma, expression of Hsp70, immunohistochemical method. (20x)

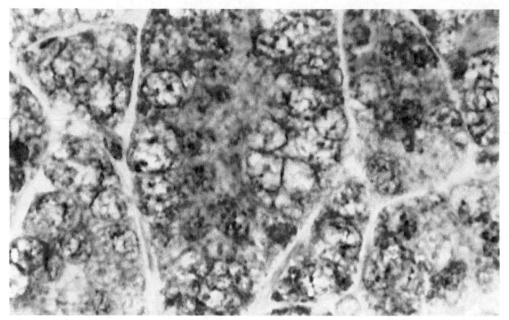

Fig. 22. Adenocarcinoma simplex, expression of Hsp70, immunohistochemical method. (100x)

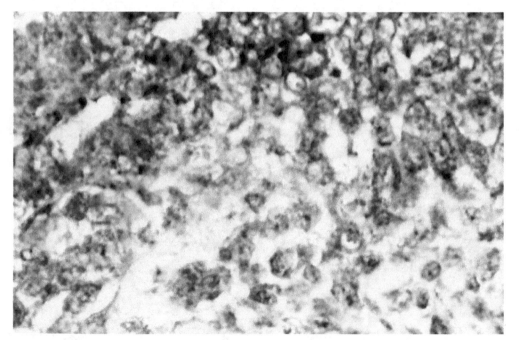

Fig. 23. Adenocarcinoma complex, expression of Hsp70, immunohistochemical method. (100x)

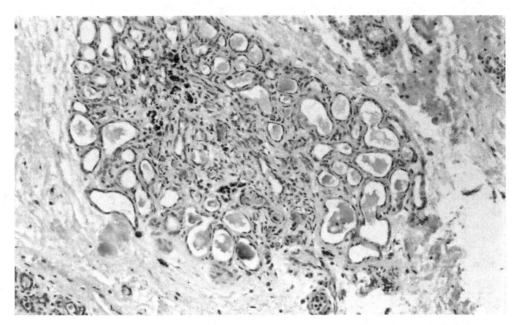

Fig. 24. Adenocarcinoma complex, expression of Hsp90, immunohistochemical method.
(10x)

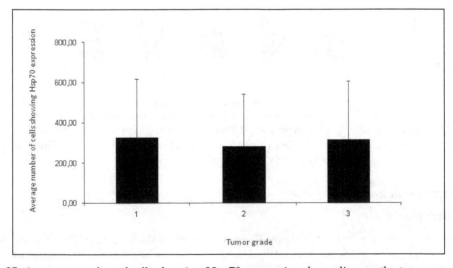

Fig. 25. Average number of cells showing Hsp70 expression depending on the tumor grade.

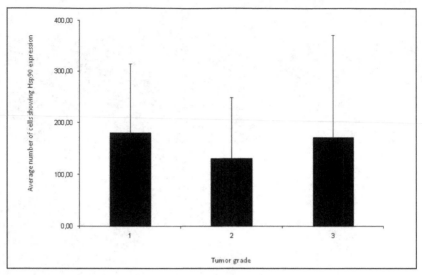

Fig. 26. Average number of cells showing Hsp90 expression depending on the tumor grade

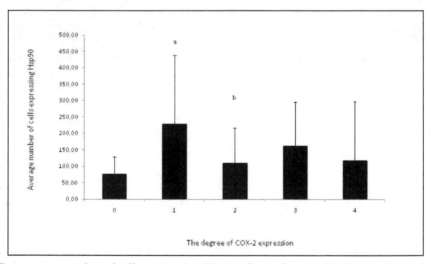

Fig. 27. Average number of cells expressing Hsp90, depending on the degree of cyclooxygenase – 2 expression. Letters (a, b) above the columns show that the difference between means was statistically significant (P≤0.05).

3. Discussion and conclusion

3.1 Discusion

In our study, cancers accounted for 89.8% of tumors of epithelial origin. This is consistent with the results of some authors, although the results of studies on the incidence and types of tumors of the mammary gland in canine females given by various authors differ.

Löhr (1997) found that 50% of the mammary gland tumors in female canines are malignant tumors (Löhr et al, 1997). Hellmén (1993) determined the incidence of malignant tumors to be 68% (Hellmén et al 1993). There are also studies showing, that about a half of tumors are benign (Bostock et al, 1992; Gilbertson et al, 1983). Moulton (1990) believes that benign tumors represent about 80% of cases and the majority of tumors studied are "benign mixed tumors" (65%) (Moulton, 1990). They are tumors in which, apart from epithelial and mesenchymal tissue, there is also cartilage and bone tissue. Their histopathological examination reveals no sign of malignancy. Nerurkar (1990) says that benign tumors represent about 27% of the mammary gland tumors in female dogs (Nerurkar et al, 1990). In our study, benign tumors of epithelial origin accounted for only 10.1% of all cases. The diversity of these results relates to the lack of uniform diagnostic criteria and lack of uniform classification of tumors of the mammary gland in dogs. In human medicine, age is a very important prognostic factor. Detection of breast cancer in women at a very young age and at the age over 60 is associated with worse prognosis (Host & Lund, 1986). In Philibert's (2003) studies there were no significant differences in survival of young and older dogs (Philibert et al, 2003). Hellmén (1993) presented completely different results (Hellmén et al, 1993). She found that age may be an important prognostic factor and showed that older bitches had a shorter survival time after surgery. Results obtained by Benjamin corresponded to that (1999) (Benjamin et al, 1999). Own results support the concept of age as an important prognostic factor, as there is very little information regarding survival or recurrence of malignancy in female dogs after surgery. Current study shows that the presence or absence of cellular inflammatory infiltrates may be a prognostic factor. Data on the incidence of cellular infiltration in mammary gland tumors in female dogs is also scarce. Gilbertson (1983) found that cell infiltration plays a role in the process of development of precancerous and invasive carcinomas (35%) (Gilbertson et al, 1983). In our study, the percentage of tumors with cellular infiltration was higher (88%). The highest intensity of cellular infiltration was observed in tumors with a high histological grade of malignancy. Skrzypczak (2004) (Skrzypczak, 2004) presented similar results in his study . Authors believe that presence of cellular infiltration plays a positive role in inhibiting tumor growth. Some studies have shown that presence of cellular infiltration is associated with good (Rilke et al, 1991) or poor (Parl & Dupont, 1982) prognosis and others, that it carries no prognostic value. In our study, no relationship was found between cellular infiltration and other tumor markers, consistent with the studies by Rodo (2007) (Rodo, 2007; Roses et al, 1982). It is worth noting the presence of necrosis in tumor foci, which may obscure the accuracy of the results. Necrosis in the tumor is the result of disparities between high proliferative activity and tumor vascularization. It may trigger cellular inflammatory reactions. We also analyzed the distribution of cellular infiltration. Our own results differ from the results of other authors, because infiltration was observed in the stroma, not scattered (Lee et al, 1996), and was more pronounced on the periphery of the tumor. The role of cellular infiltration within the tumor remains unclear and controversial. Estrogen receptors are recognized markers in the diagnosis of breast cancer in women. It is estimated that about 70-80% of breast cancers in women exhibit the expression of estrogen receptors. These tumors are characterized by slower growth, higher diversity, better prognosis with a suitable treatment regimen and correlate with the length of survival after surgical removal (Bacus et al, 1989; Barzanti et al, 2000). Study of the expression of estrogen receptors in mammary gland neoplasms in female canines was, as usual, inconclusive. Martin et. al (1984) studied 228 tumors of the mammary gland in bitches and showed the expression of estrogen receptors in only 2.1% of tumors (Martin et al, 1984). Pena et. al (1998), on the other hand, diagnosed 21 cancers with an ongoing inflammatory process and found no expression of estrogen receptors (Pena et al, 1998). According to Sartin et. al (1992) the greatest chance of long-term survival after surgery , is associated with tumors expressing ER alone or together with PgR. Indeed, in the absence of ER and PgR, researchers observed the shortest period of survival (Sartin et al, 1997). Millanta et. al (2005) study on 47 mammary gland neoplasms in bitches reported that ER and PgR expression did not correlate with survival or histological parameters of tumors (Millanta et al, 2005). Similarly, Sobczak-Filipiak and Malicka (1997) have shown no correlation between expression of ER and mitotic index (Sobczak-Filipiak & Malicka, 1997). In our study, the expression of estrogen receptors was demonstrated in 40% of the tested tumors. The highest expression of estrogen receptors was found in simple carcinomas and tumors with the highest histological grade of malignancy. There was a significant correlation between mitotic index and expression of estrogen receptors. Nowak (2007) found expression of estrogen receptors in only 6% of cancers (Nowak et al, 2007), but Mulas (2005) obtained different results- he found that estrogen receptors were expressed in benign tumors (Mulas et al, 2005). Similarly, McEwen et. al (1982) have demonstrated the expression of estrogen receptors in about 50% of cases, with a significantly higher levels of expression present in benign tumors (McEwen et al, 1982). Results obtained by Nieto et. al (2000) are different - they show a correlation between the expression of nuclear antigen Ki-67 and estrogen receptors (Nieto et al, 2000). Authors of these studies observed the highest levels of ER expression in simple and complex carcinomas, as we did in our study. Otherwise, Rutteman (1998), Sartin (1992), and Geraldes (2000), claim that high expression of ER is present in adenomas compared to adenocarcinomas, which exhibit a lower level of expression of this marker (Sartin et al, 1992; Rutteman et al, 2001; Geraldes et al, 2000). Opinions about the value of estrogen receptors as a prognostic factor are divided. Some authors consider ER expression a positive factor, but there are also voices postulating it is a negative prognostic marker. Interestingly, it seems that in our study, low expression of ER negatively correlated with high expression of nuclear antigen Ki-67. It is in agreement with the research done by Peña (1998), who led the study on the mammary gland neoplasms in canines (Peña et al, 1998). From our research we conclude, that the expression of estrogen receptors may be important in assessment of malignancy, but does not show significant correlation with other markers. An important marker of malignancy is the proliferative activity. Proper evaluation of proliferative activity of tumor cells is crucial for the evaluation of its biological activity and is used in determining the treatment of cancer. High mitotic index correlated with tumor size and presence of lymph node metastases (Niwińska, 1995; Mirecka et al, 1993). In our study, proliferative activity depended on both, the type of tumor and the degree of histological malignancy. The highest values of mitotic index were recorded in simple and solid carcinomas and in tumors with the highest histological grade of malignancy. Similar results were reported for the expression of Ki-67. The highest expression of Ki-67 was seen in solid, simple carcinomas and in 3rd grade tumors. Similar results were obtained by Nieto (2000), who confirmed that the expression of Ki-67 is high in tumors with a higher histological grade of malignancy (Nieto et al, 2000). Similar results were obtained by Peña (1998), Giziński (2003) and Szczubiał (2002) (Peña et al, 1998; Giziński et al, 2003; Szczubiał & Łopuszański, 2002). They studied the expression of nuclear antigen Ki-67 in mammary gland tumors in dogs and came to the conclusion that higher expression of Ki-67 is an important prognostic factor and is associated with a higher risk of metastasis, a shorter period to recurrence and a shorter overall survival period. The rate of tumor growth is influenced by factors related to inhibition of cell cycle and promotion of apoptosis of cancer cells., Under physiological conditions it is a function of, among others, p53 gene and its protein product. Mutation of the p53 gene plays an important role in the uncontrolled proliferation and resistance to apoptosis in cancer cells , leading to functional changes in proteins. In dogs, expression of the p53 gene was found in both benign (Muto et al, 2000) and malignant (Mayr et al, 1994; Veldhoen et al, 1999) tumors of mammary gland. Muto (2000) in his study showed no association between p53 expression and histological type of cancer, but claimed that this protein may play an important role in carcinogenesis and may be a negative prognostic factor (Muto et al, 2000). Chung-Ho (2004) came to a similar conclusion, arguing that the presence ofp53 in tumor cells is associated with their malignancy and bad prognosis in mammary gland tumors (Chun-Ho et al, 2004). In our study, p53 expression was observed in benign as well as malignant tumors. Among all tumors, more than 50% exhibited a positive reaction for 53 protein. It contradicts the data obtained in his study by Gamblin (1997), who carried out an analysis of 16 adenocarcinomas and found a positive reaction for p53 protein in only 12.5% of cases (Gamblin et al, 1994). In our study, the highest expression of p53 was observed in complex carcinomas and in 1st and 2nd grade malignant tumors. These results are consistent with the results obtained by Rungsipipata (1999), who found the highest levels of p53 expression in simple and complex carcinomas and also showed expression of this protein in adenomas (16%) (Rungspipata, 1999). Rodo (2007) obtained results on the expression of p53 , stating that there is a positive correlation between proliferative activity and the number of cells expressing p53 protein (Rodo, 2007). In our study, we found no statistically significant differences between the expression of p53 and nuclear antigen Ki-67. Obtained data in part explain why the activation of oncogenes does not always lead to uncontrolled proliferation when normal signal transduction leads to stabilization of p53 and activation of programmed cell death. There is a need for further research in this area, because the data in the literature is ambiguous and does not allow for a definite conclusion as to the importance of p53 protein and its role in mammary gland neoplasms. Varying results undermine the claim that a positive reaction for p53 protein would predict worse prognosis in cancer and that p53 mutation may be responsible for increased proliferation in tumors with advanced malignancy. Research on COX-2 expression in canine mammary cancers is scarce (Heller et al, 2005; Nowak et al, 2005; Doré et al, 2003) despite it being an attractive and motivating topic. Overexpression of COX-2 is known to occur in 56-100% of canine mammary carcinomas (Doré et al, 2003; Millanta et al, 2005; Queiroga et al, 2007; Heller et al, 2005; Mohammed et al, 2004), but there is a marked variation in the percentage of COX-2-positive tumor cells and the intensity of its expression. Doré et. al (2003) did not find any COX-2 expression in four samples of normal mammary tissue (Doré et al, 2003), whilst Mohammed et. al (2004) (Mohammed et al, 2004) and Queiroga et. al (2007) (Queiroga et al, 2007) reported expression of COX-2 in one of seven and two of four samples of normal mammary glands, respectively. Our own research demonstrated that as much as 91.7% of all carcinomas in the study displayed COX-2 expression. Doré et.al (2003) obtained similar results: he found a positive COX-2 reaction in 67% of complex cancers and in 47% of simple carcinomas (Doré et al, 2003). Our research demonstrated the highest COX-2 expression in simple cancers and the lowest in solid cancers. Similar data were presented by Heller et.al (2005), who found COX-2 expression in adenocarcinomas, whereas he failed to detect it in solid carcinomas (Heller et al, 2005). Ristimäki et. al (2002) demonstrated the relationship between COX-2 expression and certain clinical and pathological features of the tumor (Ristimäki et al, 2002). Her research into mammary gland tumours proved that COX-2 expression was positively correlated with tumour size as well as the strength of Ki-67 nuclear antigen staining and p53 protein expression. Results of our study are consistent with the results of works by Ristimäki et. al (2002) : increased COX-2 expression in carcinomas is related to higher mitotic index, i.e. with the proliferating activity (Ristimäki et al, 2002). Expression of Ki–67 nuclear antigen was demonstrated in carcinomas exhibiting increased COX-2 expression, yet research failed to prove the correlation between these markers; On the other hand, it proved the existence of statistical correlation between COX-2 expression and expression of p53 and Hsp70 proteins. Average number of cells exhibiting p53 protein expression was higher in carcinomas with higher levels of COX-2 expression. High expression level of Hsp70 protein and COX-2 was shown in carcinomas with the 3rd histological grade of malignancy, as described by low apoptotic index. Similar results were obtained by Lanza-Jacoby et. al (2004), who conducted her studies on experimental animals (Lanza-Jacoby et al, 2006), and by Liu and Rose (1996) who studied the COX-2 expression in cell cultures (Liu & Rose, 1996). Furthermore, Ristimäki et al (2002) and Dempke et al (2001) came to a conclusion that COX-2 promoted the mammary gland neoplasm growth, invasive capacity, and probability of metastasis (Ristimäki et al, 2002; Dempke et al, 2001). COX-2 expression may be relevant to a number of physiological processes within this tissue including proliferative activity, inhibition of apoptosis, increased angiogenesis and activation of matrix metalloproteinases (Dempke et al, 2001). Mammary physiology is a complex process regulated by hormones, estrogens, progesterone, growth hormone, prolactin, and epidermal growth factor (Howlin et al, 2006). As COX-2 expression is induced by different stimuli including cytokines, oncogenes, hormones and growth factors (Thomas et al, 2008), the same factors that control mammary growth and differentiation may act as trigger stimuli for COX-2 expression. The results of our work are consistent with the results obtained by other researchers. P-gp expression was discovered in epithelium and neoplasms of mesenchymal origin in dogs (Ginn, 1996). Author of these studies argues that continuation of this line of research will deliver additional prognostic data. There is a small number of works attempting to evaluate the P-gp expression in canine mammary cancers. A considerable progress in the investigation into P-gp expression in canine mammary cancers was made by Petterino et. al (2006), who attempted to define the P-gp expression in mammary gland carcinomas in female canines (Petterino et al, 2006). His study covered cases of both malignant and benign neoplasms; Petterino et al (2006) found the expression of the examined marker in two test groups and confirmed the statistical significance between the two groups (Petterino et al, 2006). Furthermore, he found that simple and complex carcinomas were the most numerous groups among the examined cancers and that P-gp expression was absent from the tissues of healthy mammary glands. We achieved similar results in our research: we found the P-gp expression in 76% of the examined canine mammary cancers. The most numerous groups exhibiting a positive P-gp immunohistochemical reaction were composed of complex carcinomas (90.9%) and simple carcinomas (73%). High expression was found in cancers with the highest histological grade of malignancy. Due to fact that there are hardly any works investigating into the P-gp expression in canine mammary cancers, we attempted not only to confirm the presence of P-gp expression and location, but also to prove the relationship between P-gp and other neoplastic markers. Statistical analysis confirmed a positive correlation between P-gp and COX-2 expression: it demonstrated a statistical significance in the case of examined characteristics ($P = 0.021$). It is worth mentioning that the expression of two markers was significant in carcinomas featuring high histological grades of malignancy. Furthermore, P-gp expression was studied in canine lymphomas; additionally, attempts were made to conduct studies on carcinomas treated by means of chemotherapy; the results were compared with the results obtained in the control group of untreated carcinomas. Higher expression was observed in the treated cancer cells. On the other hand, increased expression in untreated cancers appears to be a negative prognostic factor, given that survival rate shall decrease in such cases (Lee et al, 1996). Due to the fact that this line of research has not brought about many works, there are several questions and ambiguities concerning the role of P-gp in the process of neoplastic genesis and the importance of this factor from the clinical point of view. Additionally, the question arises whether, or not P-gp can be classified into the significant prognostic marker category. We are not aware of defensive mechanisms of the cells equipped with membrane transporters against apoptosis generated by the compounds, that are not pump substrates. There are suggestions that the phenomenon may be connected with evacuation (pumping out) of a certain important mediator of apoptosis or with the impact of P-gp on the intracellular pH (Johnson et al, 1998). Identification of a mechanism of cell resistance to apoptosis is a key instrument in selection of suitable therapy. According to studies in humans, heat shock proteins may be important predictors of breast cancer (Park & Dupont, 1982). There is not much published data in the literature on heat shock protein expression in mammary gland tumors of female dogs. The role of these proteins in carcinogenesis has not been clearly defined either. Studies have only shown that expression of heat shock proteins takes place in canine breast cancers , but the linkage between these proteins and other tumor markers was not confirmed. Seymour (1990) studied endometrial cancer in women and found that heat shock proteins were useful markers in the diagnostics of these tumors (Saymour et al, 1990). Expression of Hsp27 was also investigated in breast cancer in women (Ciocca et al, 1993). A relationship between the expression of this protein and the degree of differentiation of the tumor cells was found. Similar studies were conducted by Storm (1996), who stated that tumors with Hsp27 expression showed a higher histological grade than tumors negative for the expression of this protein (Storm et al, 1993). Kumaraguruparan (2006) studied the expression of Hsp70 and Hsp90 in breast cancer in women and found a correlation between the expression of both proteins and proliferative activity (Kumaraguruparan et al, 2006). He suggested that heat shock proteins are important prognostic factors. Presence of Hsp70 was also reported in normal gastrointestinal tissues, but an increased expression of this protein was observed in gastrointestinal tumors (Isomoto et al, 2003). Isomoto (2003) believed that Hsp70 plays an important role in the degree of cellular differentiation in tumors, which would indicate that Hsp70 is an important prognostic factor. Similar studies are conducted in veterinary medicine, but to a lesser extent (Isomoto et al, 2003). A similar study was conducted by Rommanucci (2005) in mammary gland tumors in female dogs (Romanucci et al, 2006). She found Hsp70 and Hsp90 expression in simple and complex, as well as solid-type adenocarcinomas. Expression of these proteins was observed in the cytoplasm, as well as in the nuclei of tumor cells. Rommanucci (2006), in her study of breast cancers in female dogs, has not attempted to verify the possible correlations between heat shock proteins and other tumor markers (Rommanucci et al, 2006). She focused on establishing the degree of protein expression and their localization in tumor cells. Basing on the results of her study, the author suggested that these proteins may play an important role in the process of carcinogenesis. In our study, Hsp70 protein expression was found in 86.4% of tumors, while the expression of Hsp90 was observed in 66.2% of tumors. The aim of our study was to demonstrate the relationship between the expression of heat shock proteins and other prognostic factors. When comparing the expression of Hsp70 to the expression of Hsp90 in different types of tumors, we found a high statistical significance between the expression of both proteins. Analysis of the relationship between the expression of nuclear antigen Ki-67 and the expression of heat shock proteins showed that the highest expression of Ki-67 as well as Hsp90 was present in solid tumors. The highest expression of Hsp90 protein and Ki-67 was also found in cancers of the highest histological grades. Based on these data it can be concluded that Hsp90 is an important factor, which could be considered a marker of malignancy and which may be useful in the diagnostics of cancers. Analysis of the results showed high expression of Hsp70 in cancers with grade 1 and 3 of COX-2 expression; the lowest expression of Hsp70 was found in cancers with grade 2 of COX-2 expression. Statistical significance of $P = 0.009$ was found between the expression of Hsp70 and expression of COX-2. An increased expression of COX-2 was observed in tumors with a low mean number of cells showing positive reaction to Hsp90 protein. Correlation between the expression of Hsp70 protein and p53 protein in tumors of epithelial origin was also confirmed. Based on the analysis of expression of both proteins and taking into account the mean apoptotic index, it was found that in cancers with the third (the highest) histological grade, expression of p53 protein is significantly lower than the expression of Hsp70, and the value of apoptotic index in these cancers was the lowest.

3.2 Conclusions

Occurrence of mammary tumors in female dogs and their potential use as a model in comparative pathology makes it an interesting research material. It is known that the degree of malignancy is positively correlated with proliferative activity. The relationship between expression of estrogen receptors and the degree of malignancy is not entirely clear, although most authors believe that the expression of these receptors is higher in benign tumors.

Literature concerning the expression of p53 protein in mammary tumors in canines is scarce. It deals only with the expression of p53, but leaves no answers in respect to the expression of other factors that are considered prognostic markers, such as proliferative activity, histological grade of malignancy and expression of estrogen receptors. We conclude that COX-2 is an important prognostic factor and may be applied as a marker of canine mammary neoplasm malignancy, given the fact that higher expression of COX-2 was found in adenocarcinomas and in cancers featuring the highest histological malignancy grades in comparison to simple adenomas. Obtained results suggest that cyclooxygenase-2 may be a prognostic factor, but it requires clinical confirmation. The P-gp expression is also positively correlated with the degree of histological malignancy. This suggests a prudent approach to decisions concerning chemotherapy. Expression of Hsp90 can be considered as a marker of the degree of differentiation and of histological grade of mammary gland tumors in dogs, because the highest level of expression was found in solid carcinomas and in cancers exhibiting the highest histological grades of malignancy. Hsp70 expression was confirmed, but no correlation with other factors was found. This may suggest that Hsp70 is not a useful marker in the diagnostics of breast cancers in female dogs.

4. Acknowledgments

Study was carried out at the Institute of Pathology, Department of Clinical Sciences, Faculty of Veterinary Medicine, Warsaw School of Life Sciences, 159C Nowoursynowska Street, 02-766 Warsaw. Research was conducted as a part of a doctoral dissertation, partially funded by a grant from the Ministry of Science and Information Technology, No N30800632/0667

5. References

Bacus, S.S.; Goldschmidt, R.; Chin, D.; Moran, G.; Weinberg, D.; Bacus, J.W. (1989). Biological grading of breast cancer using antibodies to proliferating cells and other markers. *The American Journal of Pathology* , Vol.135, No.5, pp. 783-792

Barzanti, F.; Dal Susino, M.; Volpi, A.; Amadori, D.; Riccobon, A.; Scarpi, E.; Medri, L.; Bernardi, L.; Naldi, S.; Aldi, M.; Gaudio, M.; Zoli, W. (2000). Comparison between different cell kinetic variables in human breast cancer. *Cell Proliferation*, Vol.33,:pp. 75-89

Benjamin, S.A.; Lee, A.C.; Saunders, W.J. (1999). Classification and behavior of canine mammary epithelial neoplasms based on life-span observations in beagles. *Veterinary Pathology*, Vol. 36, pp. 423-436

Bostock, D.E.; Moriarty, J.; Crocker, J.(1992). Correlation between histologic diagnosis mean nucleolar organizer region count and prognosis in canine mammary tumors. *Veterinary Pathology*, Vol. 29, pp. 381-385

Chung-Ho, L.; Wan-Hee, K.; Ji-Hey, L.; Min-Soo, K.; Dae-Yong, K.; Oh-Kyeong, K. (2004). Mutation and overexpression of p53 as a prognostic factor in canine mammary tumors. *Journal of Veterinary Science*, Vol.5, No.1, pp. 63-69

Ciocca, D.R.; Oesterreich, S.; Chamness, C.; Mcguire, W.L.; Fuqua, S.A. (1993). Biological and clinical implications of heat shock protein 27000 (Hsp27): a Review. *Journal of the National Cancer Institute*, Vol. 85, pp. 1558-1570

Dempke, W.; Rie, C.; Grothey, A.; Schmoll, H.J. (2001). Cyclooxygenase-2: a novel target for cancer chemotherapy? *Journal of Cancer Research & Clinical Oncology*, Vol. 127, p. 411-417

Doré, M.; Lanthier, I.; Sirois, J. (2003). Cyclooxygenase-2 expression in canine mammary tumors. *Veterinary Pathology*, Vol.40, pp. 207-212

Gamblin, R.M.; de Maria, R.; Piccoli, M. (1994). Cd44 triggering enhanced human NK cell cytotoxic function. The *Journal of Immunology*, Vol. 153, pp. 4399-4407.

Geraldes, M.; Gärtner, F.; Schmitt, F. (2000). Immunohistochemical study of hormonal receptors and cell proliferation in normal canine mammary glands and spontaneous mammary tumors. *Veterinary Record*, Vol. 146, pp. 403-406

Gilbertson, S.R.; Kurzaman, I.D.; Zachran, R.E.; Hurvitz, H.J.; Black, M.M. (1983). Canine mammary epithelial neoplasms: biologic implications of morfrologic characteristics assessed in 232 dogs. *Veterinary Pathology*, Vol. 20, pp. 127-142

Ginn, PE. (1996). Immunohistochemical detection of P-glycoprotein in formalin - fixed and paraffin-embedded normal and neoplastic canine tissues. *Veterinary Pathology*, Vol. 33, pp. 533-54

Giziński, S.; Boryczko, Z.; Katkiewicz, M.; Bostedt, H. (2003). Ki-67 protein as a prognostic indicator in breast cancer in females. *Veterinary Medicine*, Vol. 59, No. 10, pp. 888-891.

Hampe, J.F.; Misdorp, W. (1973) Tumours and dysplasias of the mammary gland. *Bull World Health Organ*, Vol. 50, pp. 111-133.

Heller, D.A,; Clifford, C.A; Goldschmidt, M.H.; Holt, D.E.; Shofer, F.S.; Smith, A.; Sorenmo, K.U. (2005). Cyclooxygenase-2 expression is associated with histologic tumor type in canine mammary carcinoma. *Veterinary Pathology*, Vol. 42, pp. 776-780.

Hellmen, E.; Bergstrom, R.; Holmberg, L.; Spanberg, I.B.; Hansson, K.; Lindgren, A. (1993). Prognostic factors in canine mammary tumors: a multivariate study of 202 consecutive cases. *Veterinary Pathology*, Vol. 30, pp. 20-27.

Host, H.; Lund, E. (2006). Age as prognostic factor in breast cancer. *Cancer*, Vol. 57, pp. 2217-2221.

Howlin, J.; McBryan, J; Martin, F. (2006) Pubertal mammary gland development: insights from mouse models. *Journal of Mammary Gland Biology and Neoplasia*, Vol. 11, pp. 283-297.

Isomoto, H.; Oka, M.; Yano, Y.; Kanazawa, Y.; Soda, H.; Terada, R.; Yasutake, T.; Nakayama, T.; Shikuwa, S.; Takeshima, F.; Udano, H.; Murata, I.; Ohtsuka, K.; Kohno, S. (2003). Expression of heat shock protein Hsp70 and Hsp40 in gastric cancer. *Cancer Letters*, Vol. 198, No.2, pp. 219-228.

Johnson, A.S.; Couto, C.G.; Weghorst, C.M. (1998). Mutation of the p53 tumor suppressor gene in spontaneously occuring osteosarcomas of the dog. *Carcinogenesis*, Vol. 19, pp. 213- 217.

Koda, M.; Reszec, J.; Sulkowska, M.; Kanczuga – Koda, L.; Sulkowska, S. (2004). Expression of the insulin-like growth factor-I receptor and proapoptotic Bax and Bak proteins in human colorectal cancer. *Annals of the New York Academy of Sciences* , Vol.1030, pp. 377-383.

Kubiak, J.Z. (2001). Cancer and cell cycle. *Advances in Cell Biology*, Vol. 28, pp. 97-307.

Kumaraguruparan, R.; Kurunagaran, D.; Balachandran, C.; Manohar, B.M.; Nagini, S. (2006). Of humans and canines: a comparative evaluation of heat shock and apoptosis-associated proteins in mammary tumors. *Clinica Chimica Acta*, Vol. 365, No.1-2, pp. 168-176.

Lanza-Jacoby, S.; Burd, R.; Rosato, F.E.J.; McGuire, K.; Little, J.; Nougbilly, N.; Miller, S. (2006). Effect of simultaneous inhibition of epidermal growth factor receptor and cyclooxygenase-2 in HER-2/neu-positive breast cancer. *Clinical Cancer Research*, Vol. 12, pp. 6161-6169.

Lee, J.; Hughes, C.S.; Fine, R.L.; Page, L.R. (1996). P-glycoprotein Expression in Canine Lymphoma a Relevant, Intermediate Model of Multidrug Resistance. *Cancer*, Vol. 77, pp. 1892-1898.

Liu, X.H.; Rose, D.P. (1996). Differential expression and regulation of cyclooxygenase-1 and –2 in two human breast cancer cell lines. *Cancer Research*, Vol. 56, pp. 5125-5127.

Lőhr C.V., Teifke, J.P.; Failing, K.; Weiss, E. (1997). Characterization the standarized AgNOR method with postfixation and immunohistologic detection of Ki-67 and PCNA. *Veterinary Pathology*, Vol. 3, No. 4, pp. 212-221.

Martin, P.M.; Cotard, M.; Mialot, J.P.; Andre, F.; Rayanaud J.P. (1984) Animal models for hormone-dependent human breast cancer. Relatioship between steroid receptor profiles in canine and feline mammary tumors and survival rate. *Cancer Chemotherapy and Pharmacology*, Vol. 12, pp. 13-70.

Mayr, B.; Schellander, K.; Schlleger, W.; Reifinger, M. (1994). Sequence of exon of the canine p53 gene-mutation in a papilloma. *British Veterinary Journal*, Vol. 150, pp. 81-84.

McEwen, E.G.; Patnaik, A.K.; Harvey, H.J.; Panko, W.B. (1092). Estrogen receptor in canine mammary tumors. *Cancer Research*, Vol. 42, pp. 2255-2259.

Millanta, F.; Calandrella, M.; Bari, G.; Niccolini, M.; Vannozzi, I.; Poli, A. (2005). Comparison of steroid receptor expression in normal, dysplastica and neoplastic canine and feline mammary tissues. *Research in Veterinary Science*, Vol. 70, No.3, pp. 225-232.

Mirecka, J.; Korabiowska, M.; Schauer, A. (1993). Correlation between the occurrence of Ki-67 antigen and clinical parameters in human breast carcinoma. *Folia Histochemica et Cytobiologica*; Vol. 31, No.2, pp. 83-86.

Misdorp, W.; Else, R.W.; Hellmen, E.; Lipscomb, T.P. (1999). Histological classification of mammary tumors of the dog and cat, *World Health Organization*, Geneva

Misdorp, W.W.; Meuten, D. (edit.). (2002). Tumors in Domestic Animals. Iowa State Press, Black Publishing Company. 4th ed., 575-606.

Mohammed, S.I.; Khan, K.N.; Sellers, R.S.; Hayek, MG.; DeNicola, D.B.; Wu, L.; Bonney, P.L.; Knapp, D.W. (2004). Expression of cyclooxygenase-1 and 2 in naturally-occurring canine cancer. *Prostaglandins Leukotrienes and Essential Fatty Acids*, Vol. 70, pp. 479-483.

Moulton, J.E. (1990). Tumors of mammary gland, W: *Tumors in Domestic Animals. 3rd ed., University of California Press*, pp. 518-549, Berkeley.

Mulas, J.M.; Millán, Y.; Dios, R. (2005). A prospective analysis of immunohistochemically determined estrogen receptor α and progesterone receptor expression and host and tumor factors as predictors of disease-free period in mammary tumors of the dog. *Veterinary Pathology*, Vol. 42, pp. 200-212.

Muto, T.; Wakui, S.; Takahashi, H.; Maekawa, S.; Masaoka, T.; Ushigome, S.; Furusato, M. (2000). p53 Gene Mutations occurring in spontaneous benign and malignant mammary tumors of the dog. *Vet Pathol*, Vol. 37, pp. 248-253.

Nerurkar, V.R.; Naik, S.N.; Lalitha, V.S.; Chitale, A.R.; Ishwad, C.S;, Jalnapurkar, B.V. (1990). Mammary tumours in dogs and their similarities with human breast cancer. W: Bamji M.S. (edit.).: *Proceedings of Symposium on Animal Information Service Center*, pp. 35-40, NIN, ICMR, India

Nieto, A.; Péna, L.; Pérez-Alenza, M.D.; Sànchez, M.A.; Flores, J.M.; Castaño, M. (2000). Immunohistologic detection of estrogen receptor alpha in canine mammary tumors: clinical and pathologic associations and prognostic significance. *Veterinary Pathology*, Vol. 37, pp. 239-247.

Niwińska, A (1995). New prognostic factors in patients with breast cancer. *Journal of Oncology*, Vol. 45, pp. 459-469.

Nowak, M.; Madej, J.A.; Dzięgiel, P. (2005). Immunohistochemical localization of cox-2 in cells of mammary adenocarcinomas in bitches as related to tumour malignancy grade. The *Bulletin of the Veterinary Institute in Pulawy*, Vol. 49, pp. 433-437.

Nowak, M.; Madej, J.A.; Dzięgiel, P. (2007). Comparison of expressions of estrogen and progesterone receptors in adenocarcinomas of the mammary gland in bitches with mitotic activity of neoplastic cells. *Veterinary Medicine*, Vol. 63, No.10, pp. 1211-1215.

Olszewski, W.(1994). Selected aspects of the pathology of breast cancer. *Journal of Oncology*, Vol. 44, No.2, pp. 10-16.

Parl, F.F.; Dupont, W.D. (1982). Retrospective cohort study of histologic risk factor in breast cancer patient. *Cancer*, Vol. 50, pp. 2410-2416.

Peña, L.; Nieto, A.; Perez-Alenza, D. (1998). Immunohistochemical detection of Ki-67 and PCNA in canine mammary tumors: Relationship to clinical and pathologic variables. *Journal of Veterinary Diagnostic Investigation*, Vol.10, pp. 237-246.

Petterino, C.; Rossetti, E.; Bertoncello, D.; Martini, M.; Zappulli, V.; Bargelloni, L.; Castagnaro, M. (2006). Immunohistochemical detection of P-glycoprotein (clone C494) in canine mammary gland tumours. *Journal of Veterinary Medicine Series A - Physiology Pathology Clinical Medic*, Vol. 53, pp. 174-178.

Philibert, J.; Snyder, P.W.; Glickman, N.; Glickman, L.T.; Knapp, D.W.; Waters D.J. (2003). Influence of host factors in survival in dogs with malignant mammary gland tumors. *Journal of Veterinary Internal Medicine*, Vol. 17, pp. 102-106.

Queiroga, FL.; Alves, A; Pires, I; Lopes, C. (2007). Expression of Cox-1 an Cox-2 in canine mammary tumours. *Journal of Comparative Pathology*, Vol. 136, pp 177-185.

Ramalho, L.N.Z.; Ribeiro-Silva, A.; Cassali, G.D. (2006). Zucoloto S. The Expression of p63 and cytokeratin 5 in mixed tumors of the canine mammary gland provides new insights into the histogenesis of these neoplasms. *Veterinary. Pathology*, Vol. 43, pp. 424-429.

Rilke, F.; Colnaghi, M.I.; Cascinelli, N.; Andreola, S.; Baldini, M.T.; Bufalino, R.; Della Porta, G.; Menard, S.; Pierotti, M.A.; Testori, A. (1991). Prognostic significance of HER-2/neu expression in breast cancer and its relationship to other prognostic factors. *International Journal of Cancer*, Vol. 49, pp. 44-49.

Ristimäki, A.; Sivula, A.; Lundin, J.; Lundin, M.; Salminen, T.; Haglund, C.; Joensuu, H.; Isola, J. (2002) Prognostic significance of elevated cyclooxygenase-2 expression in breast cancer. *Cancer Research* , Vol. 62, pp. 632-635.

Rodo, A. (2007). Expression of HER-2 receptors. E cadherin, and p53 protein in mammary gland tumors in bitches. Doctoral thesis, Agricultural University, Warsaw.

Romanucci, M.; Marinelli, A.; Giuseppe, S.; Dell Salda, L. (2006). Heat shock protein expression in canine malignant mammary tumours. *BMC Cancer*, Vol. ,6, pp. 171.

Roses, D.F.; Bell, D.A.; Flotte, T.J.; Taylor, R.; Ratech, H.; Dubin, N. (1982). Pathologic predictors of recurrence in stage 1 (T1NOMO) breast cancer. *American Journal of Veterinary Research*, Vol. 78, pp. 817-820.

Rungsipipata, A. (1999) Immunohistochemical analysis of c-yes and c-erbB-2 oncogene products and p53 tumor suppressor protein in canine mammary tumors. The *Journal of Veterinary Medical Science*; Vol.61, No.1, pp. 27-32.

Rutteman, G.R.; Withrow, S.J.; MacEwen, E.G. (2001). Tumors of the mammary gland. W: *Small Animal Clinical Oncology*. S. J. Withrow; E. G. MacEwen, (Ed.), 455-477, 3rd ed., Philadelphia

Sartin, E.A.; Barnes, S.; Kwapien, R.P.; Wolfe, L.G. (1992). Estrogen and progesterone receptor status of mammary carcinomas and correlation with clinical outcome in dogs. *American Journal of Veterinary Research*, Vol. 53, pp. 2196-2200.

Saymour, L.; Bezwoda, W.R.; Meyer, K. (1990) Tumor factors predicting for prognosis in metastatic breast cancer. The presence of P24 predicts for response to treatment and duration of survival. *Cancer*; Vol.66, No.11, pp. 2390-2394.

Skrzypczak, M. (2004). Angiogenesis in mammary gland tumors in bitches. Doctoral thesis, Agricultural University, Warsaw.

Sobczak-Filipiak, M.; Malicka, E.(1997). Diagnosis of mammary gland tumors including immumocytochemistry methods. *Materials Conference. Veterinary Oncology*. T. Rotkiewicz, (Ed.), 100-107, Olsztyn

Soslow, R.A.; Dannenberg, A.J.; Rush, D.; Werner, B.M.; Khan, K.N.; Masferrer, J.; Koki, A.T. (2000). COX-2 is expressed in human pulmonary, colonic and mammary tumours. *Cancer*, Vol. 89, pp. 2637-2645.

Storm, F.K.; Mahvi, D.M.; Gilchrist, K.W. (1993). Heat shock protein 27 overexpression in breast cancer lymph node metastasis. *Annals of Surgical Oncology*; Vol. 3, No.6, pp. 570-573

Szczubiał, M.; Łopuszański, W. (2002). Prognosis in mammary gland tumors in bitches. *Veterinary Medicine*, Vol. 58, No. 40, pp. 261-264.

Thomas, W.; Caiazza, F.; Harvey, B.J. (2008). Estrogen, phospholipase A and breast cancer. *Frontiers in Bioscience*, Vol. 13, pp. 2604-2613.

Veldhoen, N.; Watterson, J.; Brash, M. (1999). Identification of tumor-associated and germ line p53 mutation in canine mammary cancer. *British Journal of Cancer* , Vol.81, pp. 409-415.

Permissions

The contributors of this book come from diverse backgrounds, making this book a truly international effort. This book will bring forth new frontiers with its revolutionizing research information and detailed analysis of the nascent developments around the world.

We would like to thank Carlos C. Perez-Marin, for lending his expertise to make the book truly unique. He has played a crucial role in the development of this book. Without his invaluable contribution this book wouldn't have been possible. He has made vital efforts to compile up to date information on the varied aspects of this subject to make this book a valuable addition to the collection of many professionals and students.

This book was conceptualized with the vision of imparting up-to-date information and advanced data in this field. To ensure the same, a matchless editorial board was set up. Every individual on the board went through rigorous rounds of assessment to prove their worth. After which they invested a large part of their time researching and compiling the most relevant data for our readers. Conferences and sessions were held from time to time between the editorial board and the contributing authors to present the data in the most comprehensible form. The editorial team has worked tirelessly to provide valuable and valid information to help people across the globe.

Every chapter published in this book has been scrutinized by our experts. Their significance has been extensively debated. The topics covered herein carry significant findings which will fuel the growth of the discipline. They may even be implemented as practical applications or may be referred to as a beginning point for another development. Chapters in this book were first published by InTech; hereby published with permission under the Creative Commons Attribution License or equivalent.

The editorial board has been involved in producing this book since its inception. They have spent rigorous hours researching and exploring the diverse topics which have resulted in the successful publishing of this book. They have passed on their knowledge of decades through this book. To expedite this challenging task, the publisher supported the team at every step. A small team of assistant editors was also appointed to further simplify the editing procedure and attain best results for the readers.

Our editorial team has been hand-picked from every corner of the world. Their multi-ethnicity adds dynamic inputs to the discussions which result in innovative outcomes. These outcomes are then further discussed with the researchers and contributors who give their valuable feedback and opinion regarding the same. The feedback is then collaborated with the researches and they are edited in a comprehensive manner to aid the understanding of the subject.

Apart from the editorial board, the designing team has also invested a significant amount of their time in understanding the subject and creating the most relevant covers. They scrutinized every image to scout for the most suitable representation of the subject and create an appropriate cover for the book.

The publishing team has been involved in this book since its early stages. They were actively engaged in every process, be it collecting the data, connecting with the contributors or procuring relevant information. The team has been an ardent support to the editorial, designing and production team. Their endless efforts to recruit the best for this project, has resulted in the accomplishment of this book. They are a veteran in the field of academics and their pool of knowledge is as vast as their experience in printing. Their expertise and guidance has proved useful at every step. Their uncompromising quality standards have made this book an exceptional effort. Their encouragement from time to time has been an inspiration for everyone.

The publisher and the editorial board hope that this book will prove to be a valuable piece of knowledge for researchers, students, practitioners and scholars across the globe.

List of Contributors

Paulo Tomé
Algoritmi Research Center/Polytechnic Institute of Viseu, Portugal

Helena Vala
Center for Studies in Education, and Health Technologies, CI&DETS, Polytechnic Institute of Viseu, Portugal

Colette Henry and Lorna Treanor
Royal Veterinary College, University of London, Hatfield (Herts), UK

Annett Heise
Faculty of Veterinary Science, University of Pretoria, South Africa

Enio Moura and Cláudia T. Pimpão
Service of Medical Genetics, Brazil
Laboratory of Pharmacology and Toxicology, Faculty of Veterinary Medicine, Campus São José, Agricultural and Environmental Sciences Center, Pontifícia Universidade Católica do Paraná, Curitiba, Brazil

Annamaria Passantino
Department of Veterinary Public Health, Faculty of Veterinary Medicine, University of Messina, Italy

Matthew D. Stone and Alec J. Turner
Kutztown University, USA

Fábio Alessandro Pieri, Ana Paula Falci Daibert, Elisa Bourguignon and Maria Aparecida Scatamburlo Moreira
Federal University of Viçosa, Brazil

Guilherme Albuquerque de Oliveira Cavalcanti
Federal University of Minas Gerais, Brazil

Lysimachos G. Papazoglou
Department of Clinical Sciences, Faculty of Veterinary Medicine, Aristotle University of Thessaloniki, Greece

Gary W. Ellison
Department of Small Animal Clinical Sciences, Health Science Center, University of Florida Gainesville, USA

Cleuza Maria de Faria Rezende, Eliane Gonçalves de Melo and Natalie Ferreira Borges
Escola de Veterinária – UFMG, Brazil

Bruno Colaço, Maria dos Anjos Pires and Rita Payan-Carreira
CECAV, Univ. of Trás-os-Montes and Alto Douro, Portugal

Anna M. Badowska-Kozakiewicz
Department of Biophysics and Human Physiology, Medical University of Warsaw, Poland

Printed in the USA
CPSIA information can be obtained
at www.ICGtesting.com
JSHW011426221024
72173JS00004B/692

9 781632 412959